S0-AXJ-373

Third Edition

COMPLEMENTARY & ALTERNATIVE THERAPIES FOR NURSING PRACTICE

Karen Lee Fontaine

Professor, Purdue University Calumet
Hammond, Indiana

Pearson

Boston   Columbus   Indianapolis   New York   San Francisco
Upper Saddle River   Amsterdam   Cape Town   Dubai   London   Madrid
Milan   Munich   Paris   Montreal   Toronto   Delhi   Mexico City
Sao Paulo   Sydney   Hong Kong   Seoul   Singapore   Taipei Tokyo

Publisher: Julie Levin Alexander
Assistant to Publisher: Regina Bruno
Editor-in-Chief: Maura Connor
Assistant to the Editor-in-Chief: Marion Gottlieb
Executive Acquisitions Editor: Kim Mortimer
Assistant Editor: Sarah Wrocklage
Project Manager: Jillian Allison
Director of Marketing: Karen Allman
Marketing Coordinator: Michael Sirinides
Production Manager: Wanda Rockwell

Media Project Manager: Rachel Collett
Manager, Rights and Permissions: Zina Arabia
Manager, Visual Research: Beth Brenzel
Manager, Cover Visual Research & Permissions: Karen Sanatar
Image Permission Coordinator: Jan Marc Quisumbing
Creative Director: Jayne Conte
Cover Design: Suzanne Duda
Composition: Aptara®, Inc.
Printer/Binder: Bind-Rite/Robbinsville

Notice: Care has been taken to confirm the accuracy of information presented in this book. The authors, editors, and the publisher, however, cannot accept any responsibility for errors or omissions or for consequences from application of the information in this book and make no warranty, express or implied, with respect to its contents.

The authors and publisher have exerted every effort to ensure that drug selections and dosages set forth in this text are in accord with current recommendations and practice at time of publication. However, in view of ongoing research, changes in government regulations, and the constant flow of information relating to drug therapy and reactions, the reader is urged to check the package inserts of all drugs for any change in indications or dosage and for added warning and precautions. This is particularly important when the recommended agent is a new and/or infrequently employed drug.

Copyright © 2011 by Pearson Education, Inc., Upper Saddle River, New Jersey 07458.
All rights reserved. Printed in the United States of America. This publication is protected by Copyright and permission should be obtained from the publisher prior to any prohibited reproduction, storage in a retrieval system, or transmission in any form or by any means, electronic, mechanical, photocopying, recording, or likewise. For information regarding permission(s), write to: Rights and Permissions Department.

Pearson is a registered trademark of Pearson plc

Library of Congress Cataloging-in-Publication Data
Fontaine, Karen Lee
   Complementary & alternative therapies for nursing practice / Karen Lee Fontaine. —3rd ed.
      p. cm.
   Includes bibliographical references and index.
   ISBN-13: 978-0-13-510246-6
   ISBN-10: 0-13-510246-4
   1. Nursing.   2. Alternative medicine.   I. Title.   II. Title: Complementary and alternative therapies for nursing practice.
   [DNLM: 1. Complementary Therapies.   2. Nursing Care. WB 890 F678c 2010]
   RT42.F64 2011
   615.5—dc22

                                                                              2009033284

10 9 8 7 6 5 4 3 2 1

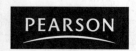

www.pearsonhighered.com

ISBN-13: 978-0-13-510246-6
ISBN-10:   0-13-510246-4

Dedication

This book is dedicated to my nursing students—past, present, and future. May you always practice your profession with great passion and an inquiring mind.

Dedication

CONTENTS

TRY THIS

PREFACE

The profession of nursing has advanced beyond the Western biomedical model to incorporate many healing tools used by our Asian, Latino, Native American, African, and European ancestors. We are rapidly rediscovering that these ancient principles and practices have significant therapeutic value. Some see this movement as a "return to our roots." Others believe it is a response to runaway health care costs, growing dissatisfaction with high-tech medicine, and increasing concern over the adverse effects and misuse of medications. The growth of consumer empowerment also fuels this movement.

As nurses, how do we begin to assimilate thousands of years of healing knowledge? How do we begin this journey of integrating practices into our own lives? In our professional practice, how do we model healthful living? How do we help consumers choose their own healing journeys? How do we break down the barriers between conventional and alternative medicine? Learning about healing practices, like anything else, is a slow process involving a steady accumulation of bits of information and skills that eventually form a coherent pattern called knowledge. While it is possible to learn a great deal about healing practices from reading, thinking, and asking questions, you must in the long run learn about healing through participation. Without hands-on experience, you can be a good student, but you can never be a great nursing practitioner of the healing arts. I trust this book will be one step in a lifelong exploration of and experiences with healing practices.

Consumers do not wish to abandon conventional medicine but they do want to have a range of options available to them including herbs, nutrition, manual healing methods, mind–body techniques, and spiritual approaches. Some healing practices, such as exercise, nutrition, meditation, and massage, promote health and prevent disease. Others, such as herbs or homeopathic remedies, address specific illnesses. Many other healing practices do both. The rise of chronic disease rates in Western society has motivated consumers to increasingly consider self-care approaches. As recently as the 1950s, we lived in a world of curable disease, largely infectious, where medical interventions were both appropriate and effective, and only 30 percent of all disease was chronic. Now, 80 percent of all disease is chronic. Western medicine, with its focus on acute disorders, trauma, and surgery, is considered to be the best high-tech medical care in the world. Unfortunately, it cannot respond adequately to the current epidemic of chronic illnesses.

Ethnocentrism, the assumption that one's own cultural or ethnic group is superior to others, has often prevented Western health care practitioners from learning "new" ways to promote health and prevent chronic illness. With consumer demand for a broader range of options, we must open our minds to the idea that other cultures and countries have valid ways of preventing and curing diseases that could be good for Western societies. Although the information may be new to us, many of these traditions are hundreds or even thousands of years old and have long been part of the medical mainstream in other cultures.

I have titled this book *Complementary & Alternative Therapies for Nursing Practice* because I believe we need to merge alternative approaches with our Western-based nursing practices. I have tried to provide enough information about alternative therapies to help guide our practice decisions. This text, as an overview and practical guide for nurses, does not pretend to be an exhaustive collection of all the facts and related research in the area of alternative medicine, nor does it offer meticulous documentation for all claims made by the various therapies. The goal of the text is to motivate you, the reader, to explore alternative approaches, increase your knowledge about factors that contribute to health and illness, and expand your professional practice appropriately.

It is possible to classify alternative practices in any number of ways. I have chosen to present more than 40 approaches categorized into seven units. In Unit One, I introduce the philosophical approaches to both Western biomedicine and alternative or complementary medicine. Concepts common to many approaches are defined and discussed such as energy, breath, spirituality, and healing. Unit Two presents a number of health care practices that have been systematized throughout the centuries and throughout the world. These typically include an entire set of values, attitudes, and beliefs that generate a philosophy of life, not simply a group of remedies. Unit Three comprises chapters relating to botanical healings used by 80 percent of the world's population. Chapter discussions cover herbs and nutritional supplements, aromatherapy, homeopathy, and naturopathy. Unit Four presents manual healing methods; some from ancient times and some developed in the latter half of the twentieth century. The chapters are chiropractic, massage, pressure point therapies, hand-mediated biofield therapies, and combined physical and biofield therapies. The chapters in Unit Five cover types of mind–body techniques for healing and include yoga, meditation, hypnotherapy and guided imagery, dreams, intuition, music therapy, biofeedback, and movement-oriented therapies. Unit Six presents two spiritual approaches to therapeutic intervention: working with shamans and the use of faith and prayer. Unit Seven includes two chapters on miscellaneous practices: bioelectromagnetics and animal-assisted therapy.

The appendix provides specific information on alternative therapies for common health problems. It is meant to provide education for the management of the types of problems that respond well to alternative therapies and lifestyle modification.

Two chapters—Chapter 3 and Chapter 21—are new to the third edition. Chapter 3, The Role of Evidence-Based Health Care in Complementary and Alternative Therapies, covers definitions, controversies, barriers, and models of evidence-based care. The rationale for the use of evidence-based practice is that it increases our confidence that nursing care and medical care will lead to better patient outcomes. Chapter 21 covers Music Therapy as the clinical and evidence-based use of music interventions to accomplish individualized goals within a therapeutic relationship.

This book does not recommend treatments but rather describes alternative practices, their backgrounds and claims, preparation of practitioners, concepts, diagnostic methods, treatments, and evidence of research studies. This section is designed to help you, the nurse, expand your practice by providing you with specific information and suggestions. Integrated nursing practice is an important section of every chapter. *Try This* features throughout the chapters provide you with examples of how these practices can be integrated into your own life and also give you ideas for client education. A list of resources is included in the chapters.

I have continued the *Using Research to Heal* feature with all new articles, each of which focuses on a significant piece of published research relating to the chapter topic. These research boxes not only present current studies, but also are designed to further critical thinking and perhaps inspire readers to design studies to answer their own questions. For each study, the following questions are answered: What is this study about? How was the study done? What were the results of the study? What additional questions might I have? And how can I use this study? Nursing is in a unique position to take a leadership role in integrating alternative healing methods into Western health care systems. We have historically used our hands, heart, and head in more natural and traditional healing interactions. As nurses, by virtue of our education and relationships with clients, we can help consumers assert their right to choose their own healing journey and the quality of their life and death experiences.

ACKNOWLEDGMENTS

I would like to express thanks to the many people who have inspired, commented on, and in other ways assisted in the writing and publication of the third edition of this book. On the publishing and production side at Prentice Hall, I was most fortunate to have an exceptional team of editors and support staff. My thanks go to Kim Mortimer, Executive Acquisitions Editor, and Sarah Wrocklage, Assistant Editor, who provided support and guidance throughout this project. Wanda Rockwell, Production Liaison kept this book on schedule and dedicated her time and skill to its completion.

   I would like to thank all those who reviewed this text and provided suggestions and guidance for the third edition.

Karen Lee Fontaine
Purdue University Calumet

Contributors

Dolores M. Huffman, RN, PhD
Associate Professor
School of Nursing
Purdue University Calumet
Hammond, IN

†Leslie Rittenmeyer, PsyD, CNS, RN
Associate Professor
School of Nursing
Purdue University Calumet
Research Associate: Northwest Indiana Center for Evidence Based Practice
A Joanna Briggs Institute Collaborating Centre
Hammond, IN

††Shelia Lewis, BScN, MHSc
Associate Lecturer
Department of Nursing, Faculty of Health
York University
Toronto, ON, Canada

---

†Contribution for Chapter 3, *The Role of Evidence-Based Health Care in Complementary and Alternative Therapies*; and Chapter 21, *Music Therapy*.
††Contribution for Chapter 14, *Hand-Mediated Biofield Therapies*.

REVIEWERS

Dot E. Baker, RN, MS(N), CNS-BC, EdD
Professor of Nursing
Wilmington University
Georgetown, DE

Lisa Capps, PhD, RN
Assistant Professor
West Suburban College of Nursing
Oak Park, IL

Cindy Kief, ND, COTA/L
Academic Fieldwork Educator, Instructor, Advisor
Cincinnati State Technical and Community College
Cincinnati, OH

Sylvia Kubsch, PhD, RN
Associate Professor Nursing
University of Wisconsin-Green Bay
Green Bay, WI

Helda Pinzon-Perez, RN, PhD, MPH
Associate Professor
California State University at Fresno
Fresno, CA

Sheila Stroman RN, APN, PhD, LMT, CHT
Assistant Professor Nursing
University of Central Arkansas
Conway, AR

Rose Utley PhD, RN, CNE
Associate Professor
Director, Nurse Educator Graduate Programs
Missouri State University
Springfield, MO

Healing Practices: Complementary/ Alternative Therapies for Nurses

We define ourselves and our deepest values by the choices we make, day by day, hour by hour, over a lifetime.

TOBIAS WOLFF

1

Integrative Healing

There is a deep yearning for a human (whole) approach to medicine.

BILL MOYERS

Who among us can predict which small and seemingly implausible observation will reveal the next great secret of the universe.

W. B. JONAS

Most of nursing education in the United States, Canada, the United Kingdom, Europe, and Australia, often referred to as Western countries, has been under the umbrella of biomedicine, and thus Western nurses are familiar and comfortable with its beliefs, theories, practices, strengths, and limitations. Fewer nurses have studied alternative medical theories and practices and as a result may lack information or even harbor misinformation about these healing practices. Unlike the medical profession in general, however, the profession of nursing has traditionally embraced two basic concepts embodied by alternative therapies—holism and humanism—in its approach with clients. Nurses have long believed that healing and caring must be approached holistically and that biological, psychological, emotional, spiritual, and environmental aspects of health and illness are equally important. Our humanistic perspective includes propositions such as the mind and body are indivisible, people have the power to solve their own problems, people are responsible for the patterns of their lives, and well-being is a combination of personal satisfaction and contributions to the larger community. This theoretical basis gives us a solid foot in each camp and places us, as nurses, in the unique position to help create a bridge between biomedicine and alternative medicine (Halcon, Chlan, Kreitzer, & Leonard, 2003; Peplau, 1952; Quinn, 2000; Shreffler-Grant, Hill, Weinert, Nichols, & Ide, 2007).

BACKGROUND

Many interesting exchanges around the world have debated the appropriate terminology of various healing practices. Some people become vested in the use of particular terms and have difficulty getting past the language limitations. For example, many people view the term *alternative medicine* as being too narrow or misleading and are concerned that the term lacks a full understanding of traditional healing practices. It would be more helpful for a common language to be developed without people being captive to it. As language evolves, the terms used today may be quite different from those used 20 years from now. For consistency purposes, the terms chosen for this text are **conventional medicine** or **biomedicine** to describe Western medical practices and the terms **alternative medicine** or **complementary medicine** to describe other healing practices. **Traditional medicine** refers to indigenous medical systems such as Traditional Chinese Medicine. There are no universally accepted terms. The following list presents commonly used words and their counterparts:

Mainstream	Complementary/Alternative
Modern	Ancient
Western	Eastern
Allopathic	Homeopathic; holistic
Conventional	Unconventional
Orthodox	Traditional
Biomedicine	Natural medicine
Scientific	Indigenous healing methods

The line between conventional and alternative medicine is imprecise and frequently changing. For example, is the use of megavitamins or diet regimes to treat disease considered medicine, a lifestyle change, or both? Can having one's pain lessened by massage be considered a medical therapy? How should spiritual healing and prayer—some of the oldest, most widely used, and least studied traditional approaches—be classified? Although the terms *alternative* and *complementary* are frequently used, in some instances they represent the primary treatment modality for an individual. Thus, conventional medicine sometimes assumes a secondary role and actually becomes a complement to the primary treatment modality.

Conventional Medicine

Biomedical or Western medicine is only about 200 years old. It is founded on the philosophical beliefs of René Descartes (1596–1650)—that the mind and body are separate—and on Sir Isaac Newton's (1642–1727) principles of physics—that the universe is like a large mechanical clock where everything operates in a linear, sequential form. This mechanistic perspective of medicine views the human body as a series of body parts. It is a *reductionistic approach* in which the person is converted into increasingly smaller components: systems, organs, cells, and biochemicals. People are reduced to patients, patients are reduced to bodies, and bodies are reduced to machines. Health is viewed as the absence of disease or, in other words, nothing being broken at the present time. The focus of sick care is on the symptoms of dysfunction. Doctors are trained to fix or repair broken parts through the use of drugs, radiation, surgery, or replacement of body parts. The approach is aggressive and militant with physicians being in a war against disease, with a take-no-prisoners attitude. Both consumers and practitioners of biomedicine believe it is better to:

• Do something rather than wait and see whether the body's natural processes resolve the problem.
• Attack the disease directly by medication or surgery rather than try to build up the person's resistance and ability to overcome the disease.

Biomedicine views the person primarily as a physical body, with the mind and spirit being separate and secondary or, at times, even irrelevant. It is powerful medicine in that it has virtually eliminated some infectious diseases such as smallpox and polio. It is based on science and technology, personifying a highly industrialized society. As a "rescue" medicine, the biomedical approach is wonderful. It is highly effective in emergencies, traumatic injuries, bacterial infections, and some highly sophisticated surgeries. In these cases, treatment is fast, aggressive, and goal oriented, with the responsibility for cure falling on the practitioner.

The priority of intervention is on opposing and suppressing the symptoms of illness. This approach is evidenced in many medications with prefixes such as *an* or *anti* as in analgesics, anesthetics, anti-inflammatories, and antipyretics. Biomedicine characterizes each disease in terms of its mechanisms of action, believing that most individuals are affected in the same way. Treatment is basically the same for most people. Because conventional medicine is preoccupied with parts and symptoms and not with whole working systems of matter, energy, thoughts, and feelings, it does not do well with long-term systemic illnesses such as arthritis, heart disease, and hypertension. In spite of the United States spending more dollars on health care than other nations, the U.S. life expectancy rate was only 13th and the infant mortality rate ranked 20th among other nations studied. The United States has failed to be a world leader in actually providing a healthier quality of life (Banks, Marmot, Oldfield, & Smith, 2006; Infant Mortality and Life Expectancy for Selected Countries, 2007).

Alternative Medicine

Alternative medicine is an umbrella term for as many as 1,800 therapies practiced all over the world. Many forms have been handed down over thousands of years, both orally and as written records. They are based on the medical systems of ancient peoples, including Egyptians, Chinese, Asian Indians, Greeks, and Native Americans. Others, such as osteopathy and naturopathy, evolved in the United States during the past two centuries. Still others, such as some of the mind–body and bioelectromagnetic approaches, are on the frontier of scientific knowledge and understanding. The National Center for Complementary and Alternative Medicine (NCCAM) at the National Institutes of Health defines alternative therapies as a broad range of healing philosophies, approaches, and therapies that conventional medicine does not commonly use, accept, study, understand, or make available (NCCAM, 2008).

Although they represent diverse approaches, alternative therapies share certain attributes. They are based on the paradigm of *whole systems* and the belief that people are more than physical bodies with fixable and replaceable parts. Mental, emotional, spiritual relationship, and environmental components of well-being are considered to play a crucial and equal role in a person's state of health. Interventions are individualized within the entire context of this person's life (Agdal, 2005; Chan & Whitehead, 2008). Even Hippocrates, the father of Western medicine, espoused a holistic orientation when he taught doctors to observe their patients' life circumstances, emotional states, stresses, living environment, inherited constitution, and the person's subjective experience of the illness. Socrates agreed, declaring, "Curing the soul; that is the first thing." In alternative medicine, symptoms are believed to be an expression of the body's wisdom as it reacts to cure its own imbalance or disease. Other threads or concepts common to most forms of alternative medicine include the following:

- An internal self-healing process exists within each person.
- People are responsible for making their own decisions regarding their health care.
- Nature, time, and patience are the great healers.

When Albert Einstein (1879–1955) introduced his theory of relativity in 1905, our way of viewing the universe changed dramatically. Einstein said that all matter is energy, energy and matter are interchangeable, and all matter is connected at the subatomic level. No single entity could be affected without all connecting parts being affected. In this view, the universe is not a giant clock, but a living web. The human body is animated by an integrated energy called the **life force**. The life force sustains the physical body but is also a spiritual entity that is linked to a higher being or infinite source of energy. When the life force flows freely throughout the body, a person experiences optimal health and vitality. When the life force is blocked or weakened, organs, tissues, and cells are deprived of the energy they need to function at their full potential, and illness or disease results.

The value of alternative medicine is especially effective for people with chronic, debilitating illnesses for which conventional medicine has few, if any, answers. It has much to offer in the arena of health promotion and disease

BOX 1.1

Paradigms of Medicine

View	Conventional Medicine	Alternative Medicine
Mind/body/spirit	are separate	are one
The body is	a machine	a living microcosm of the universe
Disease results when	parts break	energy/life force becomes unbalanced
Symptoms	dysfunctional and need to be fixed	communicators about the state of the whole person
Role of medicine	to combat disease	to restore mind/body/spirit harmony
Approach	treat and suppress symptoms	search for patterns of disharmony or imbalance
Focuses on	parts/matter	whole/energy
Treatments	attempt to "fix" broken parts; specific to disease	support self-healing; personalized for the individual
Primary interventions	drugs, surgery, diet, radiation	exercise, herbs, stress management, social support
System	sick care	health care

prevention. As costs of conventional medicine grow and people continue to suffer from chronic illnesses and degenerative diseases, the place of alternative medicine is moving closer to the mainstream. A growing number of complementary and alternative therapies are eligible for reimbursement by third-party payers in the United States. The most commonly reimbursed therapies are chiropractic, biofeedback, acupuncture, hypnotherapy, and naturopathy. Box 1.1 provides an overview of the paradigms of conventional and alternative medicine.

Integrative Medicine

Integrative medicine is a new term that embodies both conventional and alternative medicine, making use of the best available evidence of both approaches to healing. It is a multidisciplinary, collaborative approach. It is holistic and encompasses mind, body, and spirit. It stresses the relationship between the client and the practitioner as well as the human capacity for healing. Integrative practitioners believe that clients have the right to make informed choices about their health care options. The focus is on "using the least invasive, least toxic, and least costly methods to help facilitate health" (Willison, 2006, p. 255). The goal of integrative medicine is to find new solutions to prevention and treatment of health care problems.

Dr. Andrew Weil has been the driving force for integrative medicine in the United States and hopes to reform the entire medical delivery system by changing the way we look at health and disease and modifying the education of physicians. His program in integrative medicine at the University of Arizona, College of Medicine, was the first to adopt this new curriculum. Nursing must also be open to change in order to meet the goal of true integrative care (Park, 2006).

ASSUMPTIONS

In understanding conventional and alternative medicine, it is helpful to study the assumptions basic to their theories, practices, and research. These assumptions include the origin of disease, the meaning of health, the curative process, and health promotion.

Origin of Disease

Biomedicine and alternative medicine have widely divergent assumptions regarding the origin of disease. Biomedicine was shaped by the observations that bacteria were responsible for producing disease and pathologic damage and that antitoxins and vaccines could improve a person's ability to ward off the effects of pathogens. Armed with this knowledge, physicians began to conquer a large number of devastating infectious diseases. As the science developed, physicians came to believe that germs and genes caused disease and once the offending pathogen, metabolic error, or chemical imbalance was found all diseases would eventually yield to the appropriate vaccine, antibiotic, or chemical compound.

Conventional medicine has also been influenced by Darwin's concept of survival of the fittest, which says that all life is a constant struggle and that only the most successful competitors survive. When this concept is applied to medicine, it is translated that we live under constant attack by the thousands of microorganisms that, in the Western view, cause most diseases. People must defend themselves and counterattack with treatments that kill the enemy. Based on this assumption, symptoms are regarded as harmful manifestations and should be suppressed. For example, a headache is an annoyance that should be eliminated and a fever should be reduced with the use of medications.

Alternative medicine is based on the belief of a life force or energy that flows through each person and sustains life. *Balance* refers to harmony among organs in the body and among body systems, and in relationships to other individuals, society, and the environment. A balanced organism presents a strong defense against external insults such as bacteria, viruses, and trauma. When the life force or energy is blocked or weakened, the vitality of organs and tissues is reduced, oxygen is diminished, waste products accumulate, and organs and tissues degenerate. Symptoms are the body's way of communicating that the life force has been blocked or weakened, resulting in a compromised immune system. Disease is not necessarily a surprise encounter with a bacteria or virus, since these surround us constantly, but rather the end result of a series of events that began with a disruption of the life force. Based on this assumption, symptoms are not suppressed unless they endanger life, such as a headache from an aneurysm or a fever above 105°F. Rather, symptoms are cooperated with because they express the body's wisdom as it reacts to cure its own disease. For example, a headache is a signal that one's whole system needs realignment, and a fever may be the result of the breakdown of bacterial proteins or toxins. When symptoms are suppressed, they are not resolved but merely held off, gathering energy for renewed expression as soon as the outside, counteractive force is removed.

Meaning of Health

If you were to ask a healer from the Chinese, Indian, or Native American traditions about the meaning of health, you would hear answers very different from those that would be given by a Western physician. The biomedical view of health, in the past, was often described as the absence of disease or other abnormal conditions. That definition has been expanded to include the view that health is not a static condition; the body undergoes constant change and adaptation to both internal and external environmental challenges. The majority of conventional medical practitioners would define health as a state of well-being. They may disagree, however, about who determines well-being—the health professional or the individual. With some exceptions, wellness and health promotion have, for the most part, been left to the initiative of the individual.

Those practicing alternative medicine describe health as a condition of wholeness, balance, and harmony of the body, mind, emotions, and spirit. Health is not a concrete goal to be achieved; rather, it is a lifelong process that represents growth toward potential, an inner feeling of aliveness. *Physical* aspects include optimal functioning of all body systems. *Emotional* aspects include the ability to feel and express the entire range of human emotions. *Mental* aspects include feelings of self-worth, a positive identity, a sense of accomplishment, and the ability to appreciate and create. *Environmental* aspects include physical, biologic, economic, social, and political conditions. *Spiritual* aspects involve self, others, and society. Self components are the development of moral values and finding a meaningful purpose in life. Spiritual factors relating to others include the search for meaning through relationships and the feeling of connectedness with others and with an external power often identified as God or the divine source. *Societal* aspects of spiritual health can be understood as a common humanity and a belief in the fundamental sacredness and unity of all life. These beliefs motivate people toward truth and a sense of fairness and justice to all members of society.

Curative Process

The curative process is another example of divergent viewpoints. Conventional medicine promotes the view that external treatments—drugs, surgery, radiation—cure people, and practitioners are trained to fix or repair broken parts. The focus is on the disease process or abnormal condition. Alternative practitioners look at conditions that block the life force and keep it from flowing freely through the body. Healing occurs when balance and harmony are restored. The focus is on the health potential of the person rather than the disease problem. The cure model and the healing model are presented with greater detail in Chapter 2.

Health Promotion

Conventional and alternative medical systems have somewhat different foci on promotion of health. The thrust of conventional medicine is toward disease prevention. Consumers are taught how to decrease their risk of cancer, cardiac disorders, obesity, and other life-threatening diseases that kill most people prematurely in Western society. As important as these behaviors are, however, disease prevention is only one piece of health promotion. Health promotion, from the alternative perspective, is a lifelong process that focuses on optimal development of our physical, emotional, mental, spiritual, and environmental selves. An individual's worldviews, values, lifestyles, and health beliefs are considered to be of critical importance. Consumers are encouraged to adopt healthier lifestyles, to accept increased responsibility for their own well-being, and through greater self-reliance, to learn how to handle common health problems on their own. As the *Healthy People 2010* (U.S. Department of Health and Human Services, 2000; *Healthy People 2020*, due out in 2010) report illustrates, the health care delivery system of the future must make use of all approaches that effectively promote optimal health. Box 1.2 describes the goals for health care reform in the United States.

RESEARCH

Scientific beliefs rest not just on facts but on paradigms (broad views of how these facts are related and organized). Differences in views among groups of nursing and medical researchers are a reflection of the different scientific paradigms—quantitative and qualitative research—in which each group believes. Although each method results in a different type of knowledge, both provide information to researchers and consumers. Evidence-based practice is covered in Chapter 3.

Quantitative research represents the principles of Western scientific method, which include formulating and testing hypotheses and then rejecting or not rejecting the hypotheses. Every question is reduced to the smallest possible part. Results can be replicated and generalized. Outcomes can be predicted and controlled. Quantitative research is said to be objective in that the observer is separate from that which is being observed. Another part of

BOX 1.2

Ten Rules for Health Care Reform

1. **Care based on continuous healing relationships.** Health care system should be available to all people, 24 hours a day, via face-to-face visits, Internet, telephone, and other means.
2. **Customization based on patient needs and values.** The system of care should be designed to meet the most common types of needs but have the capacity to respond to individual patient choices and preferences.
3. **The patient as the source of control.** Patients should be given the necessary information and the opportunity to exercise the degree of control they choose over health care decisions that affect them.
4. **Shared knowledge and the free flow of information.** Patients should have unfettered access to their own medical information and to clinical knowledge.
5. **Evidence-based decision making.** Patient should receive care based on the best available scientific knowledge.
6. **Safety as a system property.** Patients should be safe from injury caused by the care system.
7. **The need for transparency.** The health care system should make available to patients and their families information that allows them to make informed decisions when selecting a health plan, hospital, clinical practice, or when choosing alternative treatments.
8. **Anticipation of needs.** The health system should anticipate patient needs rather than simply react to events.
9. **Continuous decrease in waste.** The health system should not waste resources or patient time.
10. **Cooperation among clinicians.** Clinicians and institutions should actively collaborate and communicate to ensure an appropriate exchange of information and coordination of care.

Source: National Institutes of Health. (2002, March). 10 Rules for health care reform. In *White House Commission on Complementary and Alternative Medicine Policy, Final Report*. Washington, DC: U.S. Government Printing Office. www.whccamp.hhs.gov/rules.html. Accessed June 11, 2008.

this objective paradigm is that all information can be derived from physically measurable data. This type of research has been extremely effective for isolating causative factors of disease and developing cures. On the other hand, it cannot explain the whole person as an integrated unit.

Qualitative research, which is currently experiencing unprecedented growth and expansion, seeks to understand events in context-specific settings. It studies the context and meaning of interactive variables as these variables form patterns reflective of the whole. Researchers observe, document, analyze, and qualify the interactive relationship of variables. In the science of physics, it is believed that objectivity is ultimately not possible. The Heisenberg uncertainty principle states that the act of observing phenomena necessarily influences the behavior of the phenomena being observed. Another part of the paradigm relates to the belief that interactions between living organisms and environments are transactional, multidirectional, and synergistic in ways that cannot be reduced. This holistic approach (the whole is greater than the parts) is basic to qualitative research.

Conventional medicine believes that procedures and substances must pass blinded randomized controlled trials (RCTs) to be proven effective. As a testing method, an RCT examines a single procedure or substance in isolated, controlled conditions and measures results against an inactive procedure of substance (called a *control* or *placebo*). This approach is based on the assumption that single factors cause and reverse illness, and that these factors can be studied alone and out of context. Alternative medicine, however, believes that no single factor causes anything, nor can a magic substance single-handedly reverse illness. Multiple factors contribute to illness, and multiple interventions work together to promote healing. RCTs are incapable of reconciling this degree of complexity and variation.

Although major alternative medical systems may not have been subjected to a great deal of quantitative research, they are generally *not* experimental therapies. They rely on well-developed clinical observational skills and experience that is guided by their explanatory models. Likewise, the majority of biomedical practices are guided by observation and experience and have *not* been tested quantitatively. New medicines must have rigorous proof of efficacy and safety before clinical use. Tests, procedures, and treatments, however, are not similarly constrained. Western physicians, like alternative practitioners, use the same well-developed clinical observational skills and experience, guided by their explanatory biomedical model. Thus the argument really becomes one of cultural turf rather than scientific method (Broom & Adams, 2007).

This text does not offer meticulous documentation for all claims that are made by the various therapies. NCCAM at the National Institutes of Health (NIH) has been mandated to explore complementary and alternative healing practices in the context of rigorous science, to train researchers, and to provide the public with authoritative information. NCCAM has established 16 research centers to explore the safety and efficacy of a wide range of therapies. In addition, NCCAM funds hundreds of research projects and grants every year. The NIH Office of Dietary Supplements is conducting scientific studies regarding the role of dietary supplements in the improvement of health care. As a result of these and other international efforts, the evidence base for alternative therapies has grown significantly during the past decade.

The results of scientific studies can be accessed at two sites. NCCAM and the National Library of Medicine (NLM) have partnered to create CAM on PubMed (http://nccam.nih.gov/research/camonpubmed/). This site provides access to citations from the MEDLINE database and links to many full-text articles at journal websites. The Cochrane Library (www.update-software.com/cochrane/), an international effort, consists of a regularly updated collection of evidence-based medicine databases, including the Cochrane Database of Systematic Reviews. It lists more than 4,000 randomized trials for various alternative therapies. This information is extremely helpful for both consumers and providers of health care. The reader is advised to access these sites for information regarding the latest research results. Chapter 3 covers evidence-based practice in more detail.

CONSUMERS

Many Americans are looking outside of conventional medicine for relief from illness and improvement of health. According to a number of random surveys, two thirds of adults in the United States use one or more types of alternative medicine, often to treat a chronic medical condition as listed in Box 1.3. Most of these consumers fail to discuss the use of alternative therapies with their primary conventional practitioner, even though the vast majority of people use both approaches simultaneously. In general, alternative therapies are more commonly used by women than men, as well as people with higher levels of education. Latinos have a higher rate of use (50%–90%) when compared to EuroAmericans (Clement, Chen, Burke, Clement, & Zazzali, 2006; Ortiz, Shields, Clauson, & Clay, 2007; Sirois, 2008).

The mainstream medical community can no longer ignore alternative therapies. The public interest is extensive and growing. One has only to look at the proliferation of popular health books, health food stores, and clinics

BOX 1.3

Frequently Reported Conditions of Those Seeking Alternative Therapies

Back pain
Head cold
Neck pain
Joint pain
Arthritis
Anxiety/depression
Stomach upset
Headache
Chronic pain
Insomnia

Source: National Center for Complementary and Alternative Medicine. 2007 Statistics on CAM Use in the United States. http://nccam.nih.gov/news/camstats/2007/index.htm. Accessed June 12, 2008.

USING RESEARCH TO HEAL

Dowd, T., Kolcaba, K., Steiner, R., & Fashinpaur, D. (2007). Comparison of Healing Touch, coaching, and a combined intervention on comfort and stress in younger college students. *Holistic Nursing Practice*, 21(4): 194–202.

What Is This Study About?

College students experience numerous concurrent challenges while pursuing their academic goals. These challenges include: academic pressures, relationship issues, financial concerns, living arrangements, and simultaneous employment. As a result of these stressors and others, students often visit their campus health center for a myriad of symptoms such as changes in eating and sleeping, anxiety, depression, and academic deficiencies. In this study, nurse researchers focused on the problem of how to help these students improve their stress management techniques through measuring and comparing the effects of three interventions. The interventions tested were three weekly sessions each of Healing Touch™ (HT), coaching, and a combination of both interventions administered in sequence.

How Was the Study Done?

This four-group experimental design study was approved by a university institutional review board. College students, aged 18–24, were recruited through fliers, pamphlets, and electronic announcements. Students meeting inclusion criteria related to age and self-identified as having stressors were randomly assigned into one of the four groups. Students with a history of mental health problems, migraine headaches, and currently receiving treatment for stress were excluded from this study. The study participants included 12 men and 40 women, and 71% were White. The mean age was 20.82. Students assigned to the Healing Touch group received 15 to 20 minutes of mind clearing (using the hands to apply gentle touch to areas of the head, shoulders, and neck region in a specific pattern). Students assigned to the coaching protocol group actively participated in 13- to 20-minute sessions to identify stress-related symptoms, assess current use of stress-reducing strategies, collaborate about new strategies to initiate at home and receive subsequent feedback about effectiveness of strategies. The students in the combined group received 30 to 40 minutes of both interventions with a nurse/coach and the HT nurse preferably in sequence. Students in the waitlist group (fourth group) were asked to complete questionnaires online at preset intervals. The interventions were done once a week for three weeks. Two measures were used for each outcome of comfort and stress for all four groups.

What Were the Results of the Study?

HT had improved immediate results on stress and comfort but coaching had better carry-over results on both outcomes. Combined treatment findings were inconsistent. Slight improvement was found in students assigned to the waitlist group.

What Additional Questions Might I Have?

Would the findings be significantly different for an older population or equal number of male participants in the study? Would the findings be dissimilar for a more culturally diverse population? How can the findings be generalized for persons living with stress associated with other health problems and attempting to balance work and school?

How Can I Use This Study?

Nurses need to be cognizant that implementing the principles of coaching and healing touch may be an effective intervention for persons living with excessive stress. Nurses may use this study in their own personal lives as they learn to adapt to stressors inherent in the discipline of nursing. The study findings support the suggestion that there are strategies to relieve stress that do not depend on medical or pharmacological intervention.

Source: Contributed by Dolores M. Huffman, RN, PhD, Associate Professor of Nursing, Purdue University Calumet.

offering healing therapies to realize that this interest cannot be dismissed. In March 2000, President Clinton ordered the establishment of the White House Commission on Complementary and Alternative Medicine Policy in an attempt to create a real integration of conventional and alternative medicine. The mission of the advisory committee was to make legislative and administrative recommendations for the education and training of health care professionals and to make suggestions for access and delivery of health care.

What are consumers seeking from alternative medicine? Some have the same goal for both types of medicine, such as the use of pain medications and acupuncture to control chronic pain. Other consumers may have a different expectation for each approach, such as seeing a conventional practitioner for antibiotics to eradicate an infection and using an alternative practitioner to improve natural immunity through a healthy lifestyle. A person receiving chemotherapy may use meditation and visualization to control the side effects of the chemotherapeutic agents. People who combine conventional and alternative therapies are making therapeutic choices on their own and assuming responsibility for their own health.

It is important for nurses to understand the reasons consumers choose alternative practitioners. Some utilize alternative healers because of financial, geographic, and cultural barriers to biomedical care. Many turn to alternative healers for a sense of hope, control, personal attention, physical contact, and regard for the whole person that seems to be overlooked in conventional medicine. Some of the common reasons for seeking alternative practitioners are listed in Box 1.4.

Because alternative therapists are rushing to meet the demand, it is increasingly difficult for consumers to figure out how and where to get the best health care. It may be problematic to find reliable information to help separate the healers from those who pretend to have medical knowledge. Consumers should *be wary* of healers who (Tiedje, 1998):

- Say they have all the answers
- Maintain that theirs is the only effective therapy

BOX 1.4

Reasons for Choosing Alternative Therapies

Pursue therapeutic benefit

Seek a degree of wellness not supported in biomedicine

Attend to quality-of-life issues

Prefer high personal involvement in decision making

Practitioners spend more time with clients

Believe conventional medicine treats symptoms not underlying cause

Find conventional medical treatments to be lacking or ineffective

Avoid toxicities and/or invasiveness of conventional interventions

Decrease use of prescribed or over-the-counter medications

Identify with a particular healing system as a part of cultural background

Sources: Clement, Chen, Burke, Clement, & Zazzali, 2006; National Center for Complementary and Alternative Medicine. 2007 Statistics on CAM Use in the United States. http://www.nccam.nih.gov/news/camstats/2007/index/.htm. Accessed June 12, 2008; Saydah & Eberhardt, 2006.

- Promise overnight success
- Refuse to include other practitioners as part of the healing team
- Seem more interested in money than in people's well-being

Some alternative specialties are more regulated and licensed than others, but none come with guarantees any more than conventional medicine comes with guarantees. Consumers may want to research the background, qualifications, and competence of any health care provider—alternative, conventional, or integrative. Most types of alternative practices have national organizations of practitioners that are familiar with legislation, state licensing, certification, or registration laws. Many of these organizations are found in the resource section at the back of each chapter in this text.

INTEGRATED NURSING PRACTICE

In the past 20 years, nursing has been moving away from a biomedical orientation that has largely defined and directed it toward a nursing–caring–healing model. Watson (1997) describes it as a shift from a *nursing qua medicine* paradigm (nurses helping doctors practice medicine) to a *nursing qua nursing* paradigm (practicing the distinct art and science of nursing). This movement has reconnected us with the finest tradition of Florence Nightingale in using our hands, heart, and head in creating healing environments. The modern nurse-healer draws on biomedical and caring-healing models by utilizing technology and focusing on caring relationships and healing processes. Dossey, Keegan, and

Guzzetta (2005) have described the modern nurse-healer as having a hybrid of scientific skills and spiritual commitment. We need scientific principles, methods, and skills, but we also need to teach people ways to become more self-reliant as we shift from caregivers to healers.

In 1979, Watson published her text *Nursing: The Philosophy and Science of Caring*, which evolved from her experiences of nursing within the limitations of traditional biomedical models. She sought to bring new meaning to the nursing paradigm of caring-healing and health. Her caritas process was developed to balance the "cure" stance of Western medicine. Watson's theory has since evolved into "clinical caritas processes." This perspective describes nurse–client relationships based on spirituality, love, caring, healing environments, wholeness, and unity of being (Watson, 2007).

The *art of nursing* is in being there, with another person or persons, in an atmosphere of caring. **Caring** involves compassion and sensitivity to each person within the context of her or his entire life. In the past, the biomedical model urged us not to care too much or get too involved. Caring, successful nurses, however, do get involved with clients as they practice nursing as an art instead of nursing as just a day-to-day job. Caring is a philosophy or context within which we practice nursing. Our practice is made caring not by the tools we use but by the attitude or perspective we bring. It is possible, of course, to use the tools of alternative therapies in the same reductionistic way of biomedicine. For example, if one knows the pressure point for headaches and simply uses this pressure point for pain relief without any further assessment, it could hardly be considered holistic or healing. The symptom of headache has been addressed, but the meaning of the headache and the person's experience of the pain has been totally ignored.

Before nurses can care for clients, they must first learn to value and care for themselves. One of your goals in reading this text might be discovering how to care for yourself more effectively because it is only when we can care first for ourselves that we have the energy to care for our patients. Caring for yourself means reducing unnecessary stress, managing conflict more effectively, communicating with family and friends more clearly, and taking time out for yourself. Caring for yourself includes developing a daily routine in practices such as relaxation, meditation, prayer, yoga, communion with nature, and other such forms of contemplation. In Watson's words, "If one is to work from a caring-healing paradigm, one must live it out in daily life" (Watson, 1997, p. 51). The following guidelines will help you maintain your self-care practices (Jahnke, 1997):

- Choose self-care activities that appeal to you and fit into your lifestyle.
- Do one or more of these practices every day. Consider them as important as you do take food and sleep.
- Seek guidance and support from teachers/practitioners if appropriate.
- Find a good spot for your practice that is physically and mentally comfortable.
- Build up your practice slowly. Success is not gained by aggressive or compulsive practice.

- Look for opportunities to practice with others.
- Focus on relaxing. The foundation of all self-healing, health enhancement, stress mastery, and personal empowerment is deep relaxation.

The plurality of the sick care, health care system may be one of its greatest strengths. It enables us to meet the diverse needs of diverse populations. The question is, "How can we combine the best ideas of conventional nursing practice and alternative healing practices?" First, we must have education. At the basic level, our nursing curricula must include courses in caring and alternative therapies. All nurses could learn Therapeutic Touch, healthy dietary plans, the use of basic herbs, as well as the use of visualization and prayer in the healing process. Since 2004, basic alternative therapies content is included in the NCLEX-RN examination. Since state boards of nursing vary in their detail of criteria for alternative therapies and nursing practice, it is critical that you check the Nurse Practice Act of your state.

The White House Commission on Complementary and Alternative Medicine (National Institutes of Health, 2002) states that "since the public utilizes both conventional health care and complementary and alternative medicine (CAM), the Commission believes that this reality should be reflected in the education and training of all health practitioners" (p. 51). The Commission goes on to say that "although there has been notable progress in introducing CAM into medical, nursing, and other fields of conventional health care education in recent years, more needs to be done" (p. 51). We must also participate in continuing education courses to expand our knowledge beyond the basic level. With additional education, we can learn such things as basic massage and reflexology, meditation, and yoga. Some nurses will choose to continue their education through master of science in nursing degrees with a holistic nursing concentration. Some schools of nursing offer certificate programs for nurse practitioners. Other nurses will choose to complete formal programs in alternative medicine such as naturopathy, Ayurveda, homeopathy, chiropractic medicine, or hypnotherapy. Advanced practice nurses should provide leadership in research and education in alternative therapies (Denner, 2007).

Next, we must provide community education. We must provide people with information, tools, skills, and support to enable them to make healthy decisions about life and negotiate their way through the health care systems. Growing immigrant populations call for more attention to a variety of health expectations, needs, and preferences. As nurses, we must also become familiar with the alternative practices they bring with them. We must also attempt to keep ourselves healthy most of the time. We should exemplify good health, since teaching by example is a powerful influence. We can teach wherever our practice is located: acute care, long-term care, community nurse-managed centers, and in areas of advanced practice nursing. And, finally, we must document our findings, utilize and participate in nursing research, keep current with evidence-based practice, and design new studies to measure the effectiveness of various healing practices.

References

Agdal, R. (2005). Diverse and changing perceptions of the body: Communicating illness, health, and risk in an age of medical pluralism. *Journal of Alternative and Complementary Medicine*, 11(1): 67–75.

Banks, J., Marmot, M., Oldfield, Z., & Smith, J. P. (2006). Diseases and disadvantage in the United States and in England. *Journal of the American Medical Association*, 295(17): 2037–2045.

Broom, A., & Adams, J. (2007). Current issues and future directions in complementary and alternative medicine (CAM) research. *Complementary Therapies in Medicine*, 15: 217–220.

Chan, O. L., & Whitehead, D. (2008). The use of CAM in a New Zealand-based general practice: A multiple case-study. *Complementary Therapies in Medicine*, 16: 36–41.

Clement, J. P., Chen, H. F., Burke, D., Clement, D. G., & Zazzali, J. L. (2006). Are comsumers reshaping hospitals? Complementary and alternative medicine in U.S. hospitals, 1999–2003. *Health Care Management Review*, I31(2): 109–118.

Denner, S. S. (2007). The advanced practice nurse and integration of complementary and alternative medicine. *Holistic Nursing Practice*, 21(3): 152–159.

Dossey, B. M., Keegan, L. G., & Guzzetta, C. E. (2005). *Holistic Nursing: A Handbook for Practice*, 4th ed. Sudburg, MA: Jones and Bartlett Publishers.

Halcon, L. L., Chlan, L. L., Kreitzer, M. J., & Leonard, B. J. (2003). Complementary therapies and healing practices: Faculty/student beliefs and attitudes and the implications for nursing education. *Journal of Professional Nursing*, 19(6): 387–397.

Infant Mortality and Life Expectancy for Selected Countries. (2007). www.infoplease.com/ipa/A0004393.html. Accessed June 11, 2008.

Jahnke, R. (1997). *The Healer Within*. San Francisco: Harper.

Keegan, L. (1994). *The Nurse as Healer*. Albany, NY: Delmar.

National Center for Complementary and Alternative Medicine. (2008). http://nccam.nih.gov. Accessed June 11, 2008.

National Institutes of Health. (2002, March). *White House Commission on Complementary and Alternative Medicine Policy, Final Report*. Washington, DC: U.S. Government Printing Office. www.whccamp.hhs.gov. Accessed June 12, 2008.

Ortiz, B. I., Shields, K. M., Clauson, K. A., & Clay, P. G. (2007). Complementary and alternative medicine use among Hispanics in the United States. *Annals of Pharmacotherapy*, 41(6): 994–1004.

Park, J. (2006). In praise of integrated health. *Complementary Therapies in Medicine*, 14: 173–174.

Peplau, H. E. (1952). *Interpersonal Relations in Nursing*. New York: Putnam.

Quinn, J. F. (2000). The self as healer: Reflections from a nurse's journey. *AACN Clinical Issues*, 11(1): 17–26.

Saydah, S. H., & Eberhardt, M. S. (2006). Use of complementary and alternative medicine among adults with chronic diseases. *Journal of Alternative and Complementary Medicine*, 12(8): 805–812.

Shreffler-Grant, J., Hill, W., Weinert, C., Nichols, E., & Ide, B. (2007). Complementary therapy and older rural women: Who uses it and who does not? *Nursing Research*, 56(1): 28–33.

Sirois, F. M. (2008). Provider-based complementary and alternative medicine use among three chronic illness groups. *Complementary Therapies in Medicine*, 16: 73–80.

Tiedje, L. B. (1998). Alternative health care: An overview. *Journal of Obstetric, Gynecologic, and Neonatal Nursing*, 27(5): 557–562.

U.S. Department of Health and Human Services. (2000). *Healthy People 2010.* Washington, DC: U.S. Government Printing Office.

Watson, J. (1979). *Nursing: The Philosophy and Science of Caring.* New York: Little, Brown and Company.

Watson, J. (1997). The theory of human caring: Retrospective and prospective. *Nursing Science Quarterly,* 10(1): 49–52.

Watson, J. (2007). Caring theory defined. University of Colorado Denver, College of Nursing. www.nursing .ucdenver.edu/faculty/theory_caring. htm. Accessed October 19, 2008.

Willison, K. D. (2006). Integrating Swedish massage therapy with primary health care initiatives as part of a holistic nursing approach. *Complementary Therapies in Medicine,* 14: 254–260.

Resources

American Holistic Health Association
   P.O. Box 17400
   Anaheim, CA 92817–7400
   714.779.6152
   www.ahha.org

American Association of Integrative
   Medicine
   2750 East Sunshine
   Springfield, MO 65804
   417.881.9995
   www.aaimedicine.com

National Center for Complementary and
   Alternative Medicine
   National Institutes of Health
   9000 Rockville Pike
   Bethesda, MD 20892
   888.644.6226
   http://nccam.nih.gov

2

Basic Concepts Guiding Alternative Therapies

*For the truly open-minded scientist,
nothing is implausible.*

J. C. WOOTTON

*For breath is life, and if you breathe well
you will live long on earth.*

SANSKRIT PROVERB

In this book, separate chapters are devoted to each of the most widely used methods in alternative medicine. Because the various methods share principles, overlap occurs in the various types of alternative practices. While practices are grouped in units, many of the practices could be placed in several units. Thus, before reading specifics on each practice, it may be helpful to introduce several concepts common to most healing practices. These are balance, spirituality, energy, and breath.

BALANCE

An expression in the Native American culture, "walking in balance," describes the philosophy of a peaceful coexistence and harmony with all aspects of life. This concept of balance is found in all cultures throughout time. Balance is viewed as a path rather than a steady state, and it is believed that each of us has a unique path as we move through life. In terms of optimal wellness, the concept of balance consists of mental, physical, emotional, spiritual, and environmental components. Not only does each component in and of itself have to be balanced, equilibrium is needed among the components. *Physical* aspects include optimal functioning of all body systems. *Emotional* aspects include the ability to feel and express the entire range of human emotions. *Mental* aspects include feelings of self-worth, a positive identity, a sense of accomplishment, and the ability to appreciate and create. *Spiritual* aspects involve moral values, a meaningful purpose in life, and a feeling of connectedness to others and a divine source. *Environmental* aspects include physical, biologic, economic, social, and political conditions. Walking in balance is a learned skill and one that must be practiced regularly to engage in the process of healthful living. This concept of balance appears again and again throughout the various alternative healing practices.

Cyclic Rhythms

The daily lives of all living things are filled with various changes that take place in cyclic patterns. **Circadian rhythms** are regular fluctuations of a variety of physiologic factors over 24 hours. Most familiar is the 24-hour temperature and sleep patterns. These include adrenal, thyroid, and growth hormone-secreting patterns, as well as temperature, sleep, arousal, energy, appetite, and motor activity patterns. **Ultradian rhythms** are regular fluctuations shorter than 24 hours and repeat more than once a day. An example of an ultradian rhythm is the 90-minute REM/non-REM sleep cycle. **Infradian rhythms** are regular fluctuations over periods longer than 24 hours, such as the menstrual cycle. The constant rhythmic processes bring about a dynamic, healthy balance in our bodies.

Rhythms may be desynchronized by external or internal factors. An example of external desynchronization is jet lag, in which rapid time zone changes result in a decreased energy level and ability to concentrate, as well as mood variations. In some individuals, internal desynchronization may result in depression. The tendency toward internal desynchronization is probably inherited, but stress, lifestyle, and normal aging influence it. Attention to the rhythmic nature of one's own being reveals an intimate relationship with the rhythms of the surrounding natural world.

Musical Rhythms

Health is about balance or harmony of body, mind, and spirit. In a state of optimal health, all frequencies are in harmony, like a finely tuned piano. In fact, music is often used in healing, from the ancient sounds of the drum, rattle, bone flute, and other primitive instruments to the current use of music as a prescription for health. Several nursing research studies demonstrate the effectiveness of music therapy for persons with mental disorders, autism, dementia, cancer, cognition disorders, and neurological problems. Chapter 21 covers music and its research in greater detail.

Dr. Andrew Weil, the leader in the new field of integrative medicine, has created the *Mindbody Tool Kit* (2005) to help people utilize self-healing techniques. *Sound therapy* consists of classical music combined with healing sound frequencies. The combination of sounds entrains your brain to theta and delta brain waves, the state of deep relaxation. It is in this state of relaxation that the body and mind can heal themselves. The benefits of sound therapy are far reaching. Beneficiaries include:

- People experiencing an illness
- People who are having or have had surgical procedures
- People who are having or have had chemotherapy infusions
- People in intensive care
- Women in labor and delivery
- People experiencing anxiety, depression, or insomnia
- People who wish to maintain a high level of wellness

Drumming and chanting are powerful ways to bring oneself in balance with self, others, and the world. The drumbeat serves as a focus for concentration and quiets the chattering mind. The pace of the drumbeat enhances theta brain wave production. One study found drumming and keyboards to be helpful in improving symptoms in young adults with severe autism (Boso, Emmanuele, Minazzi, Abbamonte, & Politi, 2007). Anna Halprin, a renowned dancer and cancer survivor, has pioneered the field of dance as a healing art. She uses movement and imagery, called **psychokinetic visualization,** as modalities for people with life-threatening illnesses. The program is detailed in her book *Returning to Health with Dance, Movement, and Imagery* (2002).

SPIRITUALITY

Spiritual healing techniques and spiritually based health care systems are among the most ancient healing practices. Spirit is the liveliness, richness, and beauty of one's life. It is who we are and how we are in the world. Spirituality is the drive to become all that one can be, and it is bound to intuition, creativity, and motivation. It is the dimension that involves relationship with oneself, with others, and with a higher power. Spirituality is that which gives people meaning and purpose in their lives. It involves finding significant meaning in the entirety of life, including illness and death (Jampolsky, 2005; Taylor, 2002).

Many people are searching for wholeness in their lives and a way to allow their innermost selves to grow and expand. Spiritual healing practices guide individuals to places within themselves they did not know existed through techniques as ancient as prayer, contemplation, meditation, drumming, storytelling, and mythology. In consciously awakening the energies of the spirit, people are able to move toward healing places and sacred moments in their lives.

During periods of stress, illness, or crisis, people search for meaning and purpose in their pain and suffering. They ask questions such as "Why am I sick?" or "Why did this bad thing happen?" This spiritual quest for meaning can lead to insight and healing or to fear and isolation. In the words of Ken Wilber:

> A person, who is beginning to sense the suffering of life, is, at the same time, beginning to awaken to deeper realities, truer realities. For suffering smashes to pieces the complacency of our normal fictions about reality, and forces us to become alive in a special sense—to see carefully, to feel deeply, to touch ourselves and our world in ways we have heretofore avoided. It has been said, and truly I think, that suffering is the first grace (quoted in Borysenko & Borysenko, 1994, p. 191).

Spirituality is often confused with religiosity, which is not surprising, because the two constructs are closely related. **Religion** involves a search for the sacred, a group identity, and a sense of belongingness. **Spirituality,** a much broader concept, is the search for wholeness and purpose that underlies the world's religions. Remove the dogma, the politics, and cultural influence from any of the world's religions, and you find the same questions, the same seeking, and the same answers. The concept of spirituality does not undermine any religion but rather enhances all religions by illuminating their commonalities and the commonality among all people. It makes us far more similar to each other than it makes us different. Chapter 23 covers faith and prayer as it relates to health and well-being.

Many traditions also speak of spiritual guides. Some of us think of them as guardian angels, others as Beings of Light who guide people through near-death experiences. Buddhists think of them as *devas*. Cherokees call them *Adawees*, the great protectors of the Four Directions. *Malakh*, or "messenger," is the Hebrew word for angel. There are the cherubim and the seraphim and the four great archangels: Uriel, Raphael, Michael, and Gabriel. The Iranian angel Vohu Manah is believed to have revealed the message of God to Zoroaster some 2,500 years ago. Similarly, the Archangel Gabriel is credited for revealing the Koran to Muhammad a thousand years later. Gabriel, honored by Jews, Christians, and Muslims, has a special role as a mediator between human consciousness and the higher realms from which spirit descends into the body. Although no Western scientific evidence supports the existence of angels, one can find phenomenological evidence. Many first-person accounts of near-death occurrences involve angels and similar experiences from people of different ages, from diverse cultures, with different personal and religious beliefs (Borysenko & Dveirin, 2007).

USING RESEARCH TO HEAL

McCaffrey, R. (2007). The effect of healing gardens and art therapy on older adults with mild to moderate depression. *Holistic Nursing Practice*, 21(2): 79–84.

What Is This Study About?

Depression is a common mental health problem among older adults in the United States. Many senior citizens are hesitant to discuss feelings and thoughts related to depression with health professionals because of the stigma attached to mental illness. This study investigated the effect of three interventions for depression in three groups of older adults living with mild to moderate depression. The interventions were (a) walking in a garden alone, (b) walking in a garden using a guided imagery leader to call attention to the garden experience through a specified script, and (c) art therapy.

How Was the Study Done?

Sixty participants meeting the inclusion criteria of a diagnosis of depression through self-identification (69%) or from a health care provider (31%), and the ability to walk and transport self to a garden twice weekly for 6 weeks were recruited for this study. Participants were randomly assigned to one of the three intervention groups, each group had 20 participants. The mean age of the participants was 75 years, 26% were married, 42% were not married, and 9% were widowed. Upon obtaining informed consent, they related stories of joy and sadness in their lives and completed the Geriatric Depression Scale. Walking groups were separated to avoid contamination of the study results. Focus group sessions were held for 2 hours on the last day of participation for each group and were asked the same set of questions.

What Were the Results of the Study?

All participants in each of the groups believed the intervention they experienced was beneficial in decreasing depression and enhancing their mood and general attitude concerning life.

What Additional Questions Might I Have?

Would older adults living with depression and using a wheelchair also benefit from these interventions? Were the older adult's responses in the focus group affected by being with other members of the group? Would 1:1 interviews at the completion of the study have obtained different results? Were participant's responses in the garden walk with a guided imagery leader influenced by having the presence of another person?

How Can I Use This Study?

Walking in a garden can be very cost effective as no special training or education is warranted. Nurses can initiate or suggest walking groups in local gardens to help older adults experiencing feelings of depression as part of their community or church activities. Guided imagery garden walks could be instituted with the use of tapes if no leader is accessible. Nurses working in residences for senior adults may suggest garden walks or art therapy for reducing mild to moderate depression.

Source: Contributed by Dolores M. Huffman, RN, PhD, Associate Professor of Nursing, Purdue University Calumet.

ENERGY

The concept of energy has been recognized for centuries and in most cultures. Many ancient and current cultures have great respect for the subtle and unseen forces in life. Most spiritual traditions share the belief that energy is the bridge between spirit and physical being. Meditation and prayer are believed to be subtle energy phenomena that represent contact with the spiritual dimension.

Chinese Taoist scholars believed that energy, not matter, was the basic building material of the universe. Albert Einstein and other physicists proved that matter and energy are the same and that energy is not only the raw material of the cosmos but the glue that holds it together. Modern scientists now look at the universe in terms of forces instead of tiny particles of matter. Their experimental findings are similar to the intuitive observations of China's ancient scholars. Everything in the world—animate and inanimate—is made of energy. People are beings of energy, living in a universe composed of energy.

Although Western scientists agree that energy comprises all things, when this notion is applied to the human body, they do not yet fully agree that a distinct energy system exists within the physical body. In order for energy to be "real," it must be measurable by scientific instruments. By this logic, of course, brain waves did not exist prior to the invention of EEG equipment! Since technology is not yet capable of measuring all the energy fields in the body, references to energy are often absent in conventional medicine.

For more than 2,000 years, various practitioners around the world have insisted that a person is more than the physical body. According to these healers, a "life force" of subtle energy surrounds and permeates every person. Energy is viewed as the force that integrates the body, mind, and spirit; it is that which connects everything. The Japanese call this energy *ki* (pronounced "key"); the Tibetans refer to it as *lung* (pronounced "loong"); the Polynesians call it *mana*; Native Americans call it *oki, orenda,* or *ton*; Americans call it *subtle energy* or bioenergy; the Greeks call it *pneuma*; and the Hindus give it the name *prana*. Prana is sometimes translated from the Sanskrit as "primary energy," "breath," or "vital force." The Chinese refer to this energy as *qi* or *chi* (pronounced "chee") and believe that it takes the form of two opposite but complementary phases, yin and yang. *Yin* is the earth, moon, night, fall and winter, cold, wetness, darkness, the feet, the left side, the female gender, and passivity. Yin is involved in tissue growth. *Yang* is the sun, day, spring and summer, heat, dryness, light, the head, the right side, the male gender, and aggressiveness. Yang is involved in tissue breakdown. It is believed that each person is a unique combination of the complementary energies of yin and yang. Wholeness is comprised of this union of opposites. Figure 2.1 shows the t'ai chi symbol, which illustrates the yin and yang of Chinese thought. The white dot on the black portion of the symbol and the black dot on the white section are reminders that each quality contains some of its opposite. Further descriptions of yin and yang are found in Chapter 4.

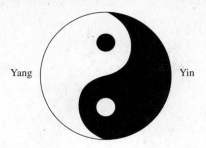

Yang   Yin

FIGURE 2.1   T'ai Chi Symbol

It is believed that qi creates qi. In other words, physical activities such as eating, work, and rest, as well as nonphysical aspects of life such as will, motivation, feelings, desires, and a sense of purpose in life, are all made possible by qi. Those same activities and aspects also create more qi. Most schools of thought basically agree on the following points regarding energy (Newman & Miller, 2006; Warber, Cornelio, Straughn, & Kile, 2004):

- Energy comes from one universal source.
- Movement of energy is the basis of all life.
- Matter is an expression of energy and vice versa.
- All things are manifestations of energy.
- The entire earth has energetic and metabolic qualities.
- People are composed of multiple, interacting energy fields that extend out into the environment.
- People's relationships with one another are shaped by the interactions of their energies.
- Qi, ki, and prana have no exact counterpart in conventional medicine, though the concept of a physical bioenergy system is under research. It is described as a weak but complex electromagnetic field that is hypothesized to involve electromagnetic bioinformation for regulating homeodynamics.

Chakras

The Hindu concept of chakras (a Sanskrit word for "spinning wheel") describes seven major energy centers within the physical body. Chakras have been described by most Eastern cultures and several South American cultures (such as Mayan) for thousands of years. **Chakras** are major centers of both electromagnetic activity and circulation of vital energy. They are usually thought of as funnels of perpetually rotating energy and are considered the gateways through which energy enters and leaves the body. Each chakra in the body is recognized as a focal point of the life force relating to physical, emotional, mental, and spiritual aspects of people and is the network through which the body, mind, and spirit interact as one holistic system. Figure 2.2 illustrates the sites of the chakras in the body.

The concept of chakras may be foreign to the Western scientific mind, but they are not completely unknown to those familiar with Judeo-Christian

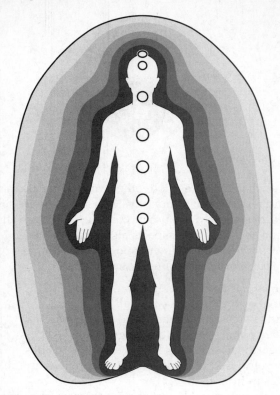

FIGURE 2.2 The Chakras and the Auric Field

culture, particularly in the artwork and sculptures passed down through the ages. For centuries, the crown chakra, which signifies a conscious awareness of the divine, has been painted as a halo over those who are consciously aware of a divine presence in their lives.

The seven main chakras are vertically aligned up the center of the body from the base of the pelvis to the top of the head. Each has its own individual characteristics and functions and each has a corresponding relationship to various organs and structures of the body, to one of the endocrine glands, as well as to one of the seven colors of the rainbow spectrum. The characteristics of the seven major chakras are described in Box 2.1. Of the many smaller chakras throughout the body, the most significant are in the palms of the hands. The hand chakras are considered extensions of the heart chakra and, as such, radiate healing and soothing energies. Spiritual healers who practice the laying on of hands concentrate energy in their hand chakras. All the chakras have purpose, function, and frequency. These are to:

- Regulate the human energy system and maintain an equilibrium of health (purpose)
- Link body, mind, and spirit and exchange energy (function)

BOX 2.1
The Chakras

1. **Root chakra**
    Location: base of the spine
    Center of: physical vitality, urge to survive
    Gland: adrenal glands
    Organs/Structures: kidneys, bladder, spine
    Color: red
2. **Sexual or navel chakra**
    Location: slightly below the navel, in front of the sacrum
    Center of: sexual energy, ego, extrasensory perception
    Gland: gonads
    Organs/Structures: reproductive organs, legs
    Color: orange
3. **Solar plexus chakra**
    Location: slightly above the navel
    Center of: unrefined emotions, urge for power
    Gland: pancreas
    Organs/Structures: stomach, liver, gallbladder
    Color: yellow
4. **Heart chakra**
    Location: middle of the chest at the height of the heart
    Center of: unconditional affection, compassion, devotion, love, spiritual growth
    Gland: thymus
    Organs/Structures: heart, liver, lungs, circulatory system
    Color: emerald
5. **Throat chakra**
    Location: throat area
    Center of: communication, self-expression, creativity
    Gland: thyroid
    Organs/Structures: throat, upper lungs, digestive tract, arms
    Color: blue
6. **Third-eye chakra**
    Location: middle of the forehead, a little higher than the eyebrows
    Center of: the will, intellect, spirit, spiritual awakening, visualization
    Gland: pituitary
    Organs/Structures: spine, lower brain, left eye, nose
    Color: purple
7. **Crown chakra**
    Location: at the top of the head at the fontanel
    Center of: highest level of consciousness or enlightenment, intuition, direct spiritual vision
    Gland: pineal
    Organs/Structures: upper brain, right eye
    Color: golden-white

Each operates at its own optimum frequency; generally the lower the chakra on the body, the lower its frequency; if one is out of sync, all others will be also (frequency).

The main purpose in working with and understanding the chakras is to create integration and wholeness within people. The chakras are the "doorways" through which the energy from within and without is distributed to cells, tissues, and organs. If chakras stop functioning properly, the intake of energy will be disturbed and the body organs served by that chakra will not get their needed supply of energy. Eventually, organ functioning will be disrupted, leading to weakened organs with a diminished immune defense. If this process continues, the end result will be dysfunction and disease (Gardner, 2006; Smith, 2008). Dr. Dean Ornish (1999), well known for his program to reverse blocked coronary arteries through diet, exercise, support groups, and meditation without surgery or drugs, believes that a closed heart chakra (unresolved anger and fear) is related to the closed coronary arteries. Consequently, the meditation technique he incorporates into his program involves opening the heart chakra. His holistic approach has now become a recognized program practiced nationwide.

Aura

Closely related to the chakras is the concept of aura. The **aura** is the energy field surrounding each person as far as the outstretched arms and from head to toe. This energy field is both an information center and a highly sensitive perceptual system that transmits and receives messages from the internal and external environments. Each of the seven layers of the auric field is associated with a chakra; the first layer is related to the first chakra, and so on. Each layer has physical, mental, emotional, and spiritual dimensions and purposes and the layers function together through the transmission of energy. Box 2.2 lists characteristics of the auric field, and Figure 2.2 shows a diagrammatic view of the auric field. Virtually every alternative healing therapy has a way of interpreting the body's subtle energy, which will be discussed throughout this text.

Meridians

A person's vital energy is not simply radiated outward but has patterns of circulation within the body, referred to as the meridian system. **Meridians** are a network of energy circuits or lines of force that run vertically through the body connecting all parts. Meridians may be understood more clearly if they are compared to a major city's highway system with entrance and exit ramps, merging roads, and connecting surface streets. If a flood blocks an exit ramp, the streets served by this ramp are inaccessible, which, in turn, affects the people who live and work on those streets. Also, the traffic may be backed up on the highway waiting for the ramp to reopen, creating a traffic jam. Meridians operate this way in a person's body. If some kind of blockage affects one's hip, for example, the pathways of energy leading to that hip get "backed up." Pain

BOX 2.2

Seven Layers of the Auric Field

Level 1. Etheric Body
Location: 1/4 inch to 2 inches beyond the physical body
Center of: physical functioning and physical sensation
Color: light blue to gray

Level 2. Emotional Body
Location: 1 to 3 inches beyond the physical body; roughly follows the outline of the physical body
Center of: emotional aspects of person
Color: all colors of the rainbow

Level 3. Mental Body
Location: 3 to 8 inches beyond the physical body
Center of: instinct, intellect, intuition
Color: bright yellow with additional colors superimposed

Level 4. Astral Body
Location: 6 to 16 inches beyond the physical body
Center of: love
Color: same colors as in level 3 but infused with the rose light of love

Level 5. Etheric Template Body
Location: 18 to 24 inches beyond the physical body
Center of: higher will connected with divine will, speaking, listening, working, taking responsibility for our actions
Color: clear lines on cobalt blue background

Level 6. Celestial Body
Location: 24 to 33 inches beyond the physical body
Center of: celestial love, spiritual ecstasy, protection and nurturance of all life
Color: shimmering pastel colors

Level 7. Causal Body
Location: 30 to 42 inches, forming an egg shape around the body
Center of: higher mind; integration of spiritual and physical body
Color: shimmering gold threads

or discomfort restricts the motion of the hip, which puts a different strain on the foot, and the foot in a different position creates a strain on other sets of muscles. These changes in the body's general posture affect the positions of the internal organs, which, in turn, restrict the nutrition to the organs, alter organ function, and thereby change the body's balance. As the body and mind are affected, the person will think and feel differently, leading to more tension and more changes (Lee, Jeong, Lee, Jeong, & Eo, 2005).

Each meridian passes close to the skin's surface at places called *hsueh*, which means "cave" or "hollow" and is translated as point or acupuncture point. Because each meridian is associated with an internal organ, the acupuncture points offer surface access to the internal organ systems. The flow of qi can be strengthened or weakened by manipulating specific points. Keeping the flow of energy open and regular contributes to a state of balance and health.

The California Institute for Human Science (www.cihs.edu) is the American center for research on a machine called the AMI, an acronym for "apparatus for meridian identification." The AMI measures the flow of ions through the body and in 10 minutes can give a complete evaluation of the condition of a person's meridian system and the corresponding internal organs related to those meridians. This stream of ions is not vital energy or qi itself. Rather, it is a secondary electromagnetic effect of qi—in a sense, its imprint in the physical domain. The AMI is now available for distribution as a diagnostic tool in alternative therapies and conventional medicine (Ahn & Martinsen, 2007).

Energy Concentration

The mind's energy, or willpower, can be developed by individuals to control their body's energy system to an extraordinary degree. Healers can concentrate and manipulate energy in remarkable ways using their energy to align and balance the electromagnetic field of the patient. In attempting to trace the source of healers' energy, studies demonstrate that it seems to come from the central body in the area between the solar plexus and the lower abdomen. The Chinese refer to this spot as the *tan dien* or the home of qi, and the Hindus refer to it as the *solar plexus chakra* or the seat of prana (Zhao, 2006).

Grounding and Centering

Two terms common in various healing practices and related to energy and balance are grounding and centering. **Grounding,** as its name suggests, relates to one's connection with the ground and, in a broader sense, to one's whole contact with reality. Being grounded suggests stability, security, independence, having a solid foundation, and living in the present rather than escaping into dreams. It means having a mature sense of responsibility for oneself. Much of the sense of grounding comes from identification with the lower half of one's body—the parts of being that are less conscious and have more instinctive functions of movement. Learning to breathe into the belly, for example, is vital for grounding, for if the breath is shallow, contact with feelings and reality is limited. Many of the practices in this text, such as biofield therapies, mind–body techniques, and spiritual therapies, help increase one's groundedness.

Centering refers to the process of bringing oneself to the center or middle. When people are centered, they are fully connected to the part of their bodies where all their energies meet. Centering is the process of focusing one's mind on the center of energy, usually in the navel or solar plexus chakra. All movement in the body originates from this center, providing the meeting point for body and mind. It is commonly considered the "earth" center, for it gathers energy from the earth rising up through the legs. Centering can be done through movement, as in t'ai chi, or can be found in stillness, as in meditation. Being centered allows one to operate intuitively, with awareness, and to channel energy throughout the body.

BREATH

Breath is at the center of all spiritual and religious traditions. In many languages, the words for *spirit* and *breath* are one and the same—Sanskrit *prana*, Hebrew *ruach*, Greek *pneuma*, and Latin *spiritus*. In Christianity, the Holy Spirit is referred to as "the breath of life." To inspire, or take in spirit, means not only to inhale but to encourage, motivate, and give hope. To expire, or lose spirit, means not only to exhale but to die, cease to exist, to end, or be destroyed.

In Eastern cultures, when air is inhaled, so is vital energy, it flows into the body to nourish and enliven. In Traditional Chinese Medicine, the exhalation is considered the yin part of the breath, and the inhalation is yang. It is impossible to only breathe in without breathing out or to breathe out without breathing in. It is the continuous dynamic balance of yin and yang that contributes to health and well-being. Most of the healing traditions worldwide believe breath is the most important function of life and that restrictions in breathing lead to dysfunction and disease.

In Western culture, the breath has been considered simply a mechanical, metabolic function of the body. Scientists are now beginning to recognize that breath can be used for healing, improving the body's self-repair processes, and reducing vulnerability to illness. Oxygen is toxic to viruses, bacteria, yeasts, and parasites in the body, and cancer cells find it more difficult to survive in an oxygen-rich environment. Andrew Weil (1995a) believes that "breath is the master key to health and wellness, a function we can learn to regulate and develop in order to improve our physical, mental, and spiritual well-being" (p. 86).

The breath is constantly adapting to accommodate the needs of the situation at hand. When people eat heavy meals or exercise rapidly, when their noses are congested or dry, or when their environment is filled with pleasant or unpleasant smells, their breathing changes. Every change in posture has an effect on the combination of muscles used to breathe. Breath does not feel the same standing or sitting as when one is lying down. Breathing also changes under stress. For example, anxious people take shallow "chest" breaths, using only their chest muscles to inhale rather than their diaphragms. As a result, only the top part of their lungs fills with air, depriving the body of the optimal amount of oxygen.

Many people, even when feeling relaxed, breathe in a shallow way that keeps them in a constant state of under-oxygenation that contributes to a decreased level of energy and increased vulnerability to illness. The typical shallow chest breath moves about half a pint of air, while a full abdominal breath can move eight to ten times that amount. Forming healthy breathing habits can produce dramatic results. Probably no other single step that people can take will so profoundly and positively affect body, mind, and spirit. Deep breathing can counter stress. Just three deep, full belly breaths can move individuals from panic to calmness by increasing their oxygen intake. Much of perceived stress is worrying about the future or the past, and deep breathing is a great way to return people to the present. Twenty minutes of deep breathing exercises a day can lower blood pressure by increasing oxygen intake, which decreases workload on the cardiovascular system (Chinese Health Qigong Association, 2008).

INTEGRATED NURSING PRACTICE

In alternative medicine, the focus of restoring health is within each person and cannot be "given" to a client by any health care practitioner. Drugs, herbs, procedures, surgeries, or mind–body techniques may be helpful or necessary, but by themselves do not cure disease. People must, and do, rebalance and repair themselves. The profession of nursing was founded on this philosophy and view of life as noted by Florence Nightingale's (1969) basic premise that healing is a function of nature that comes from within the individual. She saw the role of the nurse as putting the "patient in the best condition for nature to act on him."

In contrast, biomedicine has taught people to listen to external authorities and to view themselves as helpless victims of disease. Conventional medicine is based on the idea of cure, which usually refers to the elimination of the signs and symptoms of disease. "Curing," however, is only effective for about 15 to 20 percent of the sick population. In 80 to 85 percent of acute disruptions of health, one of three things happens with or without medical intervention: The person gets well, develops a chronic disorder for which there is no cure, or dies. When the focus is on cure, death is seen as a failure. Certainly, the curative aspects of Western medicine have allowed many people to live healthy, productive lives. But for many others, fixing the body is not enough. As they search for meaning in their illness and their lives, as well as a sense of connectedness with others, they begin the healing process. Box 2.3 compares the philosophy and beliefs of the medical-curing model with the nursing-healing model.

Most sick people eventually get better no matter what treatment is given or even if no treatment is given. If the person is given "something," recovery is even more likely because of the **placebo effect.** The concept of the "placebo effect" comes directly out of biomedicine's denial of the power of self-healing. In Western research studies, the placebo is a sham biomedical treatment with no inherent medical value. Most researchers dislike the placebo response because it complicates their experiments. In study after study, the placebo has been found effective in at least 30 to 35 percent of the cases. In fact, the rate is as high as 70 percent; typically 40 percent of individuals report excellent results and another 30 percent report good results (Benson, 1997; Harrington, 2008; Moerman, 2006). Norman Cousins, author of *Anatomy of an Illness* (1991) and *The Healing Heart* (1985), describes the placebo as the "doctor who resides within." In fact, this so-called placebo response in Western scientific literature

BOX 2.3

The Cure Versus Heal Models

Medical-Curing Model	Nursing-Healing Model
Diseases are cured	People are healed
Focus on diagnosis	Focus on meaning
Patient is dependent	Person is autonomous
Effective for 15%–20% of population; cure may or may not be possible	Effective for everyone; healing is always possible
Body is viewed as a machine; disease results when parts break	Body is a living microcosm of the universe; disease results through imbalance
Role of medicine is to combat disease; practitioners are soldiers in a war	Role of medicine is to restore harmony; practitioners are the Peace Corps, fostering learning and growth
Body is passive recipient of treatments to fix it	Body is capable of self-healing
Primary treatments are drugs, surgery, radiation	Primary treatments are diet, herbs, stress management, social support
Focus on pain	Focus on the human experience of pain, which is suffering
Caring is seen as a means to an end	Caring is the end in itself

Sources: Dossey, Keegan, & Guzzetta, 2005; Quinn, 1989; Watson, 2007.

demonstrates the unity of mind–body and provides great evidence of our self-curing capacity. Janet Quinn (1989), an outstanding nursing leader, believes that since the site of all curing is within the individual, "there are no longer any 'real' or 'placebo' treatments and effects. There are only stimuli for healing processes" (p. 554). Andrew Weil (1995b) regards the placebo response as a "pure example of healing elicited by the mind; far from being a nuisance, it is, potentially, the greatest therapeutic ally doctors can find in their efforts to mitigate disease" (p. 52).

Beliefs can also work against people. The *nocebo* is the placebo's negative counterpart. It is destructive thinking that contributes to sickness and even death. Our bodies are good at healing, but at times we inhibit this process by worrying or doubting our ability to overcome the illness. As nurses, we must routinely assess clients' beliefs and expectations for health and use them systematically in the healing process. The goal is not to deny reality, but to help people project healthy images. When a person acts "as if" the preferred reality were true, the body responds and improved health can emerge (Colloca, Sigaudo, & Benedetti, 2008).

The word *heal* comes from the Greek word *halos* and the Anglo-Saxon word *haelan*, which mean "to be or to become whole." (Interestingly, the word *holy* is derived from the same source.) Thus "healing" means "making whole"—that is, restoring balance and harmony. It is a movement toward a sense of wholeness and completion. Healing comes from surrendering to life as it is, including all feelings from anger and despair through joy and peacefulness. The irony is that in the process of accepting life as it is, most people feel more alive and live more fully, even when facing death. When the focus is on healing, success does not depend on whether the person lives. Healing can take place even as the body weakens. Through healing, people allow themselves to be everything they already are and move toward a greater sense of the meaning of their experiences. Even when nothing can be done physically to alter the course of disease, still much can be done in a caring sense to make the human experience more meaningful and understandable (Quinn, 1997; Sharoff, 2008). As Joellen Goertz Koerner (2007) states: ". . . the unifying, underlying essence of our work is the timeless and profound healing presence we offer that enhances the exploration and creation of meaning in the inevitable health challenges faced by individuals, families, and groups whose lives we are privileged to touch" (Koerner, 2007, p. xii).

Nursing has always focused on creating **healing environments** for those who have been entrusted to our care. We create healing environments when we use our hands, heart, and mind to provide holistic nursing care. We create healing environments when we empower others by providing the knowledge, skills, and support that allow them to tap into their inner wisdom and make healthy decisions for themselves. Healing environments are a synthesis of the medical-curing approach and nursing-healing approach. We need a healthy balance between technology and compassion. We create healing environments when we take the time to be with clients in deeply caring ways. It is when we stop, become still, and enter the other's subjective world that we are able to be wholly present for that person. This moment of spiritual connection is uplifting for both client and nurse. Karilee Shames (1993) described sacred healing moments that occurred when her "goal became to inspire, to share tenderness, and to help instill a will to live, or to surrender to the call of death peacefully, if that was most appropriate. In my highest vision, this is what nursing was all about" (Shames, 1993, p. 131).

Our patients come to us at the most vulnerable times of their lives. Many suffer deeply as they try to make sense of serious illness, huge losses, and unanswerable questions. Healing of spiritual suffering is as important as technical treatment of physical illness. Spirituality is also very important to the dying person's ability to complete the end-of-life task of transcending the self. Until recently, many nurses had given the spiritual health of their patients very little attention. In the area of spiritual assessment, nurses often simply write in the patient's religious affiliation. We must ask our patients about their spiritual beliefs if we are to know who they are and how they cope with their illnesses. A number of tools for assessing spirituality are available. Howden's *Spirituality Assessment Scale (SAS)* (Burkhardt and Nagai-Jacobson, 2002), the *JAREL Spiritual Well-Being Scale* (Hunglemann, Kenkel-Rossi, Klassen, & Strollenwerk, 1997), the *Spiritual Involvement and Beliefs Scale (SIBS)* (Hatch, Burg, Naberhaus, & Hellmich, 1998), and the *Spiritual Assessment Tool* (Dossey, Keegan, & Guzzetta, 2005) are available to help you gain proficiency in the area of spiritual assessment. The tools ask questions regarding relationships, sense of balance and peace, sense of meaning and purpose in life, strengths and limitations, God or a higher power, and meditation or prayer.

We must also create healing environments for ourselves. Working with people can be draining work. As nurses, we need to learn how to restore our energy and replenish ourselves. You might compare your ability to care for others to a well of fresh, healing water. If the well is never dipped into, the water becomes stagnant and brackish. If the water is constantly drawn out and given away, with no source of replenishment, the well will soon run dry. What happens to nurses who don't sincerely care for others or take the time to replenish themselves? It soon becomes obvious by their behavior that they are stagnant or depleted; they are less patient, less tolerant, more irritable, and unhappy. Their state of "burnout" contaminates all aspects of their professional and personal lives.

When you care for others, care for yourself, and allow others to care for you, your well of healing is constantly being replenished. You will find many techniques in this book that you can incorporate into your daily life. It is important that you take time for yourself, even if for only 10 minutes a day. Learning to take care of ourselves means letting go of self-defeating behaviors and attitudes. We must teach ourselves to relax without feeling guilty or selfish for taking time out. Self-renewal is a continuous process. To be there for others and care for them in their times of need, we must first look after our own well-being. It is only when we walk in balance that we can help others learn how to balance their lives.

TRY THIS

Energy

See the Aura

Find a room with a plain white background that has natural lighting or lights other than fluorescent. The lights should not be too bright and should not be shining directly on the person/subject. If you wear glasses, try the experiment with glasses on and glasses off. Ask the person to stand 18 inches in front of the white background and relax and breathe deeply. Stand 10 feet away from the person and focus on the wall, past the person's head

(continued)

and shoulders. You may notice a fuzzy white or gray field around the body, looking almost like a light behind the person. Continue to stare at the wall—DO NOT focus on the person. You may begin to see colors or sharp rays. This may take some time. Try different people as subjects.

You may want to try using your own hands. With the same background, hold your hands out at arm's length, in front of your face, with your palms facing each other. Point the fingertips of each hand until they are 1 inch apart. Soften your gaze and look past your fingers. Look for a gray, white, or other colored aura.

Energizing the Hands

Lightly oil your hands and sit in a chair with your back comfortably straight. Cup your hands slightly and bend your arms at the elbows and hold your hands up at the level of your heart. Feel the warmth or tingle as the energy enters your hands. Let the energy go through your arms into your heart. Now bring your hands together with the right hand on top of the left hand and rapidly rub the back of the left hand. Reverse the hands and rub the back of the right hand. Now rub your palms together rapidly until they feel hot. Return your hands to the original position—cupped and at the level of your heart.

Source: Tulku, T. (2003). *Tibetan Relaxation*. London: Thorsons.

References

Ahn, A. C., & Martinsen, O. G. (2007). Electrical characterization of acupuncture points. *Journal of Alternative and Complementary Medicine*, 13(8): 817–824.

Benson, H. (1997). *Timeless Healing*. New York: Fireside Books.

Borysenko, J., & Borysenko, M. (1994). *The Power of the Mind to Heal*. Carlsbad, CA: Hay House.

Borysenko, J., & Dveirin, G. (2007). *Your Soul's Compass: What Is Spiritual Guidance?* Carlsbad, CA: Hay House.

Boso, M., Emanuele, E., Minazzi, V., Abbamonte, M., & Politi, P. (2007). Effect of long-term interactive music therapy on behavior profile and musical skills in young adults with severe autism. *Journal of Alternative and Complementary Medicine*, 13(7): 709–712.

Burkhardt, M. A., & Nagai-Jacobson, M. (2002). *Spirituality: Living Our Connectedness*. Albany, NY: Delmar.

Chinese HealthChinese Health Qigong Association. (2008). *Liu Zi Jue: Six Sounds Approach to Qigong Breathing Exercises*. London: Jessica Kingsley Publisher.

Colloca, L., Sigaudo, M., & Benedetti, F. (2008). The role of learning in nocebo and placebo effects. *Pain*, 136(1–2): 211–218.

Cousins, N. (1985). *The Healing Heart*. New York: W.W. Norton.

Cousins, N. (1991). *Anatomy of an Illness*. New York: Batnam.

Dossey, B. M., Keegan, L. G., & Guzzetta, C. E. (2005). *Holistic Nursing: A Handbook for Practice*, 4th ed. Rockville, MD: Aspen.

Gardner, J. (2006). *Vibrational Healing Through the Chakras*. Berkeley, CA: Crossing Press.

Halprin, A. (2002). *Returning to Health with Dance, Movement, and Imagery*. Mendocino, CA: LifeRhythm.

Harrington, A. (2008). *The Cure Within.* New York: W.W. Norton & Company.

Hatch, R. L., Burg, M. A., Naberhaus, D. S., & Hellmich, L. K. (1998). The spiritual involvement and beliefs scale. *Journal of Family Practice*, 46: 476–486.

Hunglemann, J., Kenkel-Rossi, E., Klassen, L., & Strollenwerk, R. (1997). Focus on spiritual well-being: Harmonious interconnectedness of mind–body–spirit—Use of the JAREL spiritual well-being scale. *Geriatric Nursing*, 17: 262–266.

Jampolsky, L. (2005). *Walking Through Walls: Practical Spirituality for an Impractical World.* Berkeley, CA: Celestial Arts.

Koerner, J. G. (2007). *Healing Presence: The Essence of Nursing.* New York: Springer Publishing.

Lee, M. S., Jeong, S. Y., Lee, Y. H., Jeong, D. M., & Eo, Y. G. (2005). Differences in electrical conduction properties between meridians and non-meridians. *American Journal of Chinese Medicine*, 33(5), 723–728.

Moerman, D. E. (2006). The meaning response: Thinking about placebos. *Pain Practice*, 6(4): 233–236.

Newman, R. B., & Miller, R. L. (2006). *Calm Healing.* Berkeley, CA: North Atlantic Books.

Nightingale, F. (1969). *Notes on Nursing.* New York: Dover Press.

Ornish, D. (1999). *Love and Survival: The Scientific Basis for the Healing Power of Intimacy.* New York: HarperCollins.

Quinn, J. F. (1989). On healing, wholeness, and the haelan effect. *Nursing and Health Care*, 10(10): 553–556.

Quinn, J. F. (1997). Healing: A model for an integrative health care system. *Advanced Practice Nursing Quarterly*, 3(1): 1–7.

Shames, K. H. (1993). *The Nightingale Conspiracy.* Montclair, NJ: Enlightenment Press.

Sharoff, L. (2008). Exploring nurses' perceived benefits of utilizing holistic modalities for self and clients. *Holistic Nursing Practice*, 22(1): 15–24.

Smith, K. (2008). *Awakening the Energy Body.* Rochester, VT: Bear & Company.

Taylor, E. J. (2002). *Spiritual Care: Nursing Theory, Research, and Practice.* Upper Saddle River, NJ: Prentice Hall.

Tulku, T. (2003). *Tibetan Relaxation.* London: Thorsons.

Warber, S. L., Cornelio, M. A., Straughn, J., & Kile, G. (2004). Biofield energy healing from the inside. *Journal of Alternative and Complementary Medicine*, 10(6): 1107–1113.

Watson, J. (2007). Theoretical questions and concerns: Response from a caring science framework. *Nursing Science Quarterly*, 20(1): 13–15.

Weil, A. (1995a). *Natural Health, Natural Medicine.* Boston: Houghton Mifflin.

Weil, A. (1995b). *Spontaneous Healing.* New York: Knopf.

Weil, A. (2005). *Mindbody Tool Kit.* Boulder, CO: Sounds True.

Zhao, X. (2006). *Ancient Healing for Modern Women.* New York: Walker & Company.

Resources

American Holistic Medical Association
   One Eagle Valley Court, Suite 201
   Broadview Hts., OH 44147
   440.838.1010
   www.holisticmedicine.org

American Holistic Nurses Association
   323 N. San Francisco St., Suite 201
   Flagstaff, AZ 86001
   800.278.2462
   www.ahna.org

British Complementary Medical Association
P.O. Box 2074
Seaford England, BN25 1HQ
0845.345.5977
www.bcma.co.uk

Council of Natural Medicine College of Canada
1411-A Carling Ave., Suite 147
Ottawa, ON K1Z 1A7, Canada
www.cnmccanada.com

3

The Role of Evidence-Based Health Care in Complementary and Alternative Therapies

Science is an imaginative adventure of the mind seeking truth in a world of mystery.

Sir Cyril Herman Hinshelwood (1897–1988), English Chemist Nobel Prize 1956

Science is a way we try not to fool ourselves.

Richard Feynman 1918–1988, American Physicist

BACKGROUND

Evidence-based health care encompasses all of the health professions to include medicine, nursing, and allied health (The Joanna Briggs Institute, n.d.). The evidence-based medicine movement, influenced by scholars such as David Sackett and A. L. Cochrane, preceded evidence-based nursing and has enjoyed a rapid expansion over the past 20 years. Evidence-based medicine has been supported by the Cochrane Collaboration, which has played a leading role in promoting evidence-based practice.

The Cochrane Collaboration arose from a concern by its founder A. L. Cochrane that there was little information about the outcomes of health care practices. The emphasis of the Cochrane Collaboration was, and continues to be, the systematic review of randomized clinical trials for medical problems. A **systematic review** is the use of explicit, scientifically rigorous, and transparent research methods to critically appraise and synthesize the data from more than one research study. See Box 3.1 for the steps to systematic review.

BOX 3.1

Steps to a Systematic Review

The development of a rigorous proposal or protocol. The review protocol provides a predetermined plan to ensure scientific rigor and minimize potential bias. It also allows for periodic updating of the review if necessary. All of the stages of the review (as listed below) are described fully in the protocol, and it is usually subjected to peer review before the review commences.

Stating the questions or hypotheses that will be pursued in the review. Questions should be specific regarding the patients, setting, interventions, and outcomes to be investigated.

Identifying the criteria that will be used to select the literature. The inclusion criteria should address the participants of the primary studies, the intervention, and the outcomes. In addition to this, it should also specify what research methodologies will be considered for inclusion in the review (e.g., randomized controlled trials, clinical trials, case studies, etc.).

Detailing a strategy that will be used to identify all relevant literature within an agreed time frame. This should include databases and bibliographies that will be searched and the search terms that will be used.

Establishing how the quality of primary studies will be assessed or critically appraised and any exclusion criteria based on quality considerations.

Detailing how data will be extracted from the primary research regarding the participants, the intervention, the outcome measures and the results.

Setting out a plan of how the data extracted will be pooled. Statistical analysis (meta analysis) may or may not be used in pooling numerical data and this will depend on the nature and quality of studies included in the review. Where possible, odds ratio (for categorical outcome data) or standardized mean differences (for continuous data) and their 95% confidence intervals are calculated for each included study. If appropriate with available data, results from comparable groups of studies are then pooled in statistical meta-analysis using Review Manager software from the Cochrane Collaboration, which also tests the heterogeneity between the combined results using standard chi-square test. For textual data, the current convention is to develop a narrative summary. With the emergence of Qualitative Assessment and Review Instrument (QARI), it is anticipated that textual analysis (meta synthesis) will become the convention in reviews of this nature.

Source: Joanna Briggs Institute.

The evidence-based nursing movement, although closely aligned with the evidence-based medicine movement, has differentiated itself by its value for holistic paradigms. This has been reflected in part by the recognition that beyond the need for meta-analysis of quantitative studies, there is also a need for meta-synthesis of qualitative studies (Jensen & Allen, 1996; Sandelowski & Barroso, 2003; Walsh & Downe, 2005). This is particularly important to the discipline of nursing because as a human science, there is a large amount of qualitative research that informs our practice.

Definitions

Sackett, Rosenberg, Gray, Haynes, and Richardson (1996) provides the classic definition of **evidence-based medicine** and describes it as an explicit use of the best evidence available in making decisions about the care delivered to individual patients. It involves integrating individual clinical expertise with the best available external clinical evidence from systematic review.

There are a number of definitions of **evidence-based nursing** that can be found in the literature, and generally they all emphasize that evidence-based nursing is a set of tools, resources, and procedures for finding current best evidence from various sources and applying this evidence in order to make clinical decisions to promote positive health outcomes. This process takes into account the situation, cultural context, resources, preferences of patients, clinical expertise/judgment, and common sense. Sigma Theta Tau (n.d.) defines evidence-based nursing as the integration of the best available evidence, nursing expertise, and the values and preferences of individuals, families, and communities who are served. DiCenso, Guyatt, and Ciliska (2005) define evidence-based nursing as "the integration of best evidence with clinical expertise, and patient values to facilitate clinical decision making" (DiCenso et al., 2005, p. 4).

The Joanna Briggs Institute, an interdisciplinary, not-for-profit, international research and development agency, provides a comprehensive description of evidence-based practice and its relationship to evidence-based nursing:

> Simply defined, evidence-based practice is the melding of individual clinical judgment and expertise with the best available external evidence to generate the kind of practice that is most likely to lead to a positive outcome for a client or patient. Evidence-based nursing is nursing practice that is characterized by these attributes. Evidence-based clinical practice takes into account the context in which care takes place; the preferences of the client; and the clinical judgment of the health professional, as well as the best available evidence. (Joanna Briggs Institute, n.d.)

It is important to note that the term *best available evidence* connotes the use of the best available international evidence.

Several authors (DiCenso et al., 2005; Ingersoll, 2000; Melnyk & Fineout-Overholt, 2005; Rycroft-Malone, 2004) differentiate evidence-based practice from research utilization. Research utilization focuses on the application of individual research findings to plan and implement patient care, whereas evidence-based practice is an integration of factors such as clinical expertise, clinical context, and patient preferences with the best available international evidence identified by a transparent, systematic research process.

Controversies Related to Evidence-Based Practice

The evidence-based nursing movement is not without its controversies in the nursing literature. Fawcett, Watson, Neuman, Walker, and Fizpatrick (2001) and Upton (1999) express concern that the practice of evidence-based nursing is more focused on the science of nursing than the art of nursing. They fear this will compromise nursing's holistic roots. Melnyk and Fineout-Overholt (2005) and Mitchell (1999) caution that the practice of evidence-based nursing could lead to a kind of cookbook nursing with emphasis on only the technical side of practice. Ingersoll (2000) suggests that ethical concerns are raised if the reimbursement of health care is connected exclusively to a documented body of evidence. It has also been noted that there is not a sufficient amount of research evidence in order to plan all care.

These and other concerns have been addressed by DiCenso et al. (2005), who remind us that evidence-based practice is informed by more than just research studies but also determined by context, available resources, patient preferences, expert opinion, and feasibility. Rycroft-Malone (2004) supports this in her contention that evidence-based practice involves both quantitative and qualitative evidence, clinical expertise, patient experiences, and consideration of local and organizational influences. The scholarly debate pertaining to evidence-based nursing practice is healthy for the profession.

EVIDENCE-BASED PRACTICE

The primary rationale for the use of evidence-based practice is that it increases our confidence that medical care and nursing care will lead to better patient outcomes. Other reasons include things such as the long lag time between knowledge generation and the use of that knowledge in the planning and provision of care by clinicians. The summaries of systematic reviews in shortened forms, such as best practice sheets, provide a more expedient way for clinicians to access knowledge. It is difficult for busy clinicians to keep up when there are approximately 1,500 articles, 55 new clinical trials, 1,500 books, and over 7,000 systematic reviews produced annually.

Barriers to Evidence-Based Practice

Grol and Grimshaw (2003) and Grol and Wensing (2004) contend that one of the most consistent findings in health services research is the gap between best

BOX 3.2

Barriers to Evidence-based Practice in Nursing

Lack of knowledge regarding evidence-based practice strategies.

Misperceptions of negative views about research and evidence-based care.

Lack of belief that EBP will result in more positive outcomes than traditional care.

Voluminous amounts of information in professional journals.

Lack of time and resources to search for and appraise evidence.

Overwhelming patient loads.

Organization constraints such as lack of administrative support.

Demands by patients for a certain kind of care.

Peer pressure to continue with practices that are steeped in tradition.

Inadequate content and skills regarding evidence-based practice in educational programs.

Source: Melnyk & Fineout-Overholt, 2005.

practice and actual clinical care. A review of studies in countries such as the United States and the Netherlands indicates that 30 to 40 percent of patients do not receive care based on the best available scientific evidence. Melnyk and Fineout-Overholt (2005) have identified barriers to evidence-based practice in nursing. See Box 3.2 for a summary of these barriers.

Models of Practice

Numerous models of evidence-based practice can be found in the literature. The ACE Star Model (Academic Center for Evidence-Based Nursing, n.d.) from the University of Texas and the Iowa Model from the University of Iowa (Iowa Model for Evidence-Based Practice, n.d.) are examples of these. A discussion of all models of evidence-based practice is beyond the scope of this book but can readily be found on their websites. This chapter uses the Joanna Briggs Institute (JBI) model of evidence-based practice.

The JBI model of evidence-based health care conceptualizes evidence-based practice as "clinical decision-making that considers the best available evidence, in the context in which the care is delivered, client preference and the professional judgment of the health professional" (Pearson, Wiechula, Court, & Lockwood, 2007, p. 85). Included in the model are four major components of the evidence-based health care process, which are health care evidence generation, evidence synthesis, evidence (knowledge) transfer, and evidence utilization (Pearson et al., 2007).

The JBI Model depicts health care as a cyclical process that derives its foci from the identification of global health care needs by clinicians and or patient/consumers and addresses those needs by generating knowledge/evidence to effectively and appropriately meet those needs "in ways that are feasible and meaningful to specific populations, cultures and settings" (Pearson et al., 2007, p. 86). Lastly, the evidence is then appraised and

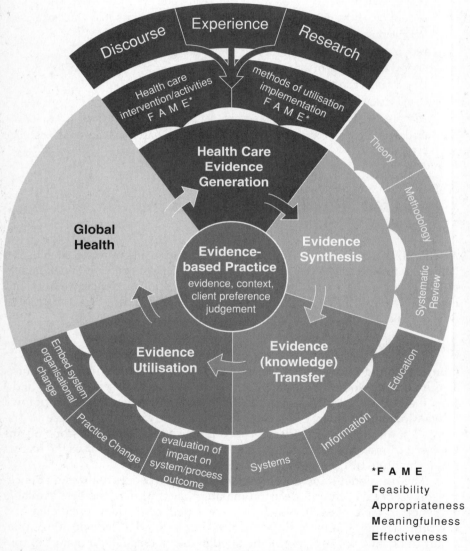

FIGURE 3.1 Joanna Briggs Institute of Evidence-Based Practice

Source: Pearson, A., Wiechula, R., Court, A., Lockwood, C. *The JBI Model of Evidence-Based Healthcare,* 2005; 3(8): 207–215.

synthesized and transferred to health care delivery systems and clinicians who utilize and evaluate its impact on health outcomes (Pearson et al., 2007). Figure 3.1 depicts the JBI Model.

EVIDENCE-BASED PRACTICE AND COMPLEMENTARY AND ALTERNATIVE THERAPIES

The use of complementary and alternative therapies is increasingly prevalent. Persons choose to pursue complementary treatment for a myriad of reasons such as quality of life issues, holistic beliefs, unresolved pain, cultural values, or simply to avoid the invasiveness of biomedical treatments. Some have contended that the use of complementary/alternative therapies has increased because patients are dissatisfied with traditional Western health care. This may be true for some, but data from a U.S. national survey do not support this view. Adults often use and seem to value both. Of 831 respondents who saw a medical doctor and used complementary therapies in the previous 12 months, 79 percent perceived the combination to be superior to either one alone (Eisenberg et al., 2001).

To apply evidence-based health care to complementary health care may seem at first glance an uncomfortable fit. It appears this is no longer true, and it is significant that the Cochrane Collaboration has a work group called the Complementary Medicine Field. The mission of this group is to facilitate the systematic review of existing randomized controlled trials (RCTs) to provide information to benefit clinical decision making and the planning of future research in the field of complementary healthcare. They also maintain a database of RCTs that pertain to complementary medicine. Manheimer and Berman (2008) report that as of 2007, there were 313 completed Cochrane complementary medicine systematic reviews in the Cochrane Collaborative Library and 180 complementary protocols. An increasing number of systematic reviews in the field of complementary interventions can be found from other sources as well. This suggests an increasing thirst by health care practitioners for knowledge generated by systematic reviews on complementary/alternative therapies.

The remaining section shows examples of systematic reviews in the area of complementary medicine. These examples are Cochrane review abstracts and plain language summaries, prepared and maintained by the Cochrane Collaboration, currently published in the Cochrane Database of Systematic Reviews. The full text of these reviews is available in the Cochrane Library. There are many reviews of this type in the Cochrane Library that can be accessed by health care practitioners. See Boxes 3.3, 3.4, and 3.5 for these examples.

Web-Based Resources in Evidence-Based Practice

The following are resources that are valuable for practitioners seeking information on evidence-based practice.

BOX 3.3
Herbal Therapy for Treating Osteoarthritis

Abstract
Background

The increasing popularity of complementary and alternative medicine appears to be particularly evident amongst people with chronic diseases. In the treatment of osteoarthritis, one therapy that has been identified as having potential benefit is plant and herbal medicine (phytotherapy).

Objectives

To determine the effectiveness of herbal therapies in treating osteoarthritis.

Search Strategy

Databases for mainstream and complementary medicine were searched using terms to include all forms of arthritis combined with herbal medicine. We searched the following electronic databases: Cochrane Musculoskeletal Group register, Cochrane Complementary Medicine Field register, Cochrane Controlled Trials Register (CCTR), MEDLINE, EMBASE, CISCOM, AMED, CINAHL, Dissertation Abstracts, and BIDS ISI. We also searched the reference lists from retrieved trials.

Selection Criteria

All randomized trials of herbal interventions in osteoarthritis, compared to placebo. Studies were included according to an a priori protocol and agreement was reached between two reviewers who independently read each selected paper for content and assessment of quality. Papers of any language were included.

Data Collection and Analysis

Data were extracted independently by the same two reviewers.

Main Results

Five studies (four different herbal interventions) met the review criteria. Two studies were suitable for data pooling. It was not possible to draw firm conclusions from the single studies but the two combined studies of avocado/soybean unsaponifiables showed beneficial effects on functional index, pain, intake of non-steroidal anti-inflammatory drugs (NSAIDs), and global evaluation. No serious side effects were reported.

Authors' Conclusions

The evidence for avocado-soybean unsaponifiables in the treatment of osteoarthritis is convincing but evidence for the other herbal interventions is insufficient to either recommend or discourage their use.

Little, Parsons, Logan, 2000.

BOX 3.4
Chinese Herbal Medicine for Schizophrenia

Abstract

Background

Traditional Chinese medicine (TCM) was the main form of treatment in China for psychiatric illnesses until the development of antipsychotic drugs in the 1950s. Antipsychotic drugs have become the primary intervention for schizophrenia, although herbal medicines can still form part of the treatment.

Objectives

To review Chinese herbal medicine, used alone or as part of a TCM approach, for people with schizophrenia and related psychoses.

Search Strategy

We undertook electronic searches of the Cochrane Schizophrenia Group's register (December 2003), the Traditional Chinese Medical Literature Analysis and Retrieval Database (TCMLARS) (October 2003), Chinese Biomedical Database (CBM) (December 2003), China National Knowledge Infrastructure Database (May 2004), Complementary Medicine Database (AMED) (December 2003). We contacted the Chinese Cochrane Centre, the Cochrane Complementary Medicine Field and first authors of included studies and inspected reference lists for additional studies.

Selection Criteria

We included all relevant randomized controlled trials involving people with schizophrenia-like illnesses, allocated to Chinese herbal medicine, including any Chinese herbs (single or mixture), compared with placebo/no treatment or antipsychotic drugs.

Data Collection and Analysis

We independently extracted data and calculated fixed effects relative risk (RR), the 95% confidence intervals (CI) for homogeneous dichotomous data and, where appropriate, the number needed to treat (NNT) on an intention-to-treat basis. For continuous data, we calculated weighted mean differences (WMD).

Main Results

Only one small trial of the seven included studies truly evaluated TCM for schizophrenia. The other trials evaluated Chinese herbs for schizophrenia. We found one study comparing Chinese herbal medicine with antipsychotic drugs. Data for the global state outcome "no change/worse" favored people allocated to antipsychotic medication (n=90, RR 1.88 CI 1.2 to 2.9, NNH 4 CI 2 to 12). Six trials compared Chinese herbal medicine in combination with antipsychotic with antipsychotic drugs alone. One trial found global state "not improved/worse" favored the herbal medicine/antipsychotic combination (n=123, RR 0.19 CI 0.1 to 0.6, NNT 6 CI 5 to 11). Two studies (n=103) also found short-term data from the

(*continued*)

Clinical Global Impression scale favored the herbal medicine plus antipsychotic group (WMD -0.46 CI -0.9 to -0.1) compared with those given only antipsychotics. Significantly fewer people in the experimental group left the study early compared with those given antipsychotics alone (n=1004, 6 RCTs, RR 0.30 CI 0.16 to 0.58, NNT 21 CI 18 to 35). Reports of constipation were significantly lower in the treatment group compared to those receiving antipsychotics (n=67, 1 RCT, RR 0.03 CI 0.0 to 0.5, NNH 2 CI 2 to 4).

Authors' Conclusions

Chinese herbal medicines, given in a Western biomedical context, may be beneficial for people with schizophrenia when combined with antipsychotics. Traditional Chinese medicine is also under-evaluated, but results from one pioneering study that attempted to evaluate TCM should encourage further trials.

Rathbone et al., 2005.

BOX 3.5

Acupuncture and hypnosis may help relieve pain during labor, but more research is needed on these and other complementary therapies.

Abstract

Background

Many women would like to avoid pharmacological or invasive methods of pain management in labor and this may contribute toward the popularity of complementary methods of pain management. This review examined currently available evidence supporting the use of alternative and complementary therapies for pain management in labor.

Objectives

To examine the effects of complementary and alternative therapies for pain management in labor on maternal and perinatal morbidity.

Search Strategy

We searched the Cochrane Pregnancy and Childbirth Group's Trials Register (February 2006), the Cochrane Central Register of Controlled Trials (*The Cochrane Library* 2006, Issue 1), MEDLINE (1966 to February 2006), EMBASE (1980 to February 2006), and CINAHL (1980 to February 2006).

Selection Criteria

The inclusion criteria included published and unpublished randomized controlled trials comparing complementary and alternative therapies (but not biofeedback) with placebo, no treatment or pharmacological forms of pain management in labor. All women whether primiparous or multiparous, and in spontaneous or induced labor, in the first and second stage of labor were included.

Data Collection and Analysis

Meta-analysis was performed using relative risks for dichotomous outcomes and mean differences for continuous outcomes. The outcome measures were maternal satisfaction, use of pharmacological pain relief, and maternal and neonatal adverse outcomes.

Main Results

Fourteen trials were included in the review with data reporting on 1,537 women using different modalities of pain management; 1,448 women were included in the meta-analysis. Three trials involved acupuncture (n = 496), one audio-analgesia (n = 24), two trials acupressure (n = 172), one aromatherapy (n = 22), five trials hypnosis (n = 729), one trial of massage (n = 60), and relaxation (n = 34). The trials of acupuncture showed a decreased need for pain relief (relative risk (RR) 0.70, 95% confidence interval (CI) 0.49 to 1.00, two trials 288 women). Women taught self-hypnosis had decreased requirements for pharmacological analgesia (RR 0.53, 95% CI 0.36 to 0.79, five trials 749 women) including epidural analgesia (RR 0.30, 95% CI 0.22 to 0.40) and were more satisfied with their pain management in labor compared with controls (RR 2.33, 95% CI 1.15 to 4.71, one trial). No differences were seen for women receiving aromatherapy, or audio analgesia.

Authors' Conclusions

Acupuncture and hypnosis may be beneficial for the management of pain during labor; however, the number of women studied has been small. Few other complementary therapies have been subjected to proper scientific study.

Smith, Collins, Cyna, & Crowther, 2006.

Evidence-Based Practice Resources

- About the Cochrane Library www.cochrane.org
- Abstracts of Cochrane Reviews www.cochrane.org/cochrane/revabstr/mainindex.htm
- Evidence-based Practice Centers www.ahrq.gov/clinic/epc
- The Joanna Briggs Institute for Evidence Based Nursing and Midwifery www.joannabriggs.edu.au/
- The NICHD Cochrane Neonatal Collaborative Review Group (alphabetical listing of systematic reviews) www.nichd.nih.gov/cochraneneonatal/cochrane.htm
- Clinical Evidence (subscription required) http://clinicalevidence.com

Guidelines

- National Guideline Clearinghouse www.guideline.gov
- American Heart Association Guidelines http://216.185.112.5/presenter.jhtml?identifier=2158
- CDC Recommends: The Prevention Guidelines System www.cdc.gov/search.do

- Society of Critical Care Medicine guidelines and practice parameters www.sccm.org
- Institute for Clinical Systems Improvement www.icsi.org/
- National Kidney Foundation Clinical Practice Guidelines www.kidney.org
- NIH Consensus Statements—Index by Date http://consensus.nih.gov
- PDQ (Physician Data Query): NCI's Comprehensive Cancer Database www.cancer.gov/cancer_information/pdq/
- Registered Nurses Association of Ontario (RNAO) www.rnao.org/ (see Best Practice Guidelines)

Implementation and Links

- The Hartford Institute for Geriatric Nursing http://hartfordign.org/
- Woundcarenetwww.woundcarenet.com/educat/links.htm
- Getting Research into Practice (how to make a change in practice) www.shef.ac.uk/scharr/ir/units/resprac/index.htm
- NMAP (part of OMNI) http://nmap.ac.uk

REFERENCES

Academic Center for Evidence Based Nursing. (n.d.). Explanation of the ACE Star Model of Knowledge Transformation. www.acestar.uthscsa.edu/Learn_model.htm. Accessed December 13, 2007.

DiCenso, A., Guyatt, G., & Ciliska, D. (2005). Introduction to evidence based nursing. In A. DiCenso, D. Ciliska, & G. Guyatt, eds., *Evidence-Based Nursing: A Guide to Clinical Practice*, pp. 3–19. St. Louis, MO: Elsevier.

Eisenberg, D. M., Kessler, R., Van Rompay, M., Kaptchuk, T., Wilkey, S., Appel, S., et al. (2001). Perceptions about complementary therapies relative to conventional therapies among adults who use both: Results from a national survey. *Annals of Internal Medicine*, 135(5): 344–351.

Fawcett, J., Watson, J., Neuman, B., Walker, P. H., & Fitzpatrick, J. J. (2001). On nursing theories and evidence. *Journal of Nursing Scholarship*, 33(2): 115–119.

Grol, R., & Grimshaw, J. (2003). From best evidence to best practice: Effective implementation of change. *Lancet*, 362: 1225–1230.

Grol, R., & Wensing, M. (2004). What drives change? Barriers to and incentives for achieving evidence-based practice. *Medical Journal of Australia*, 180: 57–60.

Ingersoll, G. L. (2000). Evidence-based nursing: What it is and what it isn't. *Nursing Outlook*, 48: 151–152.

Iowa Model of Evidence Based Practice (n.d.). Explanation of the model. www.uihealthcare.com/depts/nursing/rqom/evidencebasedpractice/iowamodel.html. Accessed December 18, 2008.

Jensen, L., & Allen, M. (1996). Metasynthesis of qualitative findings. *Qualitative Health Research*, 6(4): 553–560.

Joanna Briggs Institute. (n.d.). Definition of evidence based practice and nursing. www.joannabriggs.edu.au/. Accessed September 24, 2008.

Little, C. V., Parsons, T., & Logan, S. (2000). Herbal therapy for treating osteoarthritis. *Cochrane Database of Systematic Reviews*, Issue 4. Art. No. CD002947. DOI: 10.1002/14651858.CD002947.

Manheimer, E., & Berman, B. (2008). Cochrane complementary medicine field. *About the Cochrane Collaboration (Fields).* Cochrane Collab (2): CE000052.

Melnyk, B. M., & Fineout-Overholt, E. (2005). Making the case for evidence-based practice. In B. M. Melnyk & E. Fineout-Overhold, eds., *Evidence-Based Practice in Nursing and Healthcare: A Guide to Best Practice*, pp. 3–24. Philadelphia: Lippincott Williams & Wilkins.

Mitchell, G. J. (1999). Evidence-based practice: Critique and alternative view. *Nursing Science Quarterly*, 12(1): 30–35.

Pearson, A., Wiechula, R., Court, A., & Lockwood, C. (2007). A re-construction of what constitutes "evidence" in the healthcare professions. *Nursing Science Quarterly*, 20(1): 85–88.

Rathbone, J., Zhang, L., Zhang, M., Xia, J., Liu, X., & Yang, Y. (2005). Chinese herbal medicine for schizophrenia. *Cochrane Database of Systematic Reviews*, Issue 4. Art. No. CD003444. DOI: 10.1002/14651858.CD003444.pub2.

Rycroft-Malone, J. (2004). The PARIHS framework—A framework for guiding the implementation of evidence-based practice. *Journal of Nursing Care Quarterly*, 19(4): 297–304.

Sackett, L., Rosenberg, C., Gray, M., Haynes, B., & Richardson, S. (1996). Evidence-based medicine: What it is and what it is not. *British Medical Journal*, 312: 71–72.

Sandelowski, M. & Barroso, J. (2003). Creating metasummaries of qualitative findings. *Nursing Research*, 52(4): 226–233.

Sigma Theta Tau International. (n.d.). Position statement on evidence based nursing. www.nursingsocieity.org/research/main.html. Accessed October 5, 2008.

Smith, C. A., Collins, C. T., Cyna, A. M., & Crowther, C. A. (2006). Complementary and alternative therapies for pain management in labour. *Cochrane Database of Systematic Reviews*, Issue 4. Art. No. CD003521. DOI: 10.1002/14651858.CD003521.pub2.

Upton, D. J. (1999). How can we achieve evidence-based practice if we have a theory-practice gap in nursing today? *Journal of Advance Nursing*, 29(3): 549–555.

Walsh, D., & Downe, S. (2005). Meta-synthesis method for qualitative research: A literature review. *Journal of Advanced Nursing*, 50(2): 204–211.

Systematized Health Care Practices

Science treats all human beings alike, ignoring dissimilarities to find common features. Medicine must follow science, of course, but it also follows humanities, since a humanistic approach treats every individual as a unique person. This relationship appears totally secular, but there is a sacredness in it.

JING-BAO NIE, MD

4

Traditional Chinese Medicine

The superior physician helps before the early budding of the disease. . . . The inferior physician begins to help when [the disease] has already set in.

Yellow Emperor's Classic of Medicine

I pray for all of us, oppressor and friend, that together we succeed in building a better world through human understanding and love.

The Dalai Lama

Traditional Chinese Medicine (TCM) originated in Chinese culture more than 3,000 years ago and has spread, with variations, throughout other Asian countries, particularly Japan, Korea, Tibet, and Vietnam. As a comprehensive health system, it has a range of applications, from preventive health care and maintenance to diagnosis and treatment of acute and chronic disorders.

BACKGROUND

TCM has a long and extensive history. Shen Nong, the Fire Emperor, said to have lived from 2698 to 2598 B.C., is considered the founder of herbal medicine in China. The written history itself is more than 2,500 years old, starting with the text on internal medicine of Huang Di, the Yellow Emperor. Written long before the birth of Hippocrates, the father of Western medicine, *Yellow Emperor's Classic of Medicine* covers such principles as yin and yang, the five phases, the effects of the season, and treatments such as acupuncture and moxibustion.

TCM is associated with early Taoists and Buddhists who observed energy within themselves, in plants and animals, and throughout the cosmos. Based on a belief in the natural order of the universe and the direct correlation between the human body and the cosmos, this philosophy stresses the constant search for harmony and balance in an environment of constant change. By the close of the Han era (A.D. 220), the Chinese had a clear grasp of pathology, preventive medicine, first aid, and dietetics and had devised breathing practices to promote longevity. During the fourth and fifth centuries A.D., China's influence spread throughout Asia, and both Taoism and Buddhism had a marked impact on ideas about health. Sun Si Mian (A.D. 581–682), a famous physician, established himself as China's first medical ethicist. He advocated the need for rigorous scholarship, compassion toward patients, and high moral standards in physicians. In the eleventh century, TCM began to focus more on social phenomena, especially human relations and ethical behavior. Initially, this orientation resulted in increased scientific medical study and publications. As TCM developed further, people began to take for granted that a breakthrough in one realm of knowledge would eventually solve all problems of human existence. (As in the West, some assume that advances in technology will solve all problems.) Eventually, sociological methods were used to solve medical problems, and clinical and empirical research reached a low point. Fortunately, the core of the scientific system was never obliterated, and the past 50 years have seen a worldwide revival of TCM (Harrington, 2008; Zhao, 2006).

In China today, TCM is practiced in hospitals along with Western medicine. Physicians not only study principles of anatomy, histology, biochemistry, bacteriology, and surgery, but also acupuncture, acupressure, and herbal medicine. Patients can choose TCM or Western approaches or a combination for their particular problem. Inpatient and outpatient care is provided in large, well-equipped hospitals, as well as private clinics and pharmacies.

CONCEPTS

The focus of TCM is on the patient rather than disease with the goal to promote health and improve the quality of life. A basic understanding of TCM requires recognition of its long-lived tradition, multiple philosophies, and varied practices. It is impossible to separate the individual concepts and the specific treatment approaches from the context of a complete theoretical system. Prevention, diagnosis, and treatment of diseases are based on the concepts of qi, yin and yang, the five phases, the five seasons, and the three treasures. Often only isolated fragments of TCM emerge in the West.

Qi

The concept most central to TCM is *qi* or *chi* (pronounced "chee"), which is translated as energy. **Qi** represents an invisible flow of energy that circulates through plants, animals, and people as well as the earth and sky. It is what maintains physiologic functions and the health and well-being of the individual. In TCM theory, energy is distributed throughout the body along a network of energy circuits or meridians, connecting all parts of the body. The many different types of qi in the body are described according to their source, location, and function. *Yin qi* supports and nourishes the body, *wei qi* protects and warms the body, *jing qi* flows in the meridians, *zang qi* flows in the organs, and *zong qi* is responsible for respiration and circulation. Obstructed qi flow in the human body can cause problems ranging from social difficulties to illness. Its effects are very individual—a person gets sick, has problems at work, or fights with family—and depend on each individual's unique qi. Certain TCM treatments such as meditation, exercise, and acupuncture are ways of enhancing or correcting the flow of qi (Kong et al., 2007; Silva & Cignolini, 2005).

Yin and Yang

In the Taoist philosophy, wholeness is comprised of the union of opposites— dark and light, soft and hard, female and male, slow and fast, and so on. These opposite but complementary aspects are called *yin* and *yang*. Originally the terms designated geographical aspects such as the shady and sunny side of a mountain or the southern and northern bank of a river. In modern terms, they are used to characterize the polar opposites that exist in everything and make up the physical world.

From the health perspective, the basis of well-being is the appropriate balance of yin and yang as they interact in the body. Imbalance of yin and yang is considered to be the cause of illness. **Yin** is the general category for passivity and is like water with a tendency to be cold and heavy. Yin uses fluids to moisten and cool our bodies. It provides for restfulness as we slow down and sleep. Yin is associated more with substance than with energy. Things that are close to the ground are yin or more earthy. Yin is associated with the symptoms of coldness, paleness, low blood pressure, and chronic conditions. People with excess yin tend to catch colds easily, and are sedentary and sleepy. **Yang** is the general category for activity and aggressiveness. It is like fire with its heating and circulating characteristics. Associated with things higher up or more heavenly, yang is the energy that directs movement and supports its substance. Symptoms such as redness in the face, fever, high blood pressure, and acute conditions are associated with yang. People with excess yang tend to be nervous and agitated and cannot tolerate much heat (Ni, 2008; Zhao, 2006). It must be understood that yin and yang cannot exist independently of each other. Figure 2.1 in Chapter 2 shows the t'ai chi symbol of yin and yang. Nothing is either all yin or all yang. They are complementary and depend on each other for their very existence—without night there can be no day, without moisture there can be no dryness, and without cold there can be no heat. It is the interaction of yin and yang that creates the changes that keep the world in motion; summer leads to winter, night becomes day. Yin and yang are used in both the diagnosis and the treatment of illness.

For example, if a person is experiencing too much stress, usually understood as an excess of yang, more yin activities, such as meditation and relaxation, comprise the appropriate treatment.

Five Phases

As they studied the world around them, the Chinese perceived connections between major forces in nature and particular internal organ systems. Seeing similarities between natural elements and the body, early practitioners developed a concept of health care that encompassed both natural elements and body organs. This theory is known as the **Five Phases Theory** (*wu-hsing*). Five elements—fire, earth, metal, water, and wood—represent movement or energies that succeed one another in a dynamic relationship and in a continuous cycle of birth, life, and death. These elements do not represent static objects, since even mountains and rivers change constantly with time. In the Five Phases Theory, it is not the substances themselves that are important, but how they interact together to make up the essential life force or qi (Ni, 2008; Zhao, 2006).

The rhythm of events resembles a circle known as the *Creation Cycle*. In this cycle, burning wood feeds fire; from its ashes, fire produces earth; earth in turn gives up its ore, creating metal; from condensation on its surface, metal brings forth water; and water nourishes and creates plants and trees, creating wood. Each element is related to a pair of internal organs. The yin organ is solid and dense, like the liver, while its yang partner is hollow or forms a pocket, like the gallbladder. The proper interaction of the organ partners influences how well the entire body functions. Fire is linked to the circulation of blood, hormones, and food. Its partner organs are the heart (yin) and small intestine (yang). Earth is linked to digestion and is comprised of the spleen/pancreas (yin) and the stomach (yang). Metal is linked to respiration and elimination and is made up of the lungs (yin) and large intestine (yang). Water is linked to elimination and is comprised of the kidneys (yin) and urinary bladder (yang). Wood is linked to toxic processing and is made up of the liver (yin) and gallbladder (yang). In addition, each organ is related to a time of day of optimal functioning. If a problem occurs during those hours when an organ is most vulnerable, the timing may alert a TCM practitioner of an imbalance in that organ system. Figure 4.1 illustrates the Five Phases of the Creation Cycle and their related yin and yang organs (Zhao, 2006).

Five Seasons

The four cardinal compass directions—south, west, north, and east—are affiliated with four of the five elements: fire, metal, water, and wood. The fifth element, earth, is depicted in the center. The Chinese place so much importance on the direction south that they put it at the top of their maps and navigate from it in the same way that Westerners use north. Just as south rules the top of the compass, it also represents summer, the "high noon" of the year and is

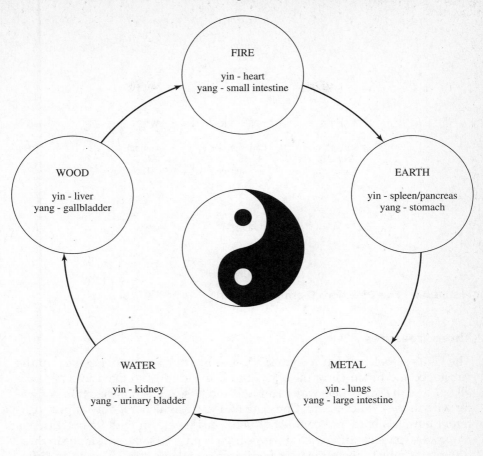

FIGURE 4.1   Creation Cycle: Five Phases and Related Organ Systems

Source: Zhao, X., (2006). *Ancient Healing for Modern Women.* New York: Walker & Company.

linked to fire. West, the direction of the setting sun, is associated with autumn and metal, which is used to make tools for harvesting. North is linked to winter and water, the opposite of the element of fire and is seen as a period of dormancy. East, the direction of the rising sun, is associated with spring and with wood, which represents all growing things. The fifth and central element, earth, is related to the late summer season and a time of maturity. Figure 4.2 illustrates the five directions as they correlate to the five seasons and the five elements.

The etiology of disease in TCM is linked to the five phases, five seasons, and five directions. It is believed that if one component is overbearing and excessive, then another becomes weak and debilitated. It is a complex system of checks and balances that is often not easily grasped by those with a Western perspective. Diagnosis and treatment of illness depends on understanding the five elements, seasons, and directions and how they interact.

SOUTH

Summer
Fire
Peak

EAST   CENTER   WEST

Spring   Late summer   Autumn
Wood   Earth   Metal
Growth   Maturity   Tools

NORTH

Winter
Water
Dormancy

FIGURE 4.2   Five Directions/Seasons/Elements

Three Treasures

The Chinese believe that a combination of life force elements makes up the substance and functions of the body, mind, and spirit, and that these three are all one and the same. One way to understand this connection is to think of water with its wet, fluid nature. Compare that to ice, which not only appears different but feels hard and cold. And then consider steam with its hot gaseous nature. Despite the differences in appearance, it is the same substance in three different forms. In the same way, body, mind, and spirit can be seen as different expressions of the same individual (Zhao, 2006).

The Taoists call body, mind, and spirit the three "vital treasures." They are *jing*, meaning basic essence; *qi*, meaning energy or life force; and *shen*, meaning spirit and mind. The balance of their abundance or deficiency influences the state of health. Jing is the essence with which people are born. It is similar to Western concepts of genes, DNA, and heredity. Essence is the gift of one's parents; it is the basic material in each cell that allows that cell to function. It is the bodily reserves that support life and must be restored by food and rest.

There are several types of qi: the hereditary qi, which is from the jing; the nutritive qi derived from food; and the cosmic qi from the air that we breathe. Wei qi is a specialized qi associated with the immune system. Wei qi circulates near the surface of the body and is the first level of protection when a bacteria or virus tries to enter the body. If the circulating wei qi is weak, it can allow a pathogen to enter the body and illness ensues.

The vital treasure known as *shen* is the gift of heaven and represents spiritual and mental aspects of life. Shen comprises one's emotional well-being, thoughts, and beliefs. It is the radiance, or inner glow, that can be perceived by others. In order for people to be healthy, their physical, emotional, mental, and spiritual aspects must be balanced (Zhao, 2006).

VIEW OF HEALTH AND ILLNESS

The Chinese regard the body as a system that requires a balance of yin and yang energy to enjoy good health. Each part of the body is also thought of as an individual system that requires its own balance of yin and yang to function properly. A headache is not just an event in the head, and it is more than just a pain. In TCM, a headache is the obstruction of energy related to the overall energy patterns in the body as well as the circumstances and lifestyle of the sufferer. TCM assumes that a balanced body has a natural ability to resist or cope with agents of disease. Symptoms are caused by an imbalance of yin and yang in some part of the body, and illness can develop if the balance is disturbed for any length of time. Therefore, health is maintained by recognizing an imbalance before it becomes a disease. It is believed that everything needed to restore health already exists in nature, and it is up to the individual, with or without the aid of a health practitioner, to free up energy and restore balance using diet, herbs, acupuncture, and other yin/yang treatments (Ni, 2008; Fan, 2006).

The Chinese believe that all living things—people, the earth, the universe—are connected by cosmic energy. Thus, the balance of qi in an individual is connected to the balance in the environment; the forces active within the world are the same forces active within the individual body. Simply put, nothing happens without consequence to something else. The concern for balance and harmony is reflected not only in the TCM approach to the individual but also in the view that the balance and well-being of the resources of the natural world and society are vital to the overall health of all who live on the earth. Practitioners never lose sight of the multifaceted relationship between individuals, communities, societies, and nature.

Because the human body is a microcosm of the universe, extremes of climate in the body can create problems, just as extreme environmental conditions can wreak havoc on the environment. Sometimes, people experience a "cold" or yin illness caused by too much coldness in the body. For example, the symptoms of a "cold" influenza include a low-grade fever, no sweating, headache, muscle aches, stuffy nose, and a cough with clear white phlegm. Some influenzas are "hot" or yang influenzas caused by too much heat in the body. Symptoms include high fever, sweating, headache, dry or sore throat, thirst, and nasal congestion with sticky or yellow mucus. Too much cold in the body requires "warming" remedies and too much heat in the body requires "cooling" remedies (Fan, 2006).

DIAGNOSTIC METHODS

The TCM practitioner has four diagnostic methods (*szu-chen*): inspection, auscultation/olfaction, inquiry, and palpation. These methods gather information about the five phases and their related body systems. The practitioner examines how the person eats, sleeps, thinks, works, relaxes, dreams, and imagines. No part of the self is considered a neutral bystander when the body is in a state of imbalance.

Inspection

Inspection refers to the visual assessment of the spirit and physical body of patients. *Spirit inspection* or observation is an assessment of the person's overall appearance, especially the eyes, the complexion, and the quality of voice. Good spirit, even in the presence of serious illness, indicates a more positive prognosis. *Tongue diagnosis* is a highly developed system of inspection of the physical body. The tongue is considered to be the visual gateway to the interior of the body. The whole body "lives" on the tongue, rather like a hologram. Different areas of the tongue correspond to the five phases and related organ systems as seen in Figure 4.3. The central area of the tongue is related to the spleen/pancreas and stomach. The very back of the tongue reflects the kidneys and urinary bladder. The sides of the tongue are related to the liver and gallbladder. The very tip of the tongue corresponds to the heart, and surrounding the heart are the lungs in the front one-third of the tongue. The practitioner inspects the color, shape, markings, and coating of the tongue to gather information about the state of balance in the person's body. For example, a moist tongue with a thin white coating may signal the presence of a

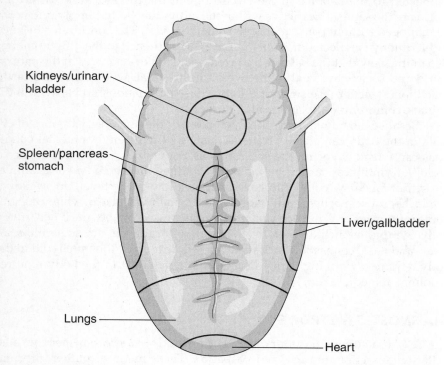

FIGURE 4.3   Tongue Map

"cold" or yin illness whereas a dry, yellow or dark tongue may signal a "hot" or yang illness (Scheid, 2007).

Auscultation/Olfaction

The second part of diagnosis, auscultation/olfaction, refers to listening to the quality of speech, breath, and other sounds, as well as being aware of the odors of breath, body, and excreta. Types of sound are associated with the five phases and organ systems. How the person is breathing is a good indication of the status of the organs. Phases and organ systems are associated with specific odors such as sickly sweet, rotten, putrid, rancid, and scorched. Odors can arise from the skin itself or from the ears, nose, genitals, urine, stool, or bodily discharges. The breath may also have a distinctive odor. Usually the stronger the odor, the more serious the imbalance has become.

Inquiry

The third part of diagnosis, inquiry, is the process of taking a comprehensive health, social, emotional, and spiritual history. The practitioner questions the person not only about the presenting complaint, but also about many other factors, including sensations of hot and cold, perspiration, excreta, hearing, thirst, sleep, digestion, emotions, sexual drive, and energy level.

Palpation

Palpation is the fourth diagnostic method and includes pulse examination, general palpation of the body, and palpation of the acupuncture points. Reading the pulses, or *pulse diagnosis*, can provide key information about the person's condition. For example, a fast pulse might indicate a problem with an overactive heart or liver; a slow pulse might indicate a sluggish digestive system; pulses described as wide, flat, and soft may indicate a spleen problem; and narrow, forceful pulses might indicate a liver dysfunction. The radial pulse is felt in three positions and two layers on both the right and left arm. The more superficial, or surface layer, belongs to the yang organs, while the deeper layer belongs to the yin organs. The locations of major points used in pulse diagnosis are illustrated in Figure 4.4. The pulse allows the practitioner to feel the quality of qi and blood at the different locations in the body. Twenty-nine pulse qualities are described according to size, rate, depth, force, and volume. Examples of qualities are surging, scattered, vacuous, slippery, stringlike, and flat (King, Walsh, & Cobbin, 2006; Shu & Sun, 2007).

All of this diagnostic information is compiled to arrive at a "pattern of disharmony," or *bian zheng*. A single biomedical disease can be associated with a large number of Chinese diagnostic patterns. A lower urinary tract infection, for example, might be related to one of four distinct diagnostic patterns. Each of these patterns would be treated in different ways, as it is said, "one disease, different treatments." Also, many different biomedical diseases may fall into one pattern, thus the saying, "different diseases, one treatment."

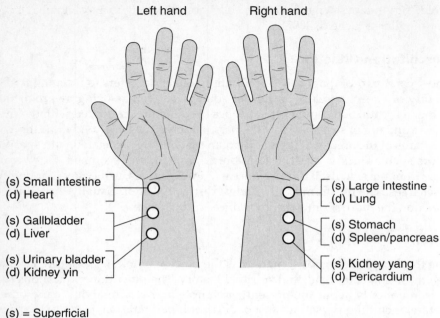

Left hand   Right hand

(s) Small intestine
(d) Heart

(s) Gallbladder
(d) Liver

(s) Urinary bladder
(d) Kidney yin

(s) Large intestine
(d) Lung

(s) Stomach
(d) Spleen/pancreas

(s) Kidney yang
(d) Pericardium

(s) = Superficial
(d) = Deep

FIGURE 4.4   Location of Major Points Used in Pulse Diagnosis

TREATMENT

Since an individual's combinations of yin and yang are unique, TCM practitioners must tailor their treatment to each client. The goal of treatment is to reestablish a balanced flow of energy in the person through diet, herbs, massage, acupuncture, qigong, and gua sha. Feng shui, although not considered an actual treatment, is employed to improve health and well-being.

Diet

The simplest and most accessible treatment is diet. Dietary interventions are individualized on the basis of the individual's pattern of disharmony. Foods are used to rebalance the body's internal "climate" by bringing warmth to coldness or by cooling off too much heat. The thermal nature of food is described by the way a person feels after ingesting it. For example, after eating watermelon or asparagus, which are cooling foods, one feels physically and emotionally cooler. An internal feeling of warmth comes after eating warming foods such as salmon, lamb, or sweet potatoes. Neutral foods do not create a specific thermal quality and are thus good diet balancers. A diet to maintain health should be varied and include a minimum of seven different fruits and vegetables a day to avoid a cold or hot imbalance. If a person is ill and the symptoms indicate a hot condition, then the diet should emphasize cooling

BOX 4.1

Thermal Food Qualities

Cooling

Pork, duck, eggs, clams, crab, millet, barley, wheat, lettuce, celery, broccoli, spinach, tomato, banana, watermelon, asparagus, ice cream, soy sauce

Neutral

Beef, beef liver, rabbit, sardines, yam, rice, corn, rye, potato, beet, turnip, carrot, lemon, apple

Warming

Tuna, turkey, salmon, lamb, venison, chicken, chicken liver, shrimp, trout, oats, cabbage, squash, kale, scallion, celery, ginger, sugar, garlic, pepper

foods, and vice versa. In addition to the overall daily diet, specific foods are used as medicines to correct hot and cold imbalances (Zhao, 2006). Box 4.1 lists common foods and their thermal effects on the body.

Foods are categorized according to one of six tastes, each taste having a specific function in the body. *Sweet* foods are often used to aid digestion and qi, and influence the spleen and stomach. *Salty* foods affect the kidney and bladder and are often used to "soften" cysts or tumors and may be tried before surgery. *Sour* foods, such as lemons or tomatoes, are used to dry mucous membranes in the intestinal, urinary, reproductive, or respiratory surfaces. *Pungent* foods such as garlic and onion are used to aid digestion, stimulate circulation, and promote sweating. *Bitter* foods, such as greens or tonic water, also help in digestion and are used to regulate the bowels. *Astringent* foods, such as beans or potatoes, stop the flow of bodily secretions such as tears, saliva, and sweat.

Each food has both yin and yang energies but often one predominates. Cooling foods and those with bitter and salty flavors are yin. Warming foods are yang, as are foods with pungent and sweet flavors. When people have an excess of yin they may be sluggish, laid back, calm, slightly overweight, and emotionally sensitive. To balance these overly yin tendencies, yang foods are added to the diet to help activate the metabolism and provide more energy. People experiencing an excess in yang may be tense, loud, hyperactive, and aggressive. Adding yin foods to the diet cools their internal tension.

TCM practitioners recommend certain foods for balancing and improving a variety of conditions. Foods can be potent healers, especially when dealing with temporary illnesses, but they are never used as a lone treatment for serious or chronic conditions.

Herbs

Herbal medicine (*ahong yao*) is an integral part of TCM. In terms of the complexity of diagnosis and treatment, it resembles the practice of Western internal medicine. Herbs may be taken in the form of tea or the substances may be powdered and made into pills, pastes, or tinctures for internal or external use. Just as in food, some herbs are warming (cinnamon) and some are cooling (mint).

With the exception of conditions that require surgery, herbs can be used to treat almost any condition in the practice of TCM. Herbs are often prescribed in complex mixtures and tend not to be used as isolated components, for example, extractions from the parent plant. TCM practitioners believe that the healing benefits of herbs result from the synergistic interactions of all the components of the plant. The same herb can be used for many different disorders. Likewise, the same disorder in different people will be treated with different herbs, depending on assessment of the individual. Herbs are used in the following ways: antiviral, antibacterial, antifungal, and anticancer. Herbs are also used to treat pain, aid digestion, lower cholesterol, treat colds and flus, increase resistance to disease, enhance immune function, improve circulation, regulate menstruation, and increase energy (Sagar & Wong, 2004; Wang, Cai, Kong, Cao, & Chen, 2005). Box 4.2 lists herbs commonly used as tonics in TCM. Chapter 7 covers the use of herbs in greater detail.

Massage

Traditional Chinese massage methods were described in texts as early as 200 B.C. *Tui na* is the forerunner of all forms of massage therapy that exist today. It differs from other forms of massage in that it is used to treat not only musculoskeletal problems but also internal diseases. Tui na practitioners must know TCM in order to make a diagnosis before beginning treatment. It is often combined with qigong exercises for building up general health, strength, and stamina. Both energizing and sedating techniques are used to treat and relieve many medical conditions. Major techniques in use are (Xiangcai, Ximing, & Xu, 2002):

- *Ma*—rubbing with palm or fingertips
- *Pai*—tapping with palm or fingertips
- *Tao*—strong pinching with thumb and fingertip
- *An*—rapid and rhythmical pressing with thumb, palm, or back of the clenched hand
- *Nie*—twisting, with both thumbs and tips of the index fingers grasping and twisting the area being treated
- *Ning*—pinching and lifting in a stationary position
- *Na*—rhythmic compression along energy channels
- *Tui*—pushing, often with slight vibratory effect

Massage increases circulation of blood and lymph to the skin and underlying muscles, bringing added nutrients and pain relief. Massage can help restore proper movement to injured limbs and joints and help restore a sense

BOX 4.2

Tonic Herbs Frequently Used in TCM

Herb	Use
Astragalus	Enhances immune function by increasing activity of WBCs and increases production of antibodies and interferon
Dong quai	Blood-building tonic that improves circulation, tones the uterus, balances female hormones
Garlic	Lowers blood pressure, lowers cholesterol and triglycerides; antiseptic, antifungal
Ginger	Warming effect; stimulates digestion, decreases nausea, relieves aches and pains
Gingko	Mediates the allergic and inflammatory reaction in asthma; not to be taken with aspirin or other anticoagulants; discontinue before surgery
Ginseng	Increases appetite and digestion, tones skin and muscles, restores depleted sexual energy
Siberian ginseng	Enhances immune function, increases energy
Green tea	Lowers cholesterol; anticancer effects, antibacterial effects
Ho shou wu	Cleans the blood, nourishes hair and teeth, increases energy; powerful sexual tonic
Licorice	Used as an expectorant in bronchitis and asthma; anti-inflammatory, antitussive
Ligusticum	Inhibits bronchospasm through bronchodilation
Ma huang	Effective for mild asthma; because it contains ephedrine, in excess it can cause hypertension, tachycardia, palpitations, headache, nervousness, and insomnia
Onion (quercetin)	Inhibits the platelet-activating factor in asthma

of balance. Massage is an effective method of reducing stress and tension that usually leads to a feeling of relaxation. Massage is the treatment modality of first choice for children. Chapter 12 covers massage in greater detail.

Acupuncture

Acupuncture involves stimulating specific anatomic points called *hsueh* where each meridian passes close to the skin surface. Puncturing the skin with very fine needles is the usual method but practitioners may also use pressure (shiatsu), friction, suction, heat, or electromagnetic energy to stimulate points. The primary goal of acupuncture is the manipulation of energy flow throughout the body following a thorough assessment by a TCM practitioner. Treatment is offered in the context of the total person and with the goal of correcting the flow of qi to restore health. Some Western health care practitioners who have learned the techniques of acupuncture miss the broader context and limit their focus to an injured or painful body part.

Acupuncture is effective in the treatment of acute and chronic pain and motion disabilities. In addition, it is used in respiratory and cardiovascular conditions (asthma, COPD, palpitations, hypertension), eye, ear, nose, and throat disorders (conjunctivitis, tinnitus, Ménière's disease, rhinitis, sore throat), gastrointestinal problems (gastritis, ulcers, colitis, constipation, irritable bowel syndrome), urogenital conditions (premenstrual syndrome, endometriosis, menopausal symptoms, prostatitis, incontinence, erectile problems), skin disorders (eczema, shingles, urticaria), psychiatric problems (anxiety, depression, schizophrenia), and in addictive disorders and withdrawal syndromes. Ear acupuncture is a complete system within itself and is quite powerful for balancing the hormones and overall energy of the body. Contraindications to acupuncture are childhood, pregnancy, hemophilia, and acute cardiovascular disorders (Lin, 2006; Sagar & Wong, 2004). Chapter 13 covers acupuncture in more detail.

Moxibustion is an application of heat from certain burning substances at acupuncture points on the body. A systematic review of moxibustion to correct breech birth presentation found it to be effective at 33 to 35 weeks of gestation. The Health Ministry of Spain has begun a multicenter, randomized controlled trial of moxibustion and breech birth (van den Berg et al., 2008; Vas et al., 2008).

Cupping is the application of suction cups on the skin. The cups create a vacuum on the skin and break up accumulated toxins. The first few applications result in painless circular areas of erythema or ecchymosis. When the toxins are successfully removed from the body, cupping no longer creates these marks (Forde, 2008).

Qigong

Qigong (pronounced "chee-gong") is the art and science of using breath, movement, self-massage, and meditation to cleanse, strengthen, and circulate vital life energy and blood. In India the comparable practice is called yoga. Both of these traditions of self-healing have been called "moving meditation" or "meditation in motion." T'ai chi, which is familiar to many Americans, is a more physical form of qigong. In China, millions of people from children, to workers, to elders, to patients in the hospital practice qigong daily. The techniques are easy to learn and simple to apply for people who are well or sick. Qigong decreases fatigue and forgetfulness and generates energy by enhancing bodily functions.

It is inevitable that taking a deep breath triggers a sense of relaxation. By adding the intention to relax with the breath, the effect is even greater. Adding gentle movements or self-massage to the deep breathing and relaxation generates increased self-healing abilities. The focus on deep and intentional relaxation allows for release of emotional stress, for a sense of tranquility, and for one's natural spirituality to arise (Shinnick, 2006).

Gua Sha

Gua sha (pronounced "gwaw saw") is a TCM technique of smearing oil on the skin and then rubbing it with a flat jade stone, spoon, or other round-edged tool to bring out impurities in the body. *Gua* means "to rub or scrape." *Sha* is the red rash that appears afterward, signifying that the impurities have been expelled through the skin. Most practitioners do gua sha on the arms, back, and chest, where many of the meridians are located. It is used to treat such problems as fibromyalgia, hypertension, arthritis, muscle aches, and early onset of colds and flu.

Feng Shui

Feng shui (pronounced "fung shway") is the ancient Chinese system of arranging the environment for living in harmony with one's surroundings. It began thousands of years ago in China and India, as a process of decorating graves. It has now gained popularity in many parts of the world. For modern practitioners, feng shui is a design system based on the flow of energy through one's home and environment. The primary objective is to control and balance surroundings in a way that brings happiness, prosperity, and health. Feng shui is based on the principles of qi, yin and yang, five phases, five seasons, and numbers and as such is an adjunct to other healing methods.

Many people are aware of the impact their surroundings have on them and use feng shui principles to improve their lives. Practitioners assess the interaction between the home's energy field and those of the people who reside there. These combined energy forces are significant factors in why and how we develop certain diseases and can be altered to improve our health status. Feng shui practitioners help people determine placement of furniture, colors, and designs that are comfortable, healthy, and supportive. For example, the entrance to the home should draw people into its nurturing space. The front door is seen as an opening for qi and obstructions near the door can block good qi, prosperity, and luck from entering the home. Feng shui describes stairway placement, front and back door alignment, bedroom arrangement, placement of electronic equipment, living room, dining room, kitchen, and bathroom arrangement, use of a fireplace, as well as the choice of art. Mirrors have many curative uses such as lighting up dark corners, slowing down the flow of qi, and deflecting unwanted influences.

Color is a vibration to which people respond both consciously and unconsciously. *Red* is stimulating and dominant and is associated with warmth and prosperity. *Yellow* is associated with intellect, decisiveness, and optimism. *Green* symbolizes growth, fertility, and harmony, while *blue* is peaceful and soothing. *Purple* is dignified and spiritual, *brown* suggests stability and safety, *pink* is linked to happiness and romance, and *orange* encourages communication. *White* symbolizes new beginnings and purity. *Black* is mysterious and independent. The aim of the feng shui is to ensure good qi flow, balance, and harmony with one's surroundings. Feng shui music is designed to help people improve their physical and mental health through naturally balancing the energy in the physical and etheric bodies (Collins, 2008).

RESEARCH

Although extensive research has been done in China through the institutions of TCM, much of this clinical research has been in the form of reports of observed results of various treatments. Many of these reports have been difficult to translate into Western languages and into the causal and analytic type of research modalities typical of the biomedical model. Research standards throughout the world are subject to cultural influences. Not all cultures require their medical practitioners to conduct randomized, double-blind clinical trials. Consequently, the research data are influenced by the location of the study. Research that is meaningful to the scientific communities of China and Japan may not have the same impact on European and North American biomedical communities.

Extensive research has been published on the pharmacology and toxicity of many traditional herbs. Researchers in China and Japan have been studying the therapeutic value of herbs in the following areas: chronic hepatitis, rheumatoid arthritis, hypertension, atopic eczema, various immunologic disorders including AIDS, and certain cancers. Herbs are also given to control the side effects of chemotherapy and radiation. It would be useful to repeat these studies using biomedical research criteria. Research on the medical effects of qigong has been continuing since the mid-1980s and is now focusing on qigong as a biophysical rather than a mystical force. Acupuncture is one of the most thoroughly researched and documented TCM practices. Research studies are covered in more detail in the chapters devoted to these specific practices. Research opportunities in the future might include studies regarding manual healing therapies, bioelectricity, magnetic physical interventions, and the use of mind–body interactions for health purposes. For the most up-to-date list of research studies available in the United States, contact the National Center for Complementary and Alternative Medicine (NCCAM) at the National Institutes of Health.

RELATED SYSTEMS

Tibet

In Tibetan Buddhism, religion and medicine are never separated from one another. The spiritual goal of Buddhism is to understand the nature of oneself and suffering and to develop compassion and compassionate action in one's life. Tibetan medicine, a sophisticated system, is based on general medical and philosophical assumptions as well as each individual's emotions, attitudes, lifestyles, and spiritual beliefs. It is believed that one's positive actions produce

USING RESEARCH TO HEAL

Ma, K., Lee, S-S., Chu, E. K.Y., Tam, D. K. P., Cheng, K. P., Kwong, V. S. C., et al. (2008).
   Popular use of Traditional Chinese Medicine in HIV patients in the HAART era. *Aids Behavior*, 12: 637–642.

What Is This Study About?

Traditional Chinese Medicine (TCM) is a commonly used practice in the Chinese popula-
tion around the world. TCM use may be even more prevalent for those living with chronic
illness. The purpose of this study was to examine the pattern of TCM use specifically by
Chinese males living with HIV while receiving highly active antiretroviral therapy (HAART).
The HAART guidelines follow the recommendations of the Panel on Clinical Practices for
Treatment of HIV Infection convened by the United States.

How Was the Study Done?

Seventy-six Chinese males living with HIV (mean age 45.36 years with a range of 25–72
years) and attending the HIV specialty service offered by the Health Department in Hong
Kong were provided a self-administered questionnaire. This anonymous survey requested
information concerning their use of TCM, beliefs and practices related to TCM, association of TCM use with HAART, and sources of advice on the use of TCM. All completed
questionnaires were coded. Additional information regarding latest clinical staging according to the Center for Disease Control and CD4 and viral load readings was obtained
for those participants providing consent to their medical records.

What Were the Results of the Study?

Fifty-nine percent of the respondents reported previous use of TCM with the majority using
over-the-counter TCM items and herbal tea intake. No specific TCM was identified as more
prevalent among the participants. Forty-three percent were categorized as "common
users" of TCM (using one or more types of TCM for more than two times within the last
6 months). Sixty-two percent of the participants had consulted specifically with a TCM practitioner. TCM users were older but age was not found to be statistically significant. There
appeared to be no difference in duration of illness for users and nonusers of TCM. No difference was found in length of diagnosis, duration of HAART, and CD4 counts between
TCM users and nonusers. Participants in stage B (symptomatic conditions) used TCM less
frequently than persons diagnosed in Stage C (AIDS indicator stage). Twenty-eight percent
had sought the services of a TCM practitioner within the last 6 months. Almost none of the
participants notified their TCM practitioner of their HIV diagnosis. None of the participants
initiated TCM use as a response to being diagnosed with HIV. In addition, the far majority
spaced their use of TCM at precise time intervals as to not potentially interfere with their
HAART protocol. Over 75% of TCM users neither consulted with the clinical staff regarding
the use of TCM nor felt that the staff would disapprove of their use of TCM.

What Additional Questions Might I Have?

Would the findings have been significantly different with Chinese men being treated
for HIV/AIDS living in other parts of the world such as the United States? What is the

(*continued*)

significance of severity of HIV/AIDS and use of TCM? Were any TCM items used by participants deemed harmful? What is the underlying rationale for not informing the professional staff (doctors, nurses) of their concurrent use of TCM?

How Can I Use This Study?

Nurses need to realize that persons living with chronic illness such as HIV/AIDS may be using a number of alternative therapies such as TCM concurrently with a Western medicine
approach to their diagnosis. Nurses need to specifically ask persons living with HIV/AIDS
about the use of supplemental therapies using a nonjudgmental communication style.
This study supports the need for nursing curricula to educate future nurses on patients'
use of complementary and alternative therapies.

Source: Contributed by Dolores M. Huffman, RN, PhD, Associate Professor of Nursing, Purdue University Calumet.

happiness and one's negative actions produce suffering. This belief in cause
and effect is referred to as **karma**.

In Tibetan medicine, disease results from two causes. The first cause is
spiritual, something brought from past life karma. Spiritual diseases are medi-
ated by a qualified teacher who uses meditation and yoga to balance body,
mind, and spirit. The process of learning how to control one's mind to function in a balanced mode with one's body is called **dharma**.

The second cause of disease involves factors from this life including seasonal changes, personal habits and behaviors, poisons, and negative spirits.
Illness is considered to be a lack of internal harmony or balance or a lack of
harmony with the larger external environment. The process of diagnosis is
similar to Traditional Chinese Medicine. Essential components in helping people mobilize their resources for self-healing are caring and compassion. As
Forde (2008) states, "The most revered healing method in Tibetan medicine is
compassion" (p. 14). We in the biomedical field should take careful note of
that philosophy.

Other treatments include dietary changes, massage, exercise, yoga, meditation, breath work, moxibustion, and acupuncture. Surgery is used only
when absolutely necessary. Herbal medicines are made from a variety of
herbs, minerals, fruits, twigs, roots, and animals. As in the Native American
tradition, the state of the practitioner's mind and the method of gathering are
important to the medication's therapeutic outcome. All preparation of medicines begins with prayer.

Korea

Chinese medicine arrived in Korea in approximately 200 B.C. The close relationship between China and Korea facilitated the exchange of ideas for hundreds of years. In the tenth century A.D., Korea established its political

independence from China but cultural and medical exchange continued. A contemporary innovative system developed in Korea in 1971 involves hand and finger acupuncture. Energy channels of the entire body are mapped onto the hands, where they are stimulated using short, fine needles and magnets. This system is rapidly gaining in popularity throughout the world (Ergil, 2001).

Japan

The history of medical information exchange dates back to the first century A.D. By the eighth century, many Chinese medical texts were translated for use in Japan. Several factors contributed to the unique adaptation of Chinese medicine. The scarcity of herbs led to an emphasis on lower prescription doses in Japan. Palpation, as a part of the diagnostic process, includes palpation of the abdominal energy pathways. A division of specialization in Japanese medicine relegates acupuncture, massage, and herbs to separately licensed practitioners. In Japanese medicine, acupuncture involves the use of somewhat finer gauge needles than those used for Chinese acupuncture and shallower insertion. Shiatsu is a holistic health care model using energy techniques to support well-being and prevent illness. Treatment is based on the relationship between the client and practitioner who uses gentle pressure along the meridians to correct energy imbalances. One study followed 948 clients over a 6-month treatment protocol with shiatsu practitioners in Austria, Spain, and the United Kingdom. There was a significant improvement in symptoms at the 3- and 6-month periods. More than 90 percent of participants felt that shiatsu helped them feel better in general (Long, 2008).

Europe

The history of Chinese medicine in Europe dates back to the middle of the sixteenth century A.D. when European physicians who traveled and studied in China and Japan wrote texts on acupuncture. In the 1950s and 1960s, two notable English acupuncturists, Dr. Felix Mann and Dr. Sidney Rose-Neil, influenced the development of acupuncture in English-speaking countries (Ergil, 2001).

United States

In 1826, Dr. Franklin Bache became one of the first American physicians to use acupuncture in his practice. When large numbers of Chinese laborers arrived in the United States, they were accompanied by TCM physicians and herbal merchants. Ah Fong Chuck became the first licensed practitioner of TCM in the United States in 1901 when he was awarded a medical license in Idaho. With the advent of World War II and the interruption of the herb supply from China, these practices disappeared or retreated into Chinatowns nationwide. In the 1970s, President Nixon reopened communication with China and the practice of TCM began to gain visibility once again throughout the United States. Now, a clear interest in acupuncture, herbs, and qigong can be found among many North American people (Ergil, 2001).

INTEGRATED NURSING PRACTICE

Although as nurses we are not educated as TCM practitioners, some principles are common to both nursing and TCM. Nursing and TCM practitioners believe that people are at once mind, body, emotions, and spirit; energy fields become unbalanced as a response to stress; energy fields are constantly interacting; people heal themselves; and the client–practitioner relationship is one of partnership.

Caring and compassion are considered to be essential components in helping people mobilize their resources for self-healing in both the practice of nursing and TCM. A critical attitude on the part of the compassionate nurse is one of *intent* to help and comfort. Even though outcomes of illness are not primarily in the hands of health care practitioners, as nurses, we must still be willing to do our best. In addition to our valuable technical skills, we must be present in the moment for each of our clients. It means grounding and centering one's self before we enter into a healing relationship with another person. It means keeping our focus on the other person rather than being distracted by our personal internal dialogue. All levels of nursing practice incorporate principles of caring as a guiding focus for nursing intervention. Some nurses will want to continue their education through in-depth study of the principles and practices of TCM. Requirements and programs of study can be obtained from the Council of Colleges of Acupuncture and Oriental Medicine, the addresses of which are found in the Resources section.

Before we can care for our clients, we must first learn to value and care for ourselves. Drawing from TCM, self-care means seeking ways to establish and maintain balance and harmony in our lives. Exercise programs might include vigorous exercise such as aerobics, running, or swimming; moderate exercise such as dancing or walking; or gentle movement exercise such as qigong, t'ai chi, or yoga. Touching and being touched are important to our sense of well-being. Self-massage, partner massage, and professional therapeutic massage contribute to a sense of balance and connection with others. Meditation, prayer, and worship are spiritual aspects of self-care. Breath work is both a physical way to increase relaxation and decrease stress and a spiritual way to connect with the universe.

Diet is another area where TCM can provide us with some practical guidelines. North Americans seem to have diets of extremes with fluctuation between overindulgence in food and starvation diets. It is often an all-or-none attitude that has neglected the principle of balance. Limiting the diet to a few fruits and vegetables may be as harmful as a steady diet of hamburgers. In TCM it is believed that illness can be avoided by eating a varied diet as much as possible. For example, avoiding a cold or hot imbalance is accomplished by eating a minimum of seven different fruits and vegetables each day.

For mild, temporary illnesses one might use a number of diet remedies. The cold type of the common cold and flu previously described as characterized by low-grade fever, no sweating, headache, muscle aches, stuffy nose, and a cough with clear white phlegm is treated with warming foods such as garlic, ginger, chives, pepper, pumpkin, apple, onion, and lamb. The hot type of the common cold and flu with its symptoms of high fever, sweating, headache, dry or sore throat, thirst, nasal congestion, and sticky or yellow mucus responds to cooling foods such as watermelon, eggplant, banana, plums, tomato, and tofu. The cold type of low back pain that is characterized by coldness and severe pain in the lower back that gradually worsens over time, is not relieved by lying down, and is aggravated by rainy days is treated with hot foods including garlic, chicken, apple, yam, celery, onion, peach, and mustard greens. The hot type of back pain that includes symptoms such as soreness of the lower back that is relieved by lying down, weakness of the legs, and frequent relapses is treated with cooling foods such as peanuts, sesame, soybeans, beef, pineapple, and grapes.

Like many other forms of alternative therapies, TCM regards breath as an important function of life. Restrictions in breathing lead to dysfunction and disease. Forming healthy breathing habits can counter stress and help balance body, mind, emotions, and spirit. See the *Try This: Relaxation* box for some suggestions you can easily incorporate into your daily life.

TRY THIS

Relaxation

Throughout the day one may find hundreds of opportunities to integrate some deep breathing, relaxation, self-massage, and gentle movement techniques into usual activities. Try this:

- You are sitting at a stoplight. Take a deep breath.
- You are in the shower washing your hair. As you apply shampoo, massage your scalp vigorously; rub your ears, relax, take several deep breaths.
- As you apply lotion or oil to your body following your bath, do so with the intent of relaxing each muscle group as you gently massage your entire body.
- You are just about to fall asleep or have just awakened. Breathe deeply and allow your whole body to become completely relaxed.
- You are about to enter a patient's room. Stop, breathe deeply, relax, and enter with an intent to help and heal.

Adapted from: Jahnke, 1997, pp. 83–98.

References

Collins, T. K. (2008). *The Western Guide to Feng Shui for Prosperity.* Carlsbad, CA: Hay House.

Ergil, K. V. (2001). China's traditional medicine. In M. S. Micozzi, ed., *Fundamentals of Complementary and Alternative Medicine,* 2nd ed., pp. 243–286. New York: Churchill Livingstone.

Fan, K. W. (2006). Foot massage in Chinese medical history. *Journal of Alternative and Complementary Medicine,* 12(1): 1–3.

Forde, R. Q. (2008). *The Book of Tibetan Medicine,* New York: Sterling Publishing Company.

Harrington, A. (2008). *The Cure Within.* New York: W.W. Norton & Company.

Jahnke, R. (1997). *The Healer Within.* San Francisco: HarperSanFrancisco.

King, E., Walsh, S., & Cobbin, D. (2006). The testing of classical pulse concepts in Chinese Medicine. *Journal of Alternative and Complementary Medicine,* 12(5): 445–450.

Kong, J., Gollub, R., Huang, T., Polich, G., Napadow, V., Hui, K., et al. (2007). Acupuncture de qi, from qualitative history to quantitative measurement. *Journal of Alternative and Complementary Medicine,* 13(10): 1059–1070.

Lin, Y. C. (2006). Perioperative usage of acupuncture. *Pediatric Anesthesia,* 16: 231–235.

Long, A. F. (2008). The effectiveness of Shiatsu. *Journal of Alternative and Complementary Medicine,* 14(8): 921–930.

Ni, M. (2008). *Secrets of Self-Healing.* New York: Penguin Group.

Sagar, S. M., & Wong, R. (2004). Chinese Medicine and supportive cancer care: A model for an evidence-based, integrative approach. *Evidence-Based Integrated Medicine,* 1(1): 11–25.

Scheid, V. (2007). Traditional Chinese medicine—What are we investigating? *Complementary Therapies in Medicine,* 15: 54–68.

Shinnick, P. (2006). Qigong: Where did it come from? Where does it fit in science? What are the advances? *Journal of Alternative and Complementary Medicine,* 12(4): 351–353.

Shu, J. J., & Sun, Y. (2007). Developing classification indices for Chinese pulse diagnosis. *Complementary Therapies in Medicine,* 15: 190–198.

Silva, L. M. T., & Cignolini, A. (2005). A medical qigong methodology for early intervention in autism spectrum disorder. *American Journal of Chinese Medicine,* 33(2): 315–327.

van den Berg, I., Bosch, J. L., Jacobs, B., Bouman, I., Duvekot, J. J., & Hunink, M. G. (2008). Effectiveness of acupuncture-type interventions versus expectant management to correct breech presentation: A systematic review. *Complementary Therapies in Medicine,* 16(2): 92–100.

Vas, J., Aranda, J. M., Baron, M., Perea-Milla, E., Mendez, C., Ramirez, C., et al. (2008). Correcting non cephalic presentation with moxibustion. *BMC Complementary and Alternative Medicine,* 8: 22.

Wang, J. F., Cai, C. Z., Kong, C. Y., Cao, Z. W., & Chen, Y. Z. (2005). A computer method for validating Traditional Chinese medicine herbal prescriptions. *American Journal of Chinese Medicine,* 33(2): 281–297.

Xiangcai, X., Ximing, H., & Xu, X. (2002). *Chinese Tui Na Massage.* Boston, MA: YMAA Publication Center.

Zhao, X. (2006). *Ancient Healing for Modern Women.* New York: Walker & Company.

Resources

Academy of Chinese Culture and Health
   Science
1601 Clay Street
Oakland, CA 94612
510.763.7787
www.acchs.edu

American Academy of Medical
   Acupuncture
1970 E. Grand Ave., Suite 330
El Segundo, CA 90245
310.364.0193
www.medicalacupuncture.org

American Association of Acupuncture
   and Oriental Medicine
P.O. Box 162340
Sacramento, CA 95816
866.455.7999
www.aaaomonline.org

Chinese Medicine and Acupuncture
   Association of Canada
154 Wellington Street
London, ON N6B 2K8, Canada
519.642.1970
www.cmaac.ca

Council of Colleges of Acupuncture and
   Oriental Medicine
3909 National Drive, Suite 125
Burtonsville, MD 20866
301.476.7790
www.ccaom.org

Guidebook provides a detailed description of all candidate and accredited schools in the
United States.

5

Ayurvedic Medicine

*Our cells are always willing to cooperate
with the mind's instructions.*

DEEPAK CHOPRA

*Healing may be defined as a miraculous
unfolding of consciousness for one's being
in the world.*

DEEPAK CHOPRA

BACKGROUND

Ayurveda, one of the oldest medical systems in the world, has
been practiced for more than 5,000 years in India. It is a holistic
and sophisticated system encompassing balance of body, mind,
and spirit as well as balance between people, their environments,
and the larger cosmos. *Ayurveda* is a Sanskrit word derived from
two roots—*ayur*, which means "life," and *veda*, or "knowledge"—
and translates literally to the science of life. Ayurveda has been
adapted by Hindu, Buddhist, and other religious groups and is
undergoing a renaissance both in India and throughout the West.

Ayurveda is an intricate system with a tradition of integrating that which is useful from other systems. This ancient system
has adapted to modern science and technology, including biomedical science and quantum physics. This blending of Ayurveda
and conventional medicine has proved very compatible (Sharma,
Chandola, Singh, & Basisht, 2007b).

CONCEPTS

Ayurveda asserts a fundamental connection between the microcosm and macrocosm. People are a creation of the cosmos and as
such are minute representations of the universe, containing

80

within them everything that makes up the surrounding world. One must understand the world in order to understand people and, conversely, understand people in order to understand the world. Ayurveda emphasizes the interdependence of the health of the individual and the quality of societal life. Therefore, measures to ensure the collective health of society, such as pollution control and appropriate living conditions, are supported. Similar to Traditional Chinese Medicine, the focus is on the person rather than disease (Tominson, 2002).

Five Elements

Ayurveda views nature and people as made up of five elements or qualities. These elements are earth, water, fire, air, and space and contain both matter and energy. As they interact, they give rise to all that exists. The *earth* element is dense, heavy, and hard. In the human body, all solid structures and compact tissues are derived from the earth element. The *water* element is liquid and soft and exists in many forms in the body, such as plasma, cytoplasm, saliva, nasal secretions, eye secretions, and cerebrospinal fluid. The *fire* element is hot and light and is believed to regulate body temperature as well as being responsible for digestion, absorption, and assimilation. The solar plexus is the seat of fire in the body. Fire manifests in the brain as the gray matter that allows one to recognize, appreciate, and comprehend the world. The *air* element is cold, mobile, and rough and in the cosmos is the magnetic field responsible for the movement of the earth, wind, and water. In the body, the air element governs cellular function, the movement of breath, and movements of the intestines. Thought, desire, and will are also governed by the air principle. The *space* element is clear and subtle and makes up most of our bodies. Space plays a unique role because it allows the existence of sound, which needs space in order to travel. Sound includes not only audible sound like music but subtler vibrations that resonate in our bodies (Atreya, 2001; Patwardhan, Warude, Pushpangadan, & Bhatt, 2005).

People are a composite of these five elements, which combine in various ways to govern mind, body, and spirit. Ayurveda sees the body as *doshas* (vital energies), *dhatus* (tissues), and *malas* (waste products). It is the dosha's job to assist with the creation of all the various tissues of the body and to remove any unnecessary waste products from the body.

Doshas

Doshas, or tridosha, are both structures and energy and are the mediators between body tissues, wastes, and the environment and are responsible for all physiological and psychological processes. The Sanskrit names for the three doshas are *Vata, Pitta,* and *Kapha.* As the driver or mover of the entire body, the Vata dosha is the most important. It is composed of the elements of air and space and is involved with all elimination, physical and mental movement, and nervous function. If Vata becomes imbalanced, it can cause the other two

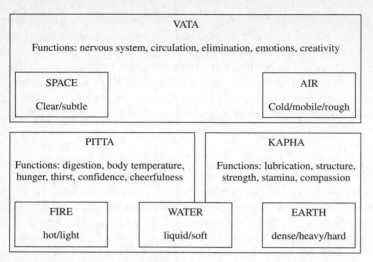

FIGURE 5.1 The Elements and the Doshas

doshas to become imbalanced. The Pitta dosha is composed of the elements fire and water, governs enzymes and hormones, and is responsible for digestion, body temperature, hunger, thirst, sight, complexion, courage, and mental activity. The Kapha dosha, composed of the elements of earth and water, is the heaviest of the three doshas. It provides the structure, strength, and stability that the body needs. It is also responsible for lubrication, sexual power, and fertility. Figure 5.1 illustrates the connections between the elements and the doshas.

Body Types

Vata, Pitta, and Kapha are present in every cell, tissue, and organ, but each person is made up of unique ratios of the three doshas. This individual constitution is determined by genetics, diet, lifestyle, and emotions. Each dosha gives an indication of physical strengths and limitations. According to Ayurveda, the ten body types are:

- *Single-dosha types.* One dosha is predominant:
  Vata
  Pitta
  Kapha
- *Two-dosha types.* One dosha is predominant with a strong secondary dosha:
  Vata–Pitta, Pitta–Vata
  Pitta–Kapha, Kapha–Pitta
  Kapha–Vata, Vata–Kapha
- *Three-dosha type.* All three doshas are in equal proportions:
  Vata–Pitta–Kapha

Knowing one's body type is the key to balancing one's life in the way that nature intended. This balance goes beyond physical and mental health and includes personal relationships, work satisfaction, spiritual growth, and social harmony. As a general rule, the strongest dosha in one's constitution has the greatest tendency to increase, making people most susceptible to illnesses associated with an increase of that dosha (Hankey, 2005).

Vatas are connected to the air and space, so they are similar to the wind—dry, cool, and capable of fast, variable movement and thought. The basic pattern of the Vata type is "changeable." Vata people are unpredictable and often start things without finishing them. Stress usually leads to anxiety or fear. They are responsive to sound and touch and dislike loud noise. Balanced Vata people are happy, enthusiastic, and energetic. When out of balance, they have a tendency to be impulsive. See Box 5.1 for characteristics of the Vata body type.

Pittas are aligned with fire and act with fervent determination. The basic pattern of the Pitta type is "intense." Pitta people are ambitious, outspoken, bold, orderly, and efficient. They tend to respond to the world visually and enjoy being surrounded by fine objects. Balanced Pitta people are sweet, joyous, and confident. Box 5.1 lists the characteristics of the Pitta body type.

Kaphas are a combination of earth and water and, therefore, move slowly and gracefully. The basic pattern of the Kapha type is "relaxed." Kapha people are stable, steady people who have a happy, tranquil view of the world. They are graceful people who wake up slowly, eat slowly, and speak slowly. They respond to the world through taste and smell and tend to place a great deal of importance on food. See Box 5.1 for characteristics of the Kapha body type.

Few people are single-dosha types. Most are two-dosha types, with one dosha predominant but not extreme. The dominant dosha gives people their primary reactions to the world, which are then moderated by the second dosha. Those with the two doshas of Vata–Pitta type are quick-moving, friendly, and talkative with a sharp intellect. They are not as unpredictable or irregular as the single Vata type. They enjoy challenges but stress makes them tense and hard driven. People who have a combination of Pitta and Kapha types are stable personalities but have a tendency toward anger and criticism. They have steady energy and good stamina but are less motivated to be active. Those whose doshas are the Kapha–Vata type may have a hard time identifying themselves since the Vata and Kapha tend to be opposites. Usually they have a thin body type but with a relaxed, easygoing manner. They tend to procrastinate but can be quick and efficient when necessary. The three-dosha type tends to have good immunity, lifelong good health, and longevity (Sharma, Chandola, Singh, & Basisht, 2007a).

Tissues/Dhatus

The seven **dhatus** or tissues are the structures of the body, are responsible for nourishment, and must be retained for health. They are *rasa* (plasma), *rakta*

BOX 5.1

Learn Your Dosha

Vata Type
- Light, thin build
- Thin, dry skin
- Dark, coarse, curly hair
- Irregular hunger and digestion
- Difficulty putting on weight
- Light, interrupted sleep
- Tendency toward constipation
- Aversion to cold weather, craves warmth
- Bursts of mental and physical energy
- Performs activity quickly
- Quick to grasp new information, also quick to forget
- Tendency for worry, anxiety, fearfulness
- Excitability, changing moods
- Enthusiasm, vivaciousness
- Fast talking

Pitta Type
- Medium build
- Fair, soft, warm skin
- Fine, soft, blond, light brown, or red hair
- Sharp hunger and thirst, strong digestion
- Cannot skip meals
- No problem gaining or losing weight
- Aversion to hot weather, craves coolness
- Moderate strength and endurance
- Sleep is sound but short
- Speech is sharp, clear, precise
- Sharp intellect, good, quick memory
- Enterprising character, likes challenges
- Busy lifestyle, achiever
- Tendency toward anger, irritability under stress, judgmental

Kapha Type
- Solid, powerful build
- Thick, pale, cold skin
- Thick, wavy, lustrous hair
- Tendency to obesity, hard to lose weight
- Slow digestion, mild hunger
- Sleep is heavy and for a long period of time
- Oily, smooth skin
- Aversion to cold, damp weather

- Steady energy, great strength and endurance
- Graceful in action
- Slow to grasp new information, good retentive memory
- Good organizer
- Affectionate, tolerant, forgiving
- Tendency to be greedy and possessive
- Tendency to be complacent
- Speech is slow, may be labored

(blood cells), *mamsa* (muscle), *meda* (adipose), *asthi* (bone), *majja* (bone marrow), and *shukra* (reproductive tissue). In general, Ayurveda practitioners work to keep these tissues intact and healthy (Sharma et al., 2007a).

Waste Products/Malas

The **malas**, or wastes, are the nonretainable substances within the body. Urine, feces, and sweat, for example, need to be released and eliminated as the body rids itself of toxins. Excretion of the malas cleanses; thus people are cautioned against inhibiting the body's natural functions, including sneezing, yawning, burping, urinating, defecating, and passing gases. Vata is the dosha that causes these urges, and suppression of them disturbs Vata. Ayurveda encourages expression of these urges in a way that is not offensive to other people (Sharma et al., 2007a).

Energy/Prana

Prana, which the Chinese call qi, in Sanskrit means "primary energy," sometimes translated as "breath" or "vital force." Prana is not only the basic life force, but also the original creative power. Prana has many levels of meaning, from the physical breath to the energy of consciousness. The five pranas are categorized according to movement, direction, and body region. The navel is considered the pranic center of the physical body. *Prana vayu*, forward-moving air, moves inward and regulates the intake of substances into the body. This prana moves energy from the head down to the navel. It is the basic energy that drives us in life. *Apana vayu*, air that moves away, moves downward and directs all forms of elimination and reproduction. It controls the movement of energy from the navel down to the root chakra at the base of the spine. *Udana vayu*, upward-moving air, brings about the transformations of life energy. It governs the growth of the body and the release of positive energy. This prana moves energy from the navel up to the head. *Samana vayu*, balancing air, moves from the periphery to the center and moves energy from the entire body back to the navel. It aids in all types of digestion—food, oxygen, and emotional and mental experiences. *Vyana vayu*, outward-moving air, moves from the center to the periphery and regulates energy out from the navel through the entire body. It directs the circulation of nutrients throughout the body (Selby, 2001).

VIEW OF HEALTH AND ILLNESS

When the doshas are balanced, individuals experience health on all levels: mental, emotional, physical, spiritual, and environmental. It is much more than the mere absence of disease. *Mentally* healthy people have good memory, comprehension, intelligence, and reasoning ability. *Emotionally* healthy people experience evenly balanced emotional states and a sense of well-being or happiness. *Physically* healthy people have abundant energy with proper functioning of the senses, digestion, and elimination. From a *spiritual* perspective, healthy people have a sense of aliveness and richness in life, are developing in the direction of their full potential, and are in good relationships with themselves, other people, and the larger cosmos. *Environmentally* healthy individuals have minimal economic, social, and political stress.

Balancing one's doshas does not mean trying to achieve an equal portion of Vata, Pitta, and Kapha. One cannot change the ratio of doshas that are present from conception. Health is the balance of each dosha that is right for that particular individual. Doshas, however, are responsive to people's habits, such as diet, exercise, and daily routines, which can either deplete or increase the doshas. While both states of imbalance lead to ill health or disease, increased doshas are more problematic than decreased doshas.

Imbalance in the doshas is the first sign that mind, body, and spirit are not perfectly coordinated. One type, called *natural imbalance*, is due to time and age. Natural imbalances are typically mild and normally do not cause problems. Each dosha becomes more predominant during certain times of day, as energy moves through six cycles in each 24-hour period: Veta predominates from 2 to 6, day and night; Kapha during the hours of 6 to 10; and Pitta from 10 until 2. Each dosha also predominates during particular seasons and stages of life. Kapha dominates during childhood and during the spring season, Pitta during summer and middle age, and Vata during fall and the latter part of one's life.

Unnatural imbalances of the doshas can be caused by a variety of factors, each of which falls into one of three broad categories of disease. Adhyatmika diseases originate *within the body* and include hereditary and congenital diseases. Adhibhautika diseases originate *outside the body* and include trauma, bacteria, and viruses. Adhidaivika diseases originate from *supernatural sources*, including those diseases that are otherwise unexplainable, such as illnesses originating from seasonal changes, divine sources, planetary influences, and curses. While some of these causes are beyond individual control, lifestyle and diet are within one's control. Preventing disease and improving overall health depends on the recognition of dosha imbalance and an understanding of the factors that increase and decrease each of the doshas (Selby, 2001).

Imbalanced Vata shows up as rough skin, weight loss, anxiety, restlessness, insomnia, decreased strength, constipation, arthritis, hypertension, rheumatic disorder, and cardiac arrhythmia. Pitta imbalance includes a yellowish complexion, excessive body heat, insufficient sleep, weak digestion, inflammation, inflammatory bowel disease, skin disease, heartburn, and peptic ulcer. Kapha imbalance presents as a pale complexion, coldness, lethargy, excessive sleep, depression, sinusitus, respiratory disease, asthma, and excessive weight gain (Atreya, 2001).

Several factors aggravate or increase each of the doshas. Factors increasing Vata are excessive exercise, wakefulness, falling, cold, late autumn and winter, fear or grief, agitation or anger, fasting, and pungent, astringent, bitter foods. Factors increasing Pitta are anger, fasting, strong sunshine, midsummer and early autumn, and pungent, sour, or salty food. Kapha is increased by factors such as sleeping during the daytime, spring and early summer, heavy food, milk products, sugar, and sweet, sour, or salty foods (Sharma et al., 2007a).

DIAGNOSTIC METHODS

The first question asked is not "What disease does this person have?" but "Who is this person?" The complete process of diagnosis takes into account physical, mental, and spiritual components integrated with the social and environmental worlds in which the person lives. In addition to using X-rays or other biomedical diagnostic tools, Ayurvedic practitioners diagnose by observing people, touching them, taking pulses, and interviewing them.

Pulse Diagnosis

Pulse diagnosis is a highly specialized skill that requires great sensitivity. The process, as shown in Figure 5.2, involves placing the index, middle, and ring fingers of the right hand on the radial arteries of the right hand of men and the left hand of women. The general feel of the pulse is related to body type. A Vata pulse, felt by the index finger, is irregular or wavering, resembling the movement of a snake. A Pitta pulse, felt at the middle finger, feels forceful and throbbing, resembling the movement of a frog. A Kapha pulse, felt at the ring finger, is said to be gliding, resembling the movement of a swan. A three-dosha pulse resembles the movement of a woodpecker. Ayurvedic doctors may also take pulse readings at other points on the body as well. These points include the brachial artery above the elbow, the femoral artery, and pulse points at the temples, ankles, and top of the feet. This basic form of pulse reading gives the practitioner a vital clue to the person's body type. Pulse diagnosis is remarkably comprehensive. Experienced physicians cannot only diagnose present diseases but can also tell what diseases the person has experienced in the past and which they are likely to develop in the future (Tominson, 2002).

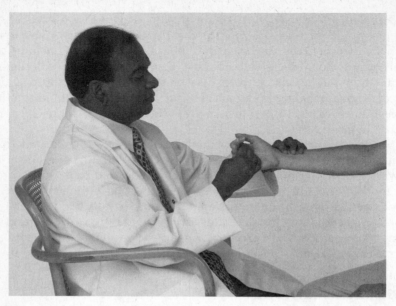

FIGURE 5.2   An Ayurvedic practitioner uses the index, middle, and ring fingers to locate three pulse points that are related to the flow of prana in the body and the three doshas.

Source: Dorling Kindersley Media Library/Andy Crawford

Tongue Diagnosis

Tongue diagnosis can also reveal the functional status of internal organs. A healthy tongue should be pink, clear, and shiny. A discoloration and/or sensitivity of a particular area of the tongue indicates dosha dysfunction. Kapha imbalance is evidenced by a whitish tongue, Pitta imbalance a yellow-green tongue, and Vata imbalance a brown to black tongue (Tominson, 2002).

Urine Diagnosis

Ayurvedic practitioners do urine examinations as another way to understand dosha imbalances. A midstream specimen is collected first thing in the morning. Healthy urine should be clear without much foam. Kapha imbalance gives the urine a cloudy appearance, Pitta imbalance imparts a dark yellow color, and pale yellow and oily urine indicates a Vata imbalance. The practitioner also puts a few drops of sesame oil in the urine and examines it in the sunlight. The shape of the drops signifies which dosha is imbalanced: A snakelike shape with wave movement indicates Vata, an umbrella shape with multiple colors, Pitta, and a pearl shape, Kapha. The movement of the oil in the urine indicates the prognosis of the disease. If the drop spreads immediately, the illness is probably easy to cure. If the oil drops to the middle of the urine sample, the illness is more difficult to cure. If the oil sinks to the bottom, the illness may be impossible to cure (Tominson, 2002).

Body Observation

The practitioner carefully examines the skin, nails, and lips. Cool, hot, rough, or dry skin indicates imbalance. Imbalance can be visualized in the nails by longitudinal striations, bumps, or a parrot beak at the end of the nail. Dry, rough lips or inflammatory patches on the lips are another sign of imbalance. Coldness, dryness, roughness, and cracking indicate Vata imbalance. Hotness and redness indicate Pitta imbalance. Kapha imbalance is indicated by wetness, whiteness, and coldness (Tominson, 2002).

TREATMENT

Specific lifestyle interventions are a major preventive and therapeutic approach in Ayurveda. Each person is prescribed an individualized diet and exercise program depending on dosha type and the nature of the underlying dosha imbalance. Care is taken to not cause new symptoms by subduing the presenting symptoms. Herbal preparations are added to the diet for preventive or regenerative purposes as well as for the treatment of specific disorders. Yoga, breathing exercises, and meditative techniques are also prescribed by the practitioner (Sharma et al., 2007a).

Nutrition

In Ayurveda, a balanced diet is different from the Western perspective of a balanced diet derived from the basic food groups of meat, dairy, fruit, grains, and vegetables. Ayurveda recognizes six tastes: sweet, sour, salty, pungent, bitter, and astringent. A balanced Ayurveda diet must contain all six tastes at every meal but in different proportions depending on dosha type. The word *taste* includes not only the perceptions on the tongue but also the immediate effect of the substances within the body. Each of the six tastes is derived from two of the five elements as illustrated in Figure 5.3. Sour, salty, and pungent have the fire element and so increase body temperature, dilate body channels, and allow energy and toxins to flow out from the body. Sweet, bitter, and astringent have no fire and thus are cooling, promoting relaxation. Sweet, sour, and salty have the water element and soften tissues, lubricate mucous membranes, and increase water retention (Sharma et al., 2007a).

Ayurveda describes the actions of each of the six tastes. *Sweet* promotes the vitality of body tissues, soothes the five senses, and adds bulk and firmness. Used in excess, sweet creates obesity, weak digestion, and a tendency to excessive sleep and heaviness. *Sour* improves the taste of food, increases digestion, and awakens the mind. In excess, sour wastes muscles and causes a buildup of toxins in the blood. *Salty* promotes digestion, moisturizes the body, softens all organs, and acts as a laxative and sedative. In excess, salty causes stagnation of blood, wasting of the muscles, wrinkling of the skin, and digestive hyperacidity. *Pungent* cleanses the mouth, opens

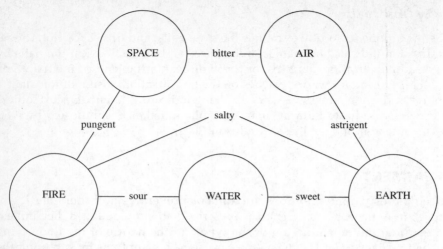

FIGURE 5.3   The Six Tastes and the Five Elements

Source: Sharma, H., Chandola, H. M., Singh, G., & Basisht, G. (2007a). Utilization of Ayurveda in health care: Part 2—Journal of Alternative and Complementary Medicine. 13(9), 1011–1019.

the vessels, improves blood flow, and cures disorders of excess fluid in the body. In excess, pungent causes fatigue, emaciation, dizziness, and thirst. *Bitter,* though it does not taste good in itself, restores the sense of taste, detoxifies, relieves thirst, and is antibacterial, germicidal, and antipyretic. In excess, bitter causes wasting away of the tissues, weakness, and dryness. *Astringent* is drying, firming, and sedating. It stops bleeding and aids in healing of wounds. In excess, astringent causes premature aging, constipation, retention of wastes, spasms, convulsions, and weakens vitality (Sharma et al., 2007a).

Three pairs of *gunas* or qualities are inherent in food: heavy or light, oily or dry, and heating or cooling. Examples are:

- *Heavy:* wheat, beef, cheese
- *Light:* barley, chicken, skim milk
- *Oily:* milk, soybeans, coconut
- *Dry:* honey, lentils, cabbage
- *Heating:* pepper, honey, eggs
- *Cooling:* mint, sugar, milk

It is not necessary to memorize which foods reduce which doshas because any number of books are available that offer long lists of foods matched to the dosha, taste, and guna. Many people seem to know naturally what their bodies need for balance. See Box 5.2 for the relationship between the doshas, tastes, and gunas. To counter an excess of *Vata,* diet recommendations consist of warm food with moderately heavy textures, salt, sour, and sweet tastes, and added oil. Examples of foods to include are asparagus, carrots, green beans, avocados, bananas, melons, rice, wheat, chicken, seafood, chickpeas, and tofu. To counter an excess of *Pitta,*

BOX 5.2

Foods in Relation to Doshas

Vata

Balances		Aggravates	
Salt	Hot	Pungent	Light
Sour	Oily	Bitter	Dry
Sweet	Heavy	Astringent	Cold

Pitta

Balances		Aggravates	
Bitter	Heavy	Pungent	Hot
Sweet	Cold	Sour	Light
Astringent	Dry	Salty	Oily

Kapha

Balances		Aggravates	
Pungent	Light	Sweet	Heavy
Bitter	Dry	Sour	Oily
Astringent	Hot	Salty	Cold

Sources: Atreya. (2001). *Perfect Balance: Ayurvedic Nutrition for Body, Mind and Soul.* New York: Avery Publishing; Selby, A. (2001). *Ayurveda.* Minnetonka, MA: Creative Publishing; Tominson, C. (2002). *Ayurveda Wisdom.* Edison, NJ: Castle Books.

diet recommendations are for cool or warm (but not hot) foods with moderately heavy textures and bitter, sweet, and astringent tastes. Examples of foods to include are broccoli, cabbage, lettuce, apples, grapes, raisins, barley, oats, ice cream, chicken, shrimp, chickpeas, and tofu. Coconut, olive, and soy oil are acceptable. For an excess of *Kapha*, diet recommendations include warm, light food, cooked without much water, pungent, bitter, and astringent tastes, and a minimum of butter and oil. Examples of foods to include are cauliflower, celery, leafy green vegetables, apricots, pears, dried fruits in general, barley, corn, rye, skim milk, chicken, shrimp, sunflower seeds, and raw honey (Chopra & Simon, 2001).

Every food can be characterized by taste and guna. In addition to a balanced diet in terms of fats, carbohydrates, and proteins, people need variety in salty, sour, sweet, pungent, bitter, and astringent foods. The goal of diet management is to avoid aggravating any of the doshas and keep them calm and balanced.

Herbs

In Ayurveda, natural medicines are primarily herbal but may include animal and mineral ingredients, and even powdered gemstones. Practitioners prescribe many thousands of herbs. Like food, herbs are classified according to the six tastes. Herbs, however, are more potent and specific in their action than is food. Some herbs, used for preventive and regenerative purposes, are readily available. The use of herbs for treating disease must be medically supervised. As in Traditional Chinese Medicine, the entire plant is used. It is believed that the plant contains other chemicals that buffer the active ingredient, thus reducing possible side effects (Sharma et al., 2007a).

Like foods, herbs balance doshas. *Vata*-balancing herbs include ginseng, licorice, Indian Penny wort, bala, and sitopladi. Aloe vera, comfrey root, Indian gooseberry, and saffron are used to balance *Pitta*, while elecampane, honey, and sitopladi balance *Kapha*. Herbs usually take longer to work than Western medications prescribed by practitioners. Historically, Ayurvedic herbs have had little exposure outside India but are now becoming more familiar with the rapid explosion of interest in herbal medicines in North America. Following are a few of the more common herbs found in health food stores. Sitopladi is a very good herbal formula for colds and flu. Indian Penny wort (brahmi) enhances a person's ability to focus mentally and learn new material. Guggulu is a powerful purifying agent, well known for lowering of blood cholesterol levels. Shilajit, with its antispasmodic qualities, is effective in acute and chronic respiratory illnesses. Bala, or Indian Country mallow, is helpful in all types of nervous system disorders and certain types of heart disease. These few examples of herbs give one an idea of how they are used as natural body medicines (Williamson, 2002). In some instances, heavy metals such as lead, mercury, and arsenic have been found in Ayurvedic herbal medicines. Thus, people have been cautioned about ordering these herbs from overseas or through the Internet (WHO Drug Information, 2007). Chapter 6 presents herbs in more detail.

Exercise

According to Ayurveda, exercise should conform to one's dosha type. *Kapha* people can perform moderately heavy exercise such as aerobics, running, dancing, and weight training. Because of their physical strength, Kaphas excel at endurance sports. *Pitta* people, who have more drive than endurance and an intense competitive spirit, should have a moderate amount of exercise. Brisk walking or jogging, hiking, swimming, and skiing are appropriate. People with a *Vata* dosha might enjoy jogging, but exercises like stretching, yoga, and t'ai chi are better choices. They have bursts of energy but tire quickly and may push themselves past their limits. Walking is probably the best exercise for all people because it calms all dosha types. Ayurveda recommends a brisk half-hour walk every day (Chopra & Simon, 2001; Selby, 2001).

For people over the age of 80 or under 10 as well as those people who have serious Vata and Pitta imbalances, exercise should be very gentle. Exercise should always leave a person ready for work as opposed to exercise being work itself. Several other exercise precautions must be noted. One should not engage in exercise sooner than half an hour before and one to two hours after a meal. Exercising in the evening is discouraged because it is better for the body to slow down and prepare for sleep. Exercise is discouraged in the wind or cold since heavy breathing of cold, damp air is unhealthy for the respiratory tract. Also discouraged is exercise during the intense heat of the day, since environmental heat causes an even greater rise in body temperature.

The key to exercise is moderation and regularity. Ayurveda suggests that all exercise should be done at one-half of one's capacity. That means working out just until sweat appears on the forehead, under the arms, and along the spinal column. This amount of exercise improves digestion, prevents constipation, improves circulation, stimulates metabolism, regulates body temperature, and maintains body weight. Exercise keeps one's senses and mind alert and attentive as well as being effective in inducing relaxation and sleep. Overexercise, as indicated by panting and heavy sweating, may cause dehydration, muscle aches, breathlessness, and even chest pain. It is believed that overexercise eventually contributes to arthritis, sciatica, or heart conditions (Atreya, 2001).

Yoga

Yoga, developed in the Ayurvedic tradition, is one of the most effective forms of exercise for the body as well as nourishment for the mind and spirit. Hatha yoga, the most familiar form of yoga in North America, is a combination of body positions, breathing exercises, and mental focus on the here-and-now. Stretching helps relax and tone the muscles, improves circulation, improves concentration, and helps one in regaining energy. Yoga is increasingly recognized for maintaining general health as well as helping people to manage chronic disorders such as headaches, insomnia, hypertension, and depression. Further information about yoga is found in Chapter 16.

Breathing

Practicing controlled breathing is a valuable technique that leads to a healthier lifestyle. Several techniques can be utilized to relax the mind and body. Simple breathing helps people become aware of their breath and often relieves tension. Simple breathing involves closing the eyes and observing the breath, becoming more aware of its pattern and changes. Slow, easy breathing is continued for several minutes until a sense of relaxation is achieved. Alternate nostril breathing, *Pranayama*, is another technique that can ease difficulty in breathing by making the respiratory rhythm

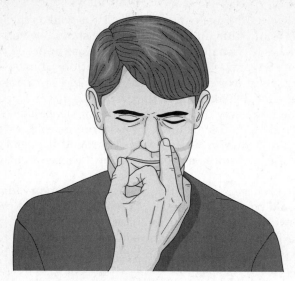

FIGURE 5.4   Pranayama/Controlled Breathing

more regular, which in turn soothes the entire nervous system. Pranayama is helpful prior to meditation because it focuses attention inward. Pranayama is performed while seated with the eyes closed. Figure 5.4 illustrates the position. The index and middle fingers of the right hand are placed on either side of the nose. The thumb closes the right nostril while the person breathes in through the left nostril. The left nostril is then closed with the ring finger and the right nostril is opened for the out-breath and the next in-breath. The right nostril is then closed and the out-breath occurs through the left nostril. After doing a couple of rounds, breathing naturally gets deeper and smoother.

Meditation

An important part of daily life in Ayurveda, meditation is considered a powerful tool to help maintain health. Meditation is a moment-to-moment awareness that is cleansing to the body, mind, and spirit. It is finding the quiet in the mind. As the mind is brought into a silent and receptive state, new energy comes into being, which is conducive to a state of health and peace. Further information about meditation is found in Chapter 17.

Massage

Marma therapy is a massage technique focusing on 107 sensitive points, called *marmas*, located on the skin. These points are similar to the acupuncture points called *hsueh* in Traditional Chinese Medicine. Marma therapy predates the Chinese approach and is likely the parent to acupuncture and acupressure. Marmas are activated through various methods. One is through yoga movements that gently stretch specific marma points. Warm oil dripped on the center of the forehead (shirodhara) on a major marma point can be profoundly soothing. A daily self-massage with oil can reach all the marmas on the skin. Once taught, these techniques can be practiced at home. Massage is covered in more detail in Chapter 12.

Aromatherapy

Aromatherapy is based on olfactory stimuli used to help balance the doshas as each responds to specific signals. Specialized olfactory cells provide instant connection of odors with the brain. The hypothalamus responds through regulation of body functions, the limbic system responds with emotions, and the hippocampus responds with memories, which explains how smells can elicit memories so vividly. In general, *Vata* is balanced with warm, sweet, and sour aromas such as basil, orange, rose geranium, clove, and other spices. *Pitta* is balanced by sweet, cool aromas like rose, mint, cinnamon, sandalwood, and jasmine. *Kapha* is balanced by warm aromas with spicy overtones such as juniper, eucalyptus, camphor, and clove. People whose doshas are out of balance are given specific oils to restore dosha balance. Aromatherapy may be used at any time but is often prescribed at night because it helps induce sleep (Tominson, 2002). Aromatherapy is discussed further in Chapter 8.

Music

India has a long tradition of merging music and medicine. Unlike most Western music in which the notes are distinct, the tones tend to blend together, creating a soothing, unifying sound. As with taste and smell, doshas can be balanced with certain tones and rhythms. The three doshas peak at different times of the day, and traditional Indian music smoothes the process of these transitions. An example of a rough transition is the inability to fall asleep because one's mind is racing with many thoughts. Ten minutes of music can be used as a gentle wakeup in the morning, after a meal to settle digestion, just before bedtime to aid sleep, and during the recovery period from an illness. Music therapy is discussed further in Chapter 21.

Purification

Panchakarma, or purification therapy, involves five procedures, any or all of which can be chosen based on the person's general condition, the season, and the nature of the disease. The five therapies of Panchakarma are experienced over a period of a week and involve purifying the body through the use of sweating, emetics, purgatives, enemas, and nasal inhalations. Commonly administered by an Ayurvedic physician with the help of a number of assistants, the benefits of Panchakarma are relief from long-standing symptoms, renewed health, and extended longevity (Sharma et al., 2007b).

RESEARCH

Many Western researchers seem to believe that they look at reality in an objective way. In contrast, Ayurvedic researchers believe that nothing happens in a vacuum. Everything that happens, happens in relationship to what is occurring around it. The principle of research is that knowledge cannot be separated from its context.

The National Center for Complementary and Alternative Medicine has supported research for a number of years. Current studies include effects of garlic on serum lipids, neuroprotective agents from oriental medicines, Ayurvedic herbals and effects on lipids and atherosclerosis, and meditation for hypertension. Funded studies related to yoga include yoga as a treatment for insomnia, for self-management of chronic obstructive pulmonary disease, and yoga and peak flow rates in pregnant asthmatics. A sampling of studies has found the following:

- Dehydrated powder of garlic showed a significant relief of some of the symptoms of depression (Sharma et al., 2007b).
- The symptoms of anxiety are lessened by herbal medications such as Brahmi and Nasya (Sharma et al., 2007b).
- Thirty-six patients with essential hypertension were divided into three groups. Group 1 received an herbal mixture, Group 2 received a purification treatment, and Group 3 received a combination treatment of herbs and purification. Results showed a significant reduction in both systolic and diastolic blood pressure in all three groups (Sharma et al., 2007b).
- The herbal formulation, Triphala, exerted a strong anti-inflammatory effect against gouty arthritis in mice (Sabina & Rasool, 2008).
- Ayurvedic oil-dripping treatment was conducted with 16 healthy women. All women had three types of treatment (plain oil, lavender oil, and control supine position) in a random order. The treatment with lavender oil resulted in the greatest reduction of anxiety (Xu et al., 2008).

INTEGRATED NURSING PRACTICE

Although most of us have not been educated in Ayurvedic medicine, as nurses we can integrate a number of principles into our professional practice. Ayurveda teaches self-discovery and self-understanding; it encourages people to learn how they maintain their health and how and when they become sick; and it advocates lifestyle changes to maximize one's well-being.

The first step to encourage self-understanding is helping people learn their dosha or body type. See Box 5.1 earlier in this chapter for a checklist and follow these steps to determine dosha type:

- Make a check mark next to the description that best describes how you have been most of your life. If you fall between two descriptions, check both of them.
- Consider the qualities carefully. There are no right or wrong answers. Be honest and check how you are, not how you would like to be.

- Look for lasting trends. For example, if your sleep has been heavy and for long periods of time most of your life but you are now sleeping light and fitfully, the change is likely to be due to imbalance rather than dosha type. Check your usual pattern.
- Notice whether each dosha has some checks because everyone has Vata, Pitta, and Kapha as part of their body type.
- Total the number of checks for each dosha. The dosha with the greatest number should be your body type. If the highest two doshas are close, you are probably a two-dosha type. If all three dosha scores are close, you have a three-dosha type.

Determining dosha type allows people to begin to understand how their health is affected by internal and external influences as they consider their unique blend of doshas. As people become more familiar with their bodies, they can observe and experience the effect of what they eat and do each day; how they think and feel; the state of their metabolism, digestion, and elimination; the relationships they engage in; their jobs; and the environment in which they find themselves. Because all of these factors are interdependent, problems in one area can cause problems in other areas.

People's dosha balance can be disrupted in a number of ways. An inappropriate diet and lifestyle for your dosha type will cause a slowly developing excess or deficiency in doshas. If you suffer significant trauma, however, the dosha levels can change immediately and dramatically. Dosha imbalance can also occur from an accumulation of toxins or when too many experiences of a particular dosha take place without enough experiences from the other doshas. Once people understand their baseline dosha type, they can assess imbalances that may contribute to disease. Remind people that the strongest dosha in their constitution has the greatest tendency to increase. For example, if you have a Kapha dosha type, you have a natural tendency to those things which have Kapha qualities, thus increasing your Kapha energy. If you have a lifestyle that includes overeating, not exercising, and sleeping excessively, and you have a desk job, your Kapha dosha can become excessive. You may need to consciously add opposite qualities to pacify or balance your Kapha energy such as decrease your food intake, eat more pungent and bitter vegetables and astringent fruits, and increase your exercise.

Achieving balance of the doshas does not happen quickly—people need to work at it consciously. In some cases, lifestyle changes may be difficult, such as the nature of your job, while others may be easier, such as a change in leisure activities. Typically, people find that diet, exercise, and leisure activities are the most amenable to change. For example, television and computers increase Vata through stimulation of the eyes and ears and increase Kapha by the passive nature of these activities. If the television program makes you angry or your computer program will not do what you wish, your Pitta may be stimulated. Limiting the time spent watching television and being selective with programs may help you balance your doshas and move toward a healthier state. Likewise, if you spend a lot of time at your computer, you need to take frequent breaks, move and stretch your body, and rest your eyes.

If your strongest dosha is *Vata*, you need to develop more regularity in your daily routines such as eating regular meals, having an established bedtime, and slowing down and taking time to think. Because you have a tendency to dry skin, oil your skin regularly. People with Vata doshas are drawn to sensory experiences involving movement, speed, and action, and you may enjoy loud music and computer games. To maintain a healthy balance, make an effort to balance those activities with quiet, creative pursuits such as writing, photography, or painting. Similarly, because you are attracted to vigorous exercise, try to engage in gentle exercise every day. Ayurveda suggests that all exercise be done at one-half of one's capacity. If you know that you are exhausted after a 40-minute aerobic class, then you should do only 20 minutes of the class. People with Vata doshas enjoy spending their vacations sightseeing, touring, and filling their days and nights with many activities and returning home exhausted. A more beneficial vacation would be in a beautiful, sunny, and warm environment where you rest and limit your activities. If you are a Vata type, your clothes are mostly dark shades that may reflect a tendency to become depressed. Bright yellow colors and pastel shades may brighten your mood.

If you are a *Pitta* type, you need to loosen up on setting and achieving goals and learn to enjoy here-and-now moments. You can learn to achieve your ambitions without pressuring yourself. Your need to organize yourself, and everyone else must be kept under control lest you should become easily frustrated when things do not go as planned. You are stimulated by competitive, mentally challenging situations that may increase your aggression or your determination to win. Learn to use constructive criticism rather than confrontation. Engaging in noncompetitive leisure activities such as gardening may help prevent an excess of Pitta. Vacations in cooler climates and water and winter sports will cool your tendency to be warm. Avoid organizing your vacations in the greatest of detail and try to enjoy whatever happens. Red clothing overstimulates Pitta and may contribute to a more aggressive approach to others. Cool, soft, pale colors are more balancing to the Pitta dosha.

If you are a *Kapha* type, you need to vary your daily experiences to avoid becoming stuck in a rut. Try to make small changes in routine every day. Get up early and go to bed late to limit your tendency to sleep many hours. Since you may prefer to sit and do nothing, find activities that are mentally and physically stimulating. Kapha is balanced by vigorous exercise but you will most likely have to force yourself. Because you have good stamina, you can exercise for a longer time than people who are Vata or Pitta. You would prefer a vacation lying on a beach doing nothing but soaking up the sun. You will find, however, that sightseeing and touring will be more stimulating and balancing for you. All colors, except greens and dark blues, balance Kapha. You will find that bright, strong colors are exciting and balancing.

Helping people understand their doshas is an ongoing process. As people observe their mind, body, spirit, and relationships, they learn how they respond to different qualities in everyday activities. After determining dosha type, have people review their lifestyles in terms of diet, work, leisure activities, exercise, daily routines, quiet times, sleep, and relationships. Applying the principles of Ayurveda, people can begin making choices about the qualities they wish to incorporate into their lives. Rather than focusing on negatives (what they want to stop doing), have them focus on positives (what they want to start doing). Suggest that they limit their exposure to those qualities they do not want and enjoy those that will aid their well-being. Change begins with small steps and is a gradual process. Some people will want to seek the advice of an Ayurvedic practitioner to individualize a lifestyle change program. Remind people that their mind and body always strive toward health and that every individual needs time, nurturing, routine, and gentle discipline to achieve a more complete level of well-being.

TRY THIS

Massage

Sesame Oil Massage

Use the refined sesame oil sold in health food stores, not the heavy Chinese sesame oil. If you wish, you may use olive oil instead. Warm a quarter cup of oil in the microwave for 10 to 15 seconds being careful not to overheat it.

Mini-Massage (1–2 minutes)

Use one tablespoon of warm oil and rub it into your scalp. Use small, circular motions with the flat of your hand. Using your palm, massage the forehead from side to side and gently massage your temples using circular motions. Gently rub the outside of the ears. Massage both the front and the back of the neck.

Use a second tablespoon of warm oil and massage both feet using the flat of the hand. Massage each toe with your fingertips. Vigorously massage the soles of your feet. Sit quietly for a few seconds to relax and then shower or bathe as usual.

Full-Body Massage (5–10 minutes)

Massage the scalp, ears, and neck with one tablespoon of warm oil as described above.

Using more oil, vigorously massage your arms using long strokes on the long parts and circular motions at the joints.

Adding oil as necessary, massage the chest, stomach, and lower abdomen using gentle circular strokes in a clockwise direction. Massage as much of your back and spine as you can reach.

Massage the legs as you did the arms using vigorous movements.

With the remaining bit of oil, massage the feet as described above. Bathe with warm water and mild soap.

Source: Chopra, D. (1991). Perfect Health. New York: Harmony Books.

References

Atreya. (2001). *Perfect Balance: Ayurvedic Nutrition for Body, Mind and Soul.* New York: Avery Publishing.

Chopra, D. (1991). *Perfect Health.* New York: Harmony Books.

Chopra, D., & Simon, D. (2001). *Grow Younger, Live Longer.* New York: Three Rivers Press.

Hankey, A. (2005). The scientific value of Ayurveda. *Journal of Alternative and Complementary Medicine,* 11(3): 221–225.

Patwardhan, B., Warude, D., Pushpangadan, P., & Bhatt, N. (2005). Ayurveda and Traditional Chinese Medicine. *Evidence-based Complementary and Alternative Medicine,* 2(4): 465–473.

Sabina, E. P., & Rasool, M. (2008). An in vivo and in vitro potential of Indian Ayurvedic herbal formulation Triphala on experimental gouty arthritis in mice. *Vascular Pharmacology,* 48: 14–20.

Selby, A. (2001). *Ayurveda.* Minnetonka, MN: Creative Publishing.

Sharma, H., Chandola, H. M., Singh, G., & Basisht, G. (2007a). Utilization of Ayurveda in health care: Part 1— Ayurveda, the science of life. *Journal of Alternative and Complementary Medicine,* 13(9): 1011–1019.

Sharma, H., Chandola, H. M., Singh, G., & Basisht, G. (2007b). Utilization of Ayurveda in health care: Part 2— Ayurveda in primary health care. *Journal of Alternative and Complementary Medicine,* 13(10): 1135–1150.

Tominson, C. (2002). *Ayurveda Wisdom.* Edison, NJ: Castle Books.

WHO Drug Information. (2007). *Journal of Alternative and Complementary Medicine,* 21(2): 91.

Williamson, E. M. (2002). *Major Herbs of Ayurveda.* New York: Churchill Livingstone.

Xu, F., Uebaba, K., Ogawa, H., Tatsuse, T., Wang, B. H., Hisajima, T., et al. (2008). Pharmaco-physio-psychologic effect of Ayurvedic oil-dripping treatment using an essential oil form lavendula angustifolia. *Journal of Alternative and Complementary Medicine,* 14(8): 947–956.

Resources

Ayurvedic Herbs—Circle of Health
2852 Willamette Street, PMB 399
Eugene, OR 97405
541.349.8680
www.ayurveda-herbs.com

Ayurvedic Medical Association, United Kingdom
59 Dulverton Rd
Selsdon, South Croydon
Surrey CR2 8PJ, UK
0208.657.6147

Bazaar of India
1810 University Avenue
Berkeley, CA 94703
800.261.7662
www.vadikherbs.com

Maharishi Ayurveda Health Center:
  The Raj
1734 Jasmine Avenue
Fairfield, IA 52556
800.248.9050

National Ayurvedic Medical Association
620 Cabrillo Avenue
Santa Cruz, CA 95065
800.669.8914
www.ayurveda-nama.org

6

Native American Healing and Curanderismo

Morning Prayer
> *I thank You for another day. I ask that*
> *You give me the strength to walk worthily*
> *this day so that when I lie down at night I*
> *will not be ashamed.*

Evening Prayer
> *At the end of each day, face west and say:*
> *Thank you for all the things that*
> *happened today, the good as well as*
> *the bad.*

For Emotional, Physical, and Mental Health
> *Lie down with your navel toward the*
> *Earth and your head to the north, saying:*
> *Grandmother Earth, please send your*
> *healing energy through this body and*
> *bring it back into balance.*

To Find an Answer to a Problem
> *Face east and think about your problem*
> *saying: Grandfather Sun, you come each*
> *day to dispel the darkness. In that same*
> *way I ask you to shed your light so that I*
> *may see where to take the next step.*

PRAYERS BY BEAR HEART, NATIVE AMERICAN SHAMAN

Although each Native American Indian–based healing system is unique, they share a number of characteristics. This chapter presents the commonalities found among tribes. The population of today's Native American tribes is only a fraction of what it was before Europeans invaded this continent. Forty-five percent of all Indians living on reservations live below the poverty level. Native Americans have the highest infant mortality rate of any group in the United States, and life expectancy among Indians is 2.4 years less than other U.S. citizens. Alcoholism is a significant problem for a variety of reasons, both social and genetic. Many customs have been lost forever. Despite these impediments, many of the traditions and ceremonies practiced by Native Americans for centuries are still in evidence today (Facts on Indian Health Disparities, 2006).

BACKGROUND

Non-Indian people can learn a great deal from the Native American approach to life and traditional healing. To learn, people must be open to the ancient wisdom and understand it in the context of the entire Indian experience. It is not something to be trivialized by simply purchasing medicine objects and trying them out at home. As one Sioux leader said, "First they took our land, now they want our pipes . . . all the wannabees, these New Agers, come with their crystals and want to buy a medicine bag to carry them around in. If you want to learn our ways, come walk the red road with us, but be silent and listen" (Johnson, 1994, p. 6).

In their earliest encounters, Euro-American physicians devalued the skills of Native healers. This association has, in a way, come full circle. Western medicine is now advancing toward a holistic point of view that Native Americans have been practicing for thousands of years. Today, medicine women and men continue with a system that is parallel to conventional medicine. Some people are traditional, meaning that they adhere strictly to the old ways of life and reject any form of biomedicine. Others have acculturated, or adapted to the mainstream culture, and use both Indian medicine and conventional medicine. A third group of Native Americans has become assimilated and has virtually abandoned all traditional ways in favor of the dominant culture and utilize only biomedicine (Shimer, 2004).

Most tribal people have one or more types of health care specialists whose treatments frequently overlap. Some Native healers use herbs, some heal with songs, and some with spiritual rituals. A midwife or a medicine woman or man might focus on natural medicines such as herbs and hands-on techniques but also use prayer and ceremony. Shamans or holy people emphasize spiritual healing but are often also knowledgeable about natural medicines. Kahunas are people, usually of Hawaiian ancestry, who have developed a level of spirituality that joins them with many of the spirit powers, allowing direct communication about the healing process. Shamans and medicine people are seen as channels the Creator has provided and trained.

Some are born into families with medical or ritual skills, while others discover this path through a dream or vision. Selection is based on signs of devotion, wisdom, humility, and honesty. Once called, the individual seeks training, usually by apprenticing to a medicine person for a number of years. All knowledge comes from the Creator, and the elders are charged with the responsibility of keeping knowledge about healing foods, herbs, and medicine and passing it on. Trusted with all secrets, rituals, and legends of their people, Native healers are considered to be inspired individuals with great importance to the tribe. Training is complete when the teacher says it is complete and when the candidate has practiced the skills publicly and with success (Bad Hand, 2002). See Chapter 24 for more information about shamans.

CONCEPTS

Spirituality

Spirituality and medicine are inseparable in Native American tradition. Essentially no distinction is made between religious and medical practices. "Making medicine" is an important part of traditional life. It is how people give thanks to the Spirit who helps, guides, nourishes, and clothes them. Medicine is the constant pipeline to the Creator. In Indian tradition, making medicine is a process for achieving a variety of positive outcomes: a good hunt, plentiful crops, connecting with someone, healing someone, a successful birthing, and so on. Medicine is the way people keep their balance; it provides them with the opportunity to grow in new and healthier ways (Hunter, Logan, Goulet, & Barton, 2006).

Native Americans believe in a singular living God, but also believe that same God may be contacted through many ways, from many cultures. In Native languages, God is given such names as Great Spirit, Creator, Great Being, Great Mystery, Above Being, The One Who Oversees All Things, and He Who Gives Life. The missionaries mistakenly thought that Indian people worshiped trees, eagles, the Pipe, and many other things. What was misinterpreted was the use of these objects as gifts from the Creator, put here to help. Using these gifts is one way to create an atmosphere conducive to addressing the Creator (Bear Heart, 1996).

Gratitude is a central aspect of Native American culture. Every day is a spiritual, sacred day. One morning prayer is "I thank You for another day. I ask that You give me the strength to walk worthily this day so that when I lie down at night I will not be ashamed" (Bear Heart, 1996, p. 164). Thanks are given to the Great Power who makes all things possible. People give thanks, not only for the good events but also for the bad things that happen throughout the day, because they believe that the more they show their appreciation, the more blessings they will receive.

Native peoples do not own or possess land but rather see themselves as caretakers of the earth for the Great Spirit. The land is considered the Mother since all things come from her body. Animals, birds, trees, and grass all come from Mother Earth and are powerful living beings, just like human beings. When Native people take something from the earth, such as herbs or even a stone, they always give an offering, usually tobacco, in return and say a prayer that the item taken will be used in a good manner (Bear Heart, 1996; O'Brien, 2008).

Healing

Medicine women and men see themselves as channels through which the Great Power helps others achieve well-being in mind, body, and spirit. The only healer is the One who created all things. Medicine people consider that they have certain knowledge to put things together to help the sick person heal and that knowledge has to be dispensed in a certain way, often through ritual or ceremony. Healers receive their knowledge through fasting and asking for guidance from Above. During the period of fasting, the Great Being might reveal a chant or the location of a particular herb and give instructions on how to use it for different illnesses (Bear Heart, 1996).

Time is often considered an ally in recovery. With the passage of time, fears and problems sometimes fade. Love is a key element in the healing process. The healer enters into the healing relationship with love and compassion. The two individuals experience a joining or merging as this process unfolds. This merger symbolizes the cementing together of people and the Divine Spirit (Forest, 2000).

Circle

The circle represents the cycles of life, which have no beginning, no end, and no time element. The Great Spirit causes everything to be round. The sun, earth, and moon are round. The sky is deep like a bowl. Things that grow from the ground like the stem of a plant or plant roots are round. The circle, symbol of infinity and interconnectedness, is seen in the sweat lodge, the bowl of the Sacred Pipe, the Sacred Hoop, and the Medicine Wheel. In addition, the camp is circular, tepees are circular, and people sit in a circle in all ceremonies. When people come together in a circle, a spirit of oneness and a sense of sacredness come upon them.

Medicine Wheel

The Medicine Wheel is both an important conceptual scheme and a major ceremonial observance. The Sacred Hoop makes up the circumference with the interior of the circle being divided into four quadrants. Each quadrant represents a direction, a totem, an element, a color, a kingdom, a quality, a season, and a gateway to the individual. The four colors—white, black, yellow, and red—represent the races of all humanity. See Figure 6.1 for an illustration of the Medicine Wheel.

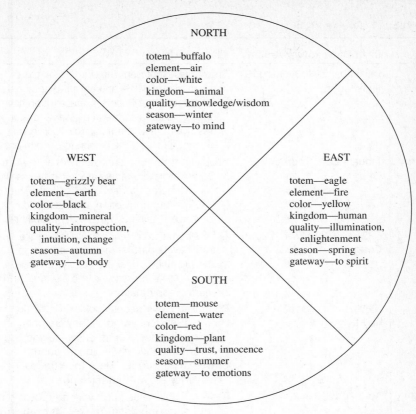

FIGURE 6.1   The Medicine Wheel

Sources: Hill, D. L. (2006). Sense of belonging as connectedness, American Indian worldview, and mental health. *Archives of Psychiatric Nursing*, 20(5): 210–216; *Medicine Wheel.* www.medicinewheel .com. Accessed July 9, 2008; Rutherford, L. (2008). *The View Through the Medicine Wheel.* Ropley, Hants, UK: John Hunt Publishing.

The four directions of the Medicine Wheel are the basis for the astrological system. Each person is represented somewhere within that circle, depending on the birth date. Table 6.1 gives a brief summary of the Twelve Moons.

Number Four

The number four is significant to Native American people and is incorporated into their daily lives through prayers, ceremonies, and activities. It is believed to be the number of completeness. Everything that grows from the earth consists of four parts: roots, stems, leaves, and fruit. Earth, air, fire, and water are the four life-giving elements. Four types of things take breath: those that crawl, those that fly, those that walk on four legs, and those that walk on two legs. There are four directions, four seasons, and four races of people—white, black, yellow, and red.

TABLE 6.1 Twelve Moons

	Birth Date/Power Animal	Characteristics
North	December 22 to January 19 Snow goose	Snow geese represent the chief at the top of the medicine wheel and have the potential for great power. People in this position have great vision and can send messages over long distances. Often just thinking of someone will be enough to get the person to call him or her.
	January 20 to February 18 Otter	People in this moon are as playful as the otter. Otter people like others as well as themselves and are humanitarian in their views. They excel in communication, intellect, and romance. They may have psychic abilities.
	February 19 to March 20 Cougar	Others come to cougar people for advice since they have a natural medicine power and psychic ability. They are deeply sensitive, hesitate to express their true feelings, and yearn for spirituality.
East	March 21 to April 19 Red-tailed hawk	Red-tailed hawk people look at the world with a sense of wonder. They are open to learning new things, enjoy life and adventure, and are passionate about everything they do. Since they are fearless, they may act without thinking.
	April 20 to May 20 Beaver	Beaver people value hard work and focus on getting the job done. The results of their work can have great impact on people far away. They strive to create and maintain an orderly and beautiful environment.
	May 21 to June 20 Deer	Deer people often have many ideas and try to accomplish them all. They may have two or three jobs at a time. They have graceful, quick movements. Deer people appreciate the beauty in themselves, others, and the environment.
South	June 21 to July 22 Flicker (large woodpecker)	People in this position are intuitive and wild in some aspects of being, but conservative in others. They have an ability to both heal and inspire. Flickers have an excellent sense of humor and a strong desire for self-expression.
	July 23 to August 22 Sturgeon	Sturgeons come into the world as teachers, with strong leadership abilities. They are always reading and studying to search for the truth. They have an outer shell that protects their inner sweetness from other people.

(continued)

TABLE 6.1 (Continued)

	Birth Date/Power Animal	Characteristics
	August 23 to September 22 Brown bear	Brown bear people have a natural creative curiosity. Their gut feelings tend to be very accurate as long as they don't overanalyze. They have good sense and make fair decisions. They are confident and well balanced.
	September 23 to October 23 Raven	Like ravens who fly together, these people tend to stay with the flock. If they can separate and follow their own convictions, they can be great leaders. They understand messages from the heart and are physically affectionate.
West	October 24 to November 21 Snake	Snake people are powerful healers who are able to travel places where others may fear to go. They are often messengers for the spiritual aspects of life. They are inquisitive and able to create change.
	November 22 to December 21 Elk	Elk people are insightful, independent, determined, and open-hearted. They are passionate about justice. They have an ability to perceive the thoughts and feelings of others and may be clairvoyant.

Source: Adapted from Brother Eagle Soaring (2003). www.spiritalk.net/naheali4.htm. Retrieved July 9, 2008.

VIEW OF HEALTH AND ILLNESS

Health is viewed as a balance or harmony of mind and body. The goal is to be in harmony with all things, which means first being in harmony with oneself. Harmony is thought to neutralize problems and help one's life to become beautiful. Good health makes it easier for all people to do their part in the universe, to serve others, and to fulfill their personal life visions.

Life is considered in all of its dualities: winter/summer, cold/hot, day/night, mind/body, spiritual/physical, work/play, and so on. Native people believe that the two sides of everything deserve equal attention and that both should be nourished with love. A healthy person who is walking in balance is energized and alert and in the presence of disease will still feel alive and fulfilled (Hunter et al., 2006).

Traditionally, Native American people lived long, happy, healthy, and balanced lives. They did everything to respect and honor Mother Earth and the Great Spirit. They ate wholesome food and considered all food to be blessed as a gift of life from the Creator. They got up with the sun and went to bed with the moon. Exercise was a natural part of their lives, integrated into daily activities. These good health habits, a sense of joy, and a purpose in life are key factors for living into old age (Sun Bear, Mulligan, Nuffer, & Wabun, 1989).

Illness occurs when balance is disrupted. It is believed that most illness begins in the head and people must get rid of ideas that predispose illness. If the mind is negative, the body will be drained, making it more vulnerable. Disease is also thought to be caused by "soul loss"—when individuals stop being generous and become selfish and dishonest. When people open up to the universe, learn what is good for them, and find ways to be happier, they can begin to work toward a longer and healthier life. Many ancient people had ways to get rid of this negativity. The Mayan people of Mexico would stand in a stream of flowing water and talk out all their angers, fears, sorrows, or troubles over the water. The moving water would take all the emotions they poured out of themselves into the current and away from them. The Bear Dance was a way the Indian people of northern California rid themselves of negativity. A man in a bear costume would dance around a circle of people who would use switches to hit him as they spoke about the things in their lives that were bothering them. When the bear had everyone's negativities, he went down into the stream, washing them away. Some Native people of the Southwest had dancers armed with swords who went through the village singing, chanting, and rattling, driving out the negative forces as they went. Behind them people came with brooms to sweep away anything that was left over. Most Indian tribes had some way of letting people get rid of negativity so that they could go on and build new positive patterns (Garrett, 2003).

Dreaming is a powerful way for people to learn what is good for them. Dreams are a personal connection to the upper, spiritual realms. Divine guidance is thought to come through dreams and visions. In a period of illness, people may actually dream the healing. Dreaming is important in the healing practices of medicine women and men since treatment information is often provided through dreams. Dream weavers, dream catchers, or dream nets are special medicine objects that catch the dream and hold it for the person.

DIAGNOSTIC METHODS

Healers must diagnose the source of the problem because they want to treat the cause, not just the effect. In a manner similar to Traditional Chinese Medicine and Ayurveda, the approach is one that takes into account all aspects of one's inner self, lifestyle, emotions, social setting, and natural surroundings when making a diagnosis. They always look at the total person whether they are treating someone for physical illness or emotional problems. They look at the overall picture, determine what is out of balance within the whole, and then pinpoint the trouble spots. Some healers diagnose by going into a trance. While in a trance, "hand tremblers" pass their shaking hands over the body of the person; when the hands stop trembling, the locale of the illness is found and the cause is usually identified. "Star gazers" also enter trance states to read cause in the stars. "Listeners" do not go into a trance but listen to the person's story and on that basis identify the cause of the illness (Struthers, Eschiti, & Patchell, 2004; Walsh, 2007).

TREATMENT

When people fall ill, they often experience anxiety and fear that may incapacitate them. The healer is not so burdened and is able to supply coherence, calmness, and hope. Power flows through the healer to the patient. Patients' preferences are always respected in determining their own path toward balance and healing. Healers use medicine objects to assist them, and treatments consist of ceremony, touch, herbs, singing, drumming, and sometimes peyote.

Items used to help make medicine are called **medicine objects.** Medicine objects can be anything that relates to the Great Spirit in a sacred way. The medicine bag contains healing objects, which vary in size and number but typically are such things as feathers, claws, bird or animal bones, an assortment of herbs or roots, smudges, or paints. The medicine bag may also contain personal items that represent the individual and personal experiences that are sacred to him or her. Native Americans are protective of their medicine bags. The bags carry a part of themselves and are among their most prized companions. The Medicine Wheel is a sacred circle usually built from stones. It is entered for the purpose of healing, giving thanks, praying, or meditating. The Pipe is one of the most sacred medicine objects and is an instrument of prayer.

The Indian art of healing is *ceremonial* or ritual in nature. Different ceremonies are conducted according to the type of illness or the severity of the person's condition. Healing ceremonies are led by medicine people or holy people. There is a communal aspect of the ceremony—as many people as possible participate to increase the power of the prayers. The primary purpose is to allow connection with the Great Healer, since physical health often fails without the aid of spiritual means. A secondary benefit is a cleansing of the body, mind, and spirit. A healing session is never a casual encounter. It is arranged through a formalized procedure after discussion by the patient, family, advisers, and healer. Acceptance by the healer is followed by instructions on preliminary actions, which may include fasting, abstinences, prayers, or the preparation of offerings or feasts.

Smudging

Smudging is a cleansing and purifying process using smoke from burning sacred herbs, usually sweet grass, sage, cedar, or tobacco. *Sweet grass* is used to bless one's self and one's home to protect from evil spirits. It is also used to purify sacred prayer instruments. *Sage* has a variety of uses. It is used in the blessing of one's home, it is part of the mixture used in the sacred smoking of the Pipe, and it is used in tea to flush out impurities. *Cedar* is considered the "tree of life" because it withstands the four elements no matter how harsh the seasons. Cedar is used in all sacred ceremonies as well as for its medicinal qualities. *Tobacco* is considered a gift from the Creator, and it is a visual representation of people's thoughts and prayers being carried to the Creator. People and all sacred objects are smudged so all can be centered and focused on the healing process. The smoke clears negativity, purifies the energy field of people and places, and is a prayer to the Creator. In addition to its use in healing ceremonies, smudging is used in the morning or evening as part of daily devotion. Smudging is a practice known to many religions; examples include the use of frankincense in Catholic churches and sticks of incense in Buddhist temples (Cohen, 2006; Hunter, Logan, Barton, Goulet, 2004).

Sweat Lodge

The **sweat lodge** or **purification ceremony** is a ritual to cleanse body, mind, heart, and spirit. It may be held as its own ceremony or in preparation for another ceremony, such as a vision quest. Typically the sweat lodge is held in a round structure covered with overlapped pieces of tarpaulin or blankets with a small door flap. When the flap is down, the place is nearly dark and almost sealed off from the outer air. Near the lodge is a fire pit, where rocks are heated and then passed into the lodge. Water from a bucket is splashed on the stones, creating a dense steam referred to as the Breath of Spirit. Depending on the illness, a variety of herbs are burned on the sweat rocks. Sacred songs and prayers go on for several hours. Everyone in the sweat lodge prays hard for the one needing healing, but it is the responsibility of the one being healed to pray that healing energies come to her or him and ask the Spirit to give guidance to the medicine person (Bear Heart, 1996).

The sweat lodge is also a powerful ceremony to keep people healthy, and many view it as the first line of defense in preventing illness. The sweat lodge raises the body's temperature well above normal, killing heat-sensitive viruses and bacteria. The lodge is also a bringing together of the four elements: earth, air, fire, and water. Through sweating and praying, the body is cleansed of toxins, the mind of negativities, the heart of hatred, and the spirit of doubt. The sweat lodge is as sacred a place as if it were a church or temple (Buhner, 2006).

Drumming and Chanting

Drumming and chanting are powerful ways to bring oneself in balance with self, others, and the world. **Drumming** harmonizes people with the heartbeat of Mother Earth. It is a pulse rather than a tempo. As people dance to the pulse of the drum, they dance in harmony with the Creator and with one another. Symbolically, the drum represents all life. The wood was once a tree, and the skin covering the drum was once life. They are related to life that has gone on, yet they are helping the lives that are still here. **Chanting** is a form of prayer through music. Holyway chants are used to attract good, to cure, and to repair. Ghostway chants are used to remove evil, and lifeway chants are used to treat injuries and accidents (Bear Heart, 1996).

Sing

A **sing** is a healing ceremony that lasts from two to nine days and nights. A highly skilled specialist called a singer guides it. Used in healing, sings are attended by as many people in the community as are able because just being present is considered healing. Some songs are only for children and call on spirits who take care of little children. Some spiritual songs take care of adults only. Other songs focus on specific problems, such as the song for small burns that will cool them and keep them from blistering. To learn a single chant can take up to several years. It takes some people 40 years of singing before they master the chants and the accompanying herbal preparations (Rutherford, 2008).

Pipe Ceremony

The Pipe ceremony takes many different forms depending on how this sacred knowledge was given to the various tribes. The **Pipe** is one of the most sacred medicine objects and represents the universe to Native American people. The bowl represents the Earth Mother and the female powers of the universe. The stem represents the plant kingdom and the male powers of the universe. When the bowl and stem are joined together, the Pipe is sacred. The tobacco smoked in the Pipe is an instrument of prayer and has come to signify the sacredness of the ritual. As the smoke of the Pipe rises, it creates an atmosphere of prayer by symbolizing prayers going up to the Creator (Sun Bear et al., 1989).

Pipes are used for private and group prayers. Prayers are transmitted in the smoke of the burning tobacco. Participants in the Pipe ceremony are as centered and focused as possible, since everything they think and feel is part of the prayers being offered. As in many other ceremonies, the number four has special significance. The Pipe is offered to the four directions and is often passed in four ritual repetitions (Bad Hand, 2002).

Sun Dance

The **sun dance** includes the sweat lodge, the Pipe ceremony, monthly prayer rituals, and a yearly ceremony. During the monthly ceremony, songs are sung to carry the prayers upward, and people come forth to be healed. The yearly three- to four-day sun dance usually takes place in July. It is a very detailed and complex ceremony. The medicine man prays on behalf of the tribe, the world, and all creation. The dancers, who spend all their time praying to the Creator, move to the drumbeat around a center pole. Since the dancers fast for the entire time, many collapse or "take a fall." This is often followed by a vision, similar to what happens on a vision quest. The sun dance ends with a purification ceremony so that tribe members can reenter the world refreshed and regenerated (Walsh, 2007).

Vision Quest

An extremely powerful ceremony is the **vision quest.** Traditionally, it is a time of fasting, praying, isolation, and exposure to the elements, all of which contribute to a mystic experience with the goal of understanding self and communicating with the Great Spirit. Questions are asked, such as "How can I best serve the people?" "How can I best serve Mother Earth?" "How can I best serve future generations?" The vision quest tells people who they are, what they are really supposed to do, what their life's goal should be, and the purpose and meaning of their lives. The vision quest begins with a sweat lodge for purification, after which the person is taken to an isolated place in nature and begins the period of silence and fasting. During the vision quest, the individual focuses only on prayer and vision and in this way is pushed into the spirit world. After the vision quest, the person returns to the sweat lodge and a Pipe ceremony is performed (Walsh, 2007).

Healing Touch/Acupressure

Native Americans have always considered touch to be therapeutic. The Creator touches patients and transfers power to them through medicine people or shamans who are healing instruments. Touching, an expression of loving care, is essential for the healing process. It cleanses the affected area and relieves pain. The willingness to touch on the part of the healer demonstrates no fear of contamination. Healing touch is a powerful way to remove barriers and create or restore relationships (Shimer, 2004).

Some tribes have used a form of acupressure since ancient times. Compared with traditional Chinese practitioners, Native Americans used fewer pressure points but the process is similar. Prior to using acupressure, medicine people warm their hands over a fire so that the Great Being can send healing warmth through them to the patient. It is believed that no harm will be done to a person as long as the pressure is applied slowly and in a relaxed way. Medicine people are taught that acupressure should only be done with the utmost gentleness and love.

Herbs

Native Americans have long used herbs in maintaining health and treating disease. Botanical remedies are supplemented with ceremony and prayer during the healing process. The beneficial properties of herbs as medicines often depend on the greenness or ripeness of the plant and the part of the plant to be used, such as roots, barks, twigs, bulbs, rhizomes, fruit seed, tubers, leaves, and flowers. Knowing the best time for cutting and digging each type of plant, for peak effectiveness, is part of the knowledge of the Native healer. Whether it be in summer, winter, spring, or autumn, the timing must be appropriate for each plant. A herb gathered with prayers, at the correct time and prepared properly, will restore a person from illness to health (Buhner, 2006).

Ancient Native people considered nature to be their pharmacy. They did not have aspirin but they did have willow bark, which contains salicylic acid. The active ingredient in squaw tea is ephedrine, the main ingredient in many cold cures now on the conventional market. The active ingredient in foxglove is digitalis, which was used to brew tea to help people with heart problems. Particular molds, similar to those forming the basis for penicillin, were used to treat infections. Purple coneflower (echinacea) is an immune system booster and antibiotic that is held in high esteem by many people today. Goldenseal, which is a good disinfectant that promotes scab formation, is one of the most important Native American medicinal plants. Currently, it is also used as a gargle for sore throat or as a mouth rinse for canker sores, tonsillitis, and infected gums (Garrett, 2003). For further information on herbs, see Chapter 7.

Peyote

A hallucinogenic herb, peyote has been used by the Indians of North America for a long time. Native people do not use peyote to "get high" but rather to see teaching visions. Using peyote is a sacrament, and it provides a connection to the sacred world. Peyote makes people highly sensitive to sight and sound and more aware of what is around and inside of them. It is used to heal all kinds of sickness, for clairvoyance, and in the worship of the Great Being. It is believed that the Creator put peyote on earth as a medicine to help people (Bad Hand, 2002; Bear Heart, 1996).

Role of Medicine Women and Men

Although they are the primary care providers in many places, the responsibilities of medicine women and men go beyond healing illness. They also evaluate advice and treatment given by other health care practitioners. They often have a strong influence on the acceptance or rejection of the treatment plans from conventional health care providers. They may also function as tribal social mediators, dispensing traditional wisdom and suggesting action. Medicine people reaffirm and strengthen tribal identity through the recounting of myth and song. They have an extensive knowledge of their communities and of family relationships and interaction. They are the formulators and teachers of the old religion and creators of the new. Medicine people are figures of authority and awe as instruments of the Creator (Struthers et al., 2004).

RESEARCH

Formal research into healing ceremonies is almost nonexistent. Native American medicine is a tradition that is subtle and difficult to document and communicate fully outside of its varied traditions and ceremonies. Anecdotally, many ailments and diseases have reportedly been cured by medicine people and shamans. These disorders range from skin rashes and asthma through heart disease, diabetes, and cancer. More current research regarding scientific data on the use of herbs is available. This information is presented in Chapter 7.

CURANDERISMO

Curanderismo (pronounced koo rahn dare ees mo), from the Spanish verb *curar*, to heal, is a cultural healing tradition found in Latin America and among many Hispanic Americans in the United States. In Mexico, many beliefs are shared with Native American cultural traditions. Curanderismo, as described here, is most characteristic of Mexican Americans. Although it is a traditional healing system, it survives by growing, changing, and incorporating Western biomedical beliefs, treatments, and practices. It is also believed, however, that in certain types of illness and healing, Native healers are more accomplished than practitioners of conventional medicine. Some professional nurses are also native healers. They combine their knowledge of nursing science with the long tradition of curanderismo (Luna, 2003).

Natural/Supernatural Illnesses

Illnesses are classified into two types: natural and supernatural. The *natural* source of illness includes genetic disorders, dysfunction of the body, improper self-care, infection, and psychological conditions. *Supernaturally* induced illnesses are said to be caused by either evil spirits or by a person practicing magic and placing a hex on the victim. Supernatural illnesses, which may look like natural illness, occur when these negative forces damage a person's health. It is believed that conventional medical practitioners are unable to intervene with supernatural illnesses (*Handbook of Texas Online*, 2008).

Healers

Curanderos (men) and curanderas (women) believe that they work by virtue of *el don*, a gift of healing, often believed to be a gift from God. In some areas, becoming a healer is a matter of inheritance, while in other areas it is a matter of being called. Healers routinely deal with physical ailments as well as with problems of a social, psychological, or spiritual nature. Healers are always one of the people. Their healing awareness comes from living with the people, feeling their pain, knowing their illnesses, and experiencing their suffering (Sobralske, 2006).

Three Levels of Healing

Three levels of care are practiced among curanderos and curanderas. These three levels are the material level, the spiritual level, and the mental level. Healers have the gift for working at only one of these levels since each requires distinct areas of knowledge, methods of diagnosis, and types of healing. The majority of the healers work at the material level and most combine shamanic healing, herbal medicine, and first-aid techniques (*Handbook of Texas Online*, 2008).

The *material level* involves the use of physical or supernatural objects to heal or to change the person's environment. Physical healers include midwives, bone setters, herbalists, and people who treat sprains and tense muscles. Objects and rituals are used for their curative powers. Objects include herbs, religious symbols (crucifix, pictures of saints, incense, holy water), and secular items (cards and ribbons). Several types of rituals are used for supernatural cures. One of the most frequently used is a cleansing ritual that includes prayers and invocations designed to remove the negative forces that are causing the illness and a purification of the environment with incense. At the same time, the patient is given the spiritual strength necessary to achieve recovery.

The *spiritual level* of healing is similar to shamanic healing rituals. It is believed that spiritual beings who exist in another dimension are interested in making contact with the physical world. These spirit entities come from once-living humans. Spiritual-level healers become a direct link or medium with these spirits. They enter a trance state and make contact with the spirit world. Some spirits have left tasks undone in their physical lives; some wish to help or harm others; and some wish to communicate with their friends and relatives. Healers believe that spirits can manipulate a person's health by directing positive or negative forces at them from the spiritual realm.

The *mental level* is the least encountered level of practice. Healers have the ability to transmit, channel, and focus mental vibrations in a way that directly affects a person's mental or physical condition. If healers are working with physical illness, such as cancer, they channel vibrations to the afflicted area to retard the growth of abnormal cells and accelerate the growth of healthy cells. If healers are working with mental conditions, they send vibrations into the person's mind to manipulate energies and modify behavior. Mental healing can be accomplished in person or over long distances (*Handbook of Texas Online*, 2008).

Most research done on curanderismo is traditional anthropological research such as participant observation and interviewing. Many of the home remedies have been tested for biochemical and therapeutic activities and have demonstrated therapeutic actions that match the healers' uses. Research regarding herbs is presented in Chapter 7.

INTEGRATED NURSING PRACTICE

Just as Native American healers see themselves as channels through which the Great Power helps others achieve a sense of wellness, some nurses see God or the Divine Being at work in their professional practice. Although clients may be unaware of this spiritual impetus, these nurses believe that the spiritual dimension provides the energy and momentum for their practice. Other nurses believe that their desire to care for others is what provides direction for their practice. The *art of nursing*, for many, is in being there, with another person or persons, in a context of caring. As we return to our nursing roots in using our hands, heart, and head in creating healing environments, we approach the Native American ideal of healing practices.

Like Native Americans, nurses have traditionally looked at the *total person* in their care. The context of people's lives is critically important to the nursing–healing model. In addition, nurses also believe that feelings or energy or caring flows from nurses to clients. People in distress or who are ill are anxious and fearful. When we are centered and balanced as nurses, we can share our sense of calmness in the face of crisis. Before entering a client's home or room, take a moment to center with a couple of deep, cleansing breaths and focus on what you are about to do with this person who is your client. When you are with the client, touch may be an appropriate intervention. For some people who are suffering or in crisis, a touch on the arm or holding his or her hand may be the most effective nursing intervention you will provide. It is important to remember that touch must always be appropriate and acceptable to the client.

Just as Native American tribes have rituals for cleansing the mind of negative thoughts and feelings that predispose to disease, we can help clients *modify unhealthy thinking* patterns. Negative thinking not only occurs in our brains, but also in our bodies; negative thoughts cause instantaneous chemical changes in every cell. Continuous cellular disruption may contribute to the onset of illness and disease. To counteract negative thinking, some people find it helpful to look at themselves in the mirror and say aloud three good things about themselves. People might say "I'm a good friend," "I'm an honest person," "I'm a caring person," "My hair looks beautiful today," "I am becoming healthier every day," and so on. The goal is to say different positive qualities about themselves each day. Keeping a journal about feelings immediately after the exercise and feelings throughout the day is helpful in evaluating the impact of positive statements on negative thinking.

Positive affirmations are another way to counteract negative thinking. In this nursing intervention you encourage people to make a list of positive things that are occurring in their lives or things that they would like to have occur. Affirmations are always stated as if they were a fact, even when they are still a dream. For example, if you have financial problems, instead of thinking "I'm never going to get ahead. My debts are just too big," you might make affirmations such as "I am financially secure," "I pay my bills easily," "Money comes in when I need it," "I am at ease about the subject of money." Affirmations can be made about work, school, relationships, feelings, commitments, future goals, and even pleasurable activities. Encourage clients to write a list of affirmations over a period of several days. People often record their affirmations and listen to them every day. Some people find that it makes a commute to work more pleasant. Other people find a time and place to say them aloud every day. Since people tend to live their lives according to their expectations, changing expectations from negative to positive can improve the level of wellness.

Although it might not be reasonable to find a stream of flowing water to take away angers, fears, sorrows, or troubles, you can teach people to *visualize* that process. Direct clients through the relaxation process and have them mentally walk into a stream or actually stand in a shower that is comfortable in terms of temperature and force of the flow. As they stand in the stream, have them visualize the water washing out all their physical, mental, emotional, or relational problems. Similar to the Indian art of healing, this nursing intervention may be beneficial for clients who feel weighted down with their problems or sorrows.

Gratitude is important in Native American culture. As a nurse, you can help others become more grateful for their life experiences. Many people find it extremely beneficial to keep a gratitude journal. At the close of every day, they write at least three things that happened during the day for which they are thankful. They may be thankful for a beautiful sunrise, a smile from a stranger, a hug from a child, an A on an exam, a wonderful dinner, an intimate moment with a partner, and so on. Focusing on gratitude is another way to become more in harmony with oneself and is thought to neutralize problems and negative thinking.

A number of substance abuse programs, both Native American and non-Native American, have added drumming groups to their programs. In addition, drumming is being studied in the treatment of soldiers with posttraumatic stress disorder. *Drumming* enhances hypnotic susceptibility, increases relaxation, improves meditation, and synchronizes brain wave patterns. It facilitates an outlet for rage and a way to regain self-control. Drumming groups may also enhance recovery by encouraging social support and social networks. As a nurse, you can encourage the study and practice of drumming groups in these types of programs (Bensimon, Amir, & Wolf, 2008; Weatherup, 2006).

Most people have *objects* that are significant to them. Although these objects are not medicine objects in the Native American tradition, they may bring with them a sense of comfort and perhaps protection. Encourage and support clients to have religious symbols or holy books around them if those items are important. Secular items can also be of great comfort, such as pictures of family and friends, get-well cards, poems, beloved books, and so on. Most of us may not have sweat lodges or sings as part of our healing practices, but many clients have a *community* of family or friends who may be sending their love and concern or praying for their healing. Actively support those activities that provide love and hope to counteract the fears and doubts that accompany illness.

Like Native Americans, nurse psychotherapists find the *circle* to be a beneficial design. Group therapy typically occurs with all the participants sitting in a circle, which contributes to the group's sense of oneness and connectedness. Circle arrangements foster cooperation rather than competition. It is often helpful to use a circle arrangement for nursing team conferences or interdisciplinary clinical conferences.

Integrated nursing practices related to herbs are covered in Chapter 7, those related to acupressure in Chapter 13, and those related to dreams in Chapter 19.

TRY THIS
Positive Thoughts

Often we endure such runs of negative thoughts that we are unaware of the process until we have been "beating ourselves up" for 10 to 15 minutes. To become more aware of this habitual process, tap your left finger on a firm surface for every negative thought. When your finger becomes quite sore, you will have another level of awareness of your negativity. Negative thoughts can be countered with positive ones. When you catch yourself thinking and feeling a negative thought, such as how fat your body is or how dumb you are, STOP. Now look for and substitute a positive thought or feeling in the place of the one you removed, such as how lovely your hair looks or how well you have succeeded at something. Now listen to yourself saying the positive phrase out loud. Continue in this way, adding other phrases and wishes for yourself.

USING RESEARCH TO HEAL

Gallagher, M. R., Gill, S., & Reifsnider, E. (2008). Child health promotion and protection among Mexican mothers. *Western Journal of Nursing Research*, 30: 588–604.

What Is This Study About?
Mexican children experience many health disparities for a variety of reasons. One plan for addressing the disparities is to increase the health promotion and protection behaviors used by Mexican-descent mothers in caring for their preschool children. The purpose of this study was to examine the health promotion and protection practices used by Mexican mothers in caring for preschool children.

How Was the Study Done?
An ethnographic approach using Spradley's development of research sequence was used in this study. Nine Mexican mothers (all born in Mexico) now living in San Antonio, Texas, responded to two to three interviews in their homes. The face-to-face taped interviews lasted from 45 to 90 minutes, and Spanish was the dialogue of choice. The first interview questions were "What kinds of things do you do to help your child be healthier?" "What kinds of things do you do to keep your child from getting sick?" and "What kinds of things do you do to keep your child from getting physically hurt?" The second interview questions focused on structural and contrast questions to gain a better understanding of

their children's health promotion and protection practices. Examples of questions were "What are the different kinds of foods you give your child to provide a good food intake?" and contrast questions such as "What is the difference between junk foods and nutritious foods?" The focus of the third interview was to confirm findings from the previous two interviews with the participants.

What Were the Results of the Study?

Upon in-depth analysis of the interviews, three main cultural themes emerged in promoting and protecting the health of their young children. The themes were body, mind, and soul as components of child health; *al cuidado* (taking care); and *al pendiente* (being mindful). These mothers incorporated these themes in their children's daily lives to *balance* the body, mind, and soul despite confronting economic and environmental challenges. The mothers felt that an imbalance in one or two of these themes would cause a disruption in the children's health. They believed the themes were linked and could not be separated for the welfare of their children.

What Additional Questions Might I Have?

Would the findings be similar for mothers of Mexican descent not born in Mexico? What are the most common traditions Mexican mothers use in attaining body, mind, and soul balance for their children's health?

How Can I Use This Study?

Nurses can use the findings of this study as a framework for teaching and implementing health promotion strategies with mothers of Mexican descent. For example, healthy snacks can be taught or demonstrated by incorporating how good nutrition affects the mind–body–soul for the health of the child. In addition, the cultural themes of al cuidado and al pendiente could be integrated in discussions of anticipatory guidance when teaching health promotion to mothers.

Source: Contributed by Dolores M. Huffman, RN, PhD, Associate Professor of Nursing, Purdue University Calumet.

References

Bad Hand, H. P. (2002). *Native American Healing*. Chicago: Keats Publishing.

Bear Heart. (1996). *The Wind Is My Mother*. New York: Berkeley Books.

Bensimon, M., Amir, D., & Wolf, Y. (2008). Drumming through trauma: Music therapy with post-traumatic soldiers. *The Arts in Psychotherapy*, 35: 34–48.

Buhner, S. H. (2006). *Sacred Plant Medicine: The Wisdom in Native American Herbalism*. Rochester, VT: Bear & Company.

Cohen, K. (2006). *Honoring the Medicine: The Essential Guide to Native American Healing*. New York: Ballantine Books.

Facts on Indian Health Disparities. (2006). Indian Health Service. info.ihs.gov/Files/DisparitiesFacts-Jan2006.pdf. Accessed July 21, 2008.

Forest, O. S. (2000). *Dreaming the Council Ways*. York Beach, MA: Samuel Weiser.

Garrett, J. T. (2003). *The Cherokee Herbal*. Rochester, VT: Bear & Company.

University of Texas. (2008). Curanderismo. In *Handbook of Texas Online*. www.tshaonline.org/handbook/online/articles/CC/sdcl.html. Accessed July 9, 2008.

Hunter, L., Logan, J., Barton, S., & Goulet, J. G. (2004). Linking aboriginal healing traditions to holistic nursing practice. *Journal of Holistic Nursing*, 22(3): 267–285.

Hunter, L. M., Logan, J., Goulet, J. G., & Barton, S. (2006). Aboriginal healing: Regaining balance and culture. *Journal of Transcultural Nursing*, 17(1): 13–22.

Johnson, S. (1994). *The Book of Elders*. San Francisco: HarperSanFrancisco.

Luna, E. (2003). Nurse-Curanderas. *Journal of Holistic Nursing*, 12(4): 326–342.

O'Brien, S. J. C. (2008). *Religion and Healing in Native America*. Westport, CT: Praeger Publishers.

Rutherford, L. (2008). *The View Through the Medicine Wheel: Shamanic Maps of How the Universe Works*. Ropley, Hants, UK: John Hunt Publishing.

Shimer, P. (2004). *Healing Secrets of the Native Americans*. New York: Black Dog & Leventhal Publishers.

Sobralske, M. (2006). Machismo sustains health and illness beliefs of Mexican American men. *Journal of the American Academy of Nurse Practitioners*, 18: 348–350.

Struthers, R., Eschiti, V. S., & Patchell, B. (2004). Traditional indigenous healing: Part 1. *Complementary Therapies in Nursing & Midwifery*, 10: 141–149.

Sun Bear, Mulligan, C., Nuffer, P., & Wabun. (1989). *Walk in Balance*. New York: Simon & Schuster.

Walsh, R. (2007). *The World of Shamanism*. Woodbury, MN: Llewellyn Publications.

Weatherup, K. (2006). *Practical Shamanism, A Guide for Walking in Both Worlds*. San Diego, CA: Hands Over Heart Publishing.

Resources

Association of American Indian Physicians
1225 Sovereign Row, Suite 103
Oklahoma City, OK 73108
405.946.7072
www.aaip.org

Dance of the Deer Foundation, Center for Shamanic Studies
P.O. Box 699
Soquel, CA 95073
831.475.9560
www.shamanism.com

Feathered Pipe Ranch Foundation
Box 1682
Helena, MT 59624
406.442.8196
www.featheredpipe.com

The School of Lost Borders
P.O. Box 796
Big Pine, CA 93513
530.305.4414
www.schooloflostborders.com

Singing with the Wheel (compact disc)
West Winds
P.O. Box 16729
Mobile, AL 36616

Botanical Healing

The Lord hath created medicines out of the earth:
and he that is wise will not abhor them.

ECCLESIASTICUS 38:4

7

Herbs and Nutritional Supplements

Physicians pour drugs, about which they know little, to cure diseases, about which they know less, into humans, about whom they know nothing.

VOLTAIRE

The Great Spirit is our father, but the earth is our mother. She nourishes us; that which we put into the ground, she returns to us, and healing plants she gives us likewise.

BIG THUNDER

Also known as *botanical medicine* or *phytotherapy* (*phyto* means "plant"), **herbal medicine** is used by 80 percent of the world's population. Herbs are also the most popular alternative therapy in the United States, with more than 750 herbs now on the market. It is estimated that Americans spend over $18.8 billion a year on herbal remedies and dietary supplements, while Australians spend AUS$200 million a year. For many conditions, herbs are the treatment of choice because they are milder and have fewer side effects than prescription drugs (Bardia, Nisly, Zimmerman, Gryzlak, & Wallace, 2007). Vitamins, minerals, diet supplements, and specialized diets are beyond the scope of this text. Entire books are devoted to each of those topics, to which the reader is referred.

BACKGROUND

Throughout history, almost all societies have used plants for therapeutic purposes. For example, the oldest surviving garlic prescription, carved into a clay tablet, dates from 3000 B.C. Over thousands of years, a medical pharmacopoeia developed in every culture, from Asia to the Americas, to Europe and Africa. Over an extensive period of time, Chinese herbalists documented the healing properties of more than 7,000 herbs and thousands of herbal combinations. St. John's wort has a 2,500-year history of safe and effective use and was prescribed as medicine by Hippocrates (460–377 B.C.) himself. Galen (A.D. 129–200) described 130 herbal antidotes and medicines, and Dioscorides (first century A.D.) wrote about the medicinal properties of 500 plants and described how to prepare 1,000 simple remedies. The ancient Egyptians used peppermint and spearmint to relax the digestive tract, while Chinese and Ayurvedic doctors used mint to treat colds, coughs, and fevers (Castleman, 2001).

When Europeans came to the Americas, they found that Native Americans had a vast pharmacopoeia of medicinal plants such as birch, blackberry, coneflower, ginseng, goldenseal, and ginger, handed down from generation to generation. Early Jesuit missionaries in Canada discovered American ginseng in the early 1700s and exported it to Asia, where it became a highly revered tonic. The Shakers (Church of the United Society of Believers), who were great friends of Native Americans, were the first to cultivate medicinal plants in mass quantities and became the first reputable pharmaceutical manufacturers in the United States. Until the Civil War disrupted their efforts, they sold 354 varieties of therapeutic herbs. During the early twentieth century, tincture of echinacea was highly valued for its antibiotic properties until synthetic antibiotics became available. Kava, used to calm the nervous system and decrease anxiety, was even sold during the 1920s in the Sears, Roebuck and Co. catalog. Many herbs used in ancient times are still in use today throughout the world. Herbal medicine has generally been more widely accepted outside the United States, where health care providers often combine it with conventional therapy (Castleman, 2001).

Researchers are intensifying their efforts to collect and screen more natural products for their medicinal properties. Gordon Cragg, chief of the National Cancer Institute's natural-products branch, states, "Nature produces chemicals that no chemist would ever dream of at the laboratory bench" (Hallowell, 1997, p. 19). A great variety of some of the most concentrated healing herbs is found in a wide band around the equator. Unfortunately, destruction of these natural plant habitats, especially tropical rain forests, is driving many species to extinction before they can be found and studied.

In the 1960s, the Food and Drug Administration (FDA) developed the current U.S. regulations regarding medications. At that time, herbal medicine had little popularity and thus was virtually ignored by the FDA. Herbs are viewed as dietary supplements and are controlled by the 1994 Dietary Supplement Health and Education Act. Under this act, dietary supplements cannot make specific medical claims as can prescription and over-the-counter (OTC) drugs. General statements such as "improves memory" or "promotes regularity" can be used as long as a disclaimer notes that the herb is not approved by the FDA and that the product is not intended to diagnose, treat, cure, or prevent any disease.

It is unlikely that most herbal medicines will ever win FDA approval since the process costs approximately $100 million per drug. Large pharmaceutical companies are willing to invest this fortune in new drugs that can be patented and sold at high profits. In contrast, granting exclusive rights or patents to most herbs, such as garlic or ginseng, is nearly impossible, which takes away the financial incentive to get them approved for medicinal use. The lack of profit, rather than the lack of efficacy of herbs, keeps drug companies from advocating change toward FDA approval of herbs.

Much of what is known about herbs comes from Germany, where an expert panel called Commission E, set up in 1978, has reviewed all available literature on 650 medicinal herbs, issuing recommendations for their use. The National Center for Complementary and Alternative Medicine is actively involved in researching healing herbs. In addition, the National Cancer Institute (NCI) is screening plants for compounds active against the AIDS virus and nine major types of cancer. Since 1986, the NCI has received samplings of thousands of plants from ethnobotanists throughout the world. Indigenous people have been testing and using healing plants for thousands of years, but only recently have Western researchers sought their knowledge.

CONCEPTS

Synergism

The active chemicals in herbs work *synergistically*; that is, the action of two or more substances achieves an effect of which each is individually incapable. Most herbal medicines rely on the complex interplay of many chemicals for their therapeutic action and many lose their activity when purified and isolated. For example, a number of antimicrobial compounds are found in tea tree oil, but studies indicate that no single compound in the oil accomplishes its remarkable germ-fighting ability; rather, the interaction of at least eight distinct chemicals in the oil seems to produce the effects. This complexity makes it nearly impossible for an infectious microbe to build up resistance to tea tree oil. One of the primary problems with conventional antibiotics is the ability of many microbes to develop resistance, thus rendering the drug useless. Antioxidant defenses also operate synergistically. For example, a number of carotenoids working together have higher anticancer properties than a single carotenoid. Thus beta-carotene supplements may not provide the same protection as eating fruits and vegetables rich in beta-carotene. Other substances in the plant may help the body to assimilate its benefits as well as buffer any side effects. Including the whole plant in the final product often ensures that some measure of the natural "checks and balances" will be retained (Castleman, 2001; Duke, 2002).

Various herbs and other substances may also work synergistically with one another. A rather dramatic example of this effect occurred during the testing of plant samples from the rain forest of Ecuador for chemicals that could be used to treat diabetes. The leaves from the plant were immersed in an alcohol extract and then a water extract. The debate among the researchers concerned whether to throw a live crab into the extract, just as native healers did. Some believed it might make a difference, while others believed the crab was simply ritualistic. Amazingly, the only extract that showed therapeutic effect was the one with the crab in it. It turns out that a component in a crab's shell is needed to extract the active chemical compound from the plant (Cray, 1997).

Phytonutrients

Phytonutrients are chemicals present in plants that make the plants biologically active and are responsible for giving plants their color, flavor, and natural disease resistance. Phytonutrients are products of photosynthesis or are substances that serve as defense mechanisms against attacks by insects and other predators. These active components of plants usually occur in groups that complement the protective and healing effects of each other. Descriptions of the most important phytonutrients and their uses are found in Table 7.1.

Antioxidants

Antioxidants are a group of vitamins, minerals, enzymes, and herbs that help protect the body from naturally occurring free radicals. As the body goes through its normal processes and oxygen is used to provide cellular fuel, some of the oxygen molecules lose one of their pair of electrons. When they do, the formerly stable oxygen molecules become dangerous **free radicals** that try to stabilize themselves by stealing another electron from stable molecules, thus damaging them and creating more free radicals. Because free radicals react so easily with other compounds, they can effect significant changes in the body. Many different factors can lead to the production of free radicals. *Internal sources*, in addition to oxygen consumption, include emotional stress and strenuous exercise. *External sources* include air pollution, cigarette smoke, factory and car exhaust, smog, pesticides, herbicides, food contaminants, chemotherapy, and radiation. All cause the overproduction of free radicals. Oxidative damage can be visualized when one bites into an apple, leaves it for a few minutes, and then notices that the exposed part becomes brown or oxidized. Humans, however, cannot "see" the damage being done by free radicals in the body. An excess of free radicals is, in

TABLE 7.1 Phytonutrients

Name	Properties	Use/Effects
Alkaloids	Group of nitrogen-containing compounds. Analgesic, local anesthetic, sedating, antispasmodic, hallucinatory; poisonous to varying degrees.	Affect both the nervous and circulatory systems. Most familiar are atropine, caffeine, cocaine, morphine, nicotine, and quinine.
Bitter principles	Group of chemicals that have an extremely bitter taste.	Through a reflex action via taste buds, stimulate appetite and flow of digestive juices, stimulate liver activity and flow of bile; some act as diuretics. Viewed as overall tonics.
Carbohydrates	Main energy source and structural support of plants.	In some herbs, such as coltsfoot and marshmallow, the cellulose combines with other chemicals to form mucilage, a gummy substance, which, when ingested by humans, soothes and protects irritated or inflamed internal tissue.
Carotenoids	Yellow, orange, or red pigments in photosynthetic plants; converted to vitamin A in liver.	Three most important to humans: Beta-carotene may aid in cancer prevention by neutralizing free radicals. Used in conjunction with topical sunscreens, better prevention of sunburn and skin damage. Lycopene may prevent prostate cancer and decrease risk of heart attacks. Lutein may be useful in prevention of macular degeneration, a leading cause of blindness in the elderly.
Essential oils	Vaporize when heated; combinations give plants their particular smell.	Garlic is an antiseptic, thyme is an expectorant, chamomile relieves gaseous distention and painful intestinal spasms.
Fatty oils	Mixture of triglycerides, glycerol, fatty acids.	Omega-3 fatty acids are used against cardiovascular disease and depression; improve cognition.

(continued)

TABLE 7.1 Phytonutrients (*Continued*)

Name	Properties	Use/Effects
Glycosides	Complex organic substances; some of the most potent herbal remedies and among the most toxic substances known.	Cardiac glycosides include foxglove and lily of the valley, which affect cardiac contractions; used to correct arrhythmias. Mustard glycosides are used externally and have antiseptic and analgesic effects. Cyanogenic glycosides release hydrogen cyanide when chewed or digested, resulting in antispasmodic, purgative, and sedative effects. Found in some nuts, vegetables, and the seeds of some fruits. Hydrogen cyanide, sometimes called prussic acid, is highly poisonous. Phenolic glycosides include salicylic derivatives found in willow and other plants and is the main ingredient in aspirin—antiseptic, analgesic, and anti-inflammatory effects. Coumarine glycosides strengthen capillary walls and act as an anticoagulant. Anthraquinone glycosides are used as laxatives. Flavonoid glycosides, known as bioflavonoids or flavonoids, improve circulation, stimulate bile production, lower cholesterol levels, and strengthen the liver.
Isoflavones	Compounds similar to human estrogen; found primarily in soy products.	May prevent hormone-related cancers; lower cholesterol, relieve menopausal symptoms, prevent osteoporosis by increasing bone density.
Tannins	Chemical substances with astringent and antiseptic properties.	Form a protective layer on the skin and mucous membranes and are useful in treatment of burns and local inflammation; used for eye and mouth infections.

part, responsible for the effects of aging and is implicated in cancer and a variety of chronic and degenerative conditions, including arthritis and heart disease (Atsumi & Tonosaki, 2007; Duke & Castleman, 2001).

Free radicals are normally kept under control through the production of enzymes—**antioxidants**—that act as free-radical scavengers to search out and neutralize dangerous free radicals. As people age, they produce fewer of these enzymes, and they may benefit from dietary antioxidants such as vitamin C, vitamin E, carotenoids, the mineral selenium, and the hormone melatonin. Herbs with antioxidant properties include bilberry, ginkgo, grape seed extract, green tea, and flavonoids. Fruits and vegetables are the primary sources for antioxidants, though they are also available in the form of supplements.

Plant-Derived Products

Herbal medicines were in use even before pharmaceutical companies came into existence. In many parts of the world, treating illness with herbs is still the only medicine available. Even though only a tiny fraction of plants have been studied for medicinal benefits, conventional physicians use plant-derived products regularly. Fifty percent of all prescription and over-the-counter drugs sold in the United States are derived from plants. Examples of herbal remedies that have been synthesized into modern drugs are reserpine from Indian snakeroot, digoxin from foxglove, quinine from Peruvian bark, aspirin from willow tree bark, morphine from opium poppy, cocaine from coca leaves, and atropine from deadly nightshade. Recently, researchers discovered taxol, found in Pacific yew bark, which is currently being used in the treatment of early and advanced breast cancer and ovarian tumors. Another recent advance is the drug vincristine, which has been isolated from the Madagascar periwinkle. Vincristine has been found to arrest cell division so dramatically that it is being used to treat acute leukemia and Hodgkin's disease (Bowden, 2008; O'Malley, Trimble, & Browning, 2005).

Safety

Not all plant life is beneficial. Most plant-related poisonings are due to accidental consumption of toxic ornamental plants such as jade, holly, poinsettia, schefflera, philodendron, and dieffenbachia rather than from herbs. Data compiled by the American Association of Poison Control indicate that medications such as analgesics, sedatives, antipsychotics, cold/cough preparations, and cardiovascular drugs are much more likely to cause adverse reactions and fatalities than are herbs (Bronstein et al., 2007).

The vast majority of herbal medicines presents no danger if taken appropriately. Some can, however, cause serious side effects if taken in excess or, for some, if taken over a prolonged period of time. For example, comfrey, a digestive remedy; coltsfoot, used to treat cough; and kava, used for anxiety, can cause liver damage if taken in large doses. Herbs can also interact with drugs, and caution should be used when combining herbs with prescription and OTC medications (see Table 7.2). Pregnant and lactating

TABLE 7.2 Herb Interactions

Herb/Supplement	May Interact with	Potential Effects
Black cohosh	Hormone replacement medications	May potentiate one another
Capsicum	Anticoagulants, aspirin	May prolong bleeding time
	Theophylline	Increases absorption, may cause toxicity
Echinacea	Immunosuppressants	Reduces effectiveness of immunosuppressants
	Antifungals; drugs known to elevate liver enzymes	May cause liver damage
Evening primrose oil	Phenothiazine medications, Wellbutrin	May increase risk of seizures
Feverfew	Anticoagulants, aspirin	May increase anticoagulant effects
Garlic	Anticoagulants, aspirin	May increase anticoagulant effects
	Hypoglycemics	May cause hypoglycemia
	Antihypertensives	May need increased dose of antihypertensive
	HIV medications	May increase or decrease effectiveness of medications
Ginger	Anticoagulants, aspirin	May increase anticoagulant effects
Ginkgo	Anticoagulants, aspirin	May increase anticoagulant effects
	Anticonvulsants	May decrease effectiveness of anticonvulsants
Ginseng	Oral contraceptives	Increases the potency of estrogen in oral contraceptives causing side effects such as weight gain, breast pain, and vaginal bleeding
	MAO inhibitors	May result in mania
	Caffeine	May cause irritability
	Glaucoma medications	May decrease effectiveness of glaucoma medications
Goldenseal	Anticoagulants, aspirin	Decreases effectiveness of anticoagulants
	Diuretics	Increases diuretic effect
	General anesthetics	May increase hypotensive effect of anesthetic
Licorice	Hypoglycemics	May interfere with regulation of blood sugar levels
	Lanoxin, Lasix, Hygroton, Lozol, Bumex	Licorice depletes potassium; may cause hypokalemia
	Thyroid replacement medication	May need higher doses of thyroid replacement

TABLE 7.2 *(Continued)*

Herb/Supplement	May Interact with	Potential Effects
	Oral contraceptives	May cause high blood pressure, fluid retention, hypokalemia
	Antihypertensives	Decreases effectiveness of antihypertensives
Ma huang	Most antihypertensives	May increase blood pressure and risk of cardiac arrhythmia
	Antidepressants	May increase blood pressure and risk of cardiac arrhythmia
	Decongestants	May increase blood pressure and risk of cardiac arrhythmia
	Lanoxin	Increases risk of cardiac arrhythmia
	Hypoglycemics	May interfere with regulation of blood sugar levels
Milk thistle	Oral contraceptives	Reduces effectiveness of oral contraceptives
Psyllium	Laxatives	Effects may be increased
St. John's wort	Oral contraceptives	Reduces effectiveness of oral contraceptives
	Tetracyclines, sulfa drugs, Feldane, Prilosec, Prevacid	Extreme photosensitivity may occur; increasing risk for severe sunburn
	Antidepressants	May potentiate one another, causing severe agitation, nausea, confusion, and possible cardiac problems
	Anticonvulsants	May decrease effectiveness of anticonvulsants
	Dioxin, immunosuppressants, protease inhibitors	May reduce effectiveness of these medications
	Theophylline	May decrease serum theophylline levels
	General anesthetics	May prolong effect of anesthesia
Saw palmetto	Proscar	May potentiate each other resulting in overdose
Valerian	Antianxiety medication, Benadryl, Vistaril, anticonvulsants	May increase sedative effects
	General anesthetics	Prolongs anesthesia
Vitamin A	Accutane for acne	Toxicity may occur, resulting in severe headaches, dry eyes and skin, hair loss, and possible liver damage
Vitamin B_6	Carbidopa, levodopa	May decrease effectiveness, resulting in breakthrough symptoms such as tremors

women should be cautioned not to take herbs internally except for mild herb teas. Any herbs that act as anticoagulants or those that potentiate anesthesia must be discontinued before surgery if at all possible (Lynch & Berry, 2007).

TREATMENT

Medicinal herbs are available at health food stores, herb shops, supermarkets, and pharmacies. They can be used as a preventive, a tonic, or a treatment. Herbs can be prepared and used in a number of ways. **Extracts** or **tinctures** are made by pressing herbs with a heavy press and soaking them in alcohol or water, which after evaporation yields a concentrated extract. Extracts are generally measured in drops and diluted in a small amount of water for ingestion. A preparation of the delicate parts of plants—that is, leaves, flowers, and seeds—is called an **infusion**, a process similar to making tea. Hot water is poured over the herb, steeped for 3 to 5 minutes, and strained before drinking. Honey or lemon may be added to taste. **Decoction** is the preparation of the more resilient parts of plants, such as the bark, roots, and berries. These parts of the herb are usually boiled for 10 to 20 minutes and strained before drinking. A *compress* is a cloth soaked in a warm or cool herbal solution and applied directly to an injured area. An herbal *poultice* is made by mixing powered herbs with enough hot water to make a thick paste that is then applied directly to the skin. Poultices are used to reduce swelling, relieve pain, decrease muscle spasms, draw out toxins from the body, increase circulation, and speed healing. Table 7.3 lists some of the more common herbs as well as their action, dosage, and side effects.

RESEARCH

Most herbal medicines have not been tested as thoroughly as prescription drugs in the United States, although the National Center for Complementary and Alternative Medicine funds many herbal research trials. South Africa has more than 20,000 plant species, several thousand of which are used by traditional healers. Research teams from the United States are teaming up with the South African Herbal Science and Medicine Institute to study the medicinal properties, safety, and effectiveness of several of these African plants. In contrast, many scientific studies have been conducted outside the United States on a variety of herbal remedies. Commission E in Germany has reviewed all available literature on 650 medicinal herbs and issued recommendations for their use. In the coming years, we are likely to learn more about which herbs are helpful and which are not, since research in the field of herbal medicine is on the rise worldwide.

In 1995, the American Herbal Pharmacopoeia was organized as an educational foundation to disseminate information regarding the pharmacology,

TABLE 7.3 Common Herbs

Name	Properties/Use	Form/Dose	Contraindications/Side Effects
Black cohosh	Menopause, dysmenorrheal, PMS	80–120 mg/day	Nausea, dizziness, decreased pulse rate, increased perspiration NOT to be used with hormone replacement therapy
Capsaicin	Tenderness and pain of osteoarthritis, fibromyalgia, periphera neuropathy, shingles	Topical cream	May be brief burning or stinging sensation with first use Wash hands after applying. Avoid touching eye
Chamomile	Anxiety, stomach distress or ulcers, mouth ulcers, infant colic, drug withdrawal	2–3 teaspoons in one cup of hot water Tincture: 1 teaspoon TID	NOT for those with extreme allergy to ragweed NOT for pregnant and lactating women
Chondroitin	Helps slow cartilage degradation in osteoarthritis	400 mg TID	Headache, indigestion NOT for pregnant and lactating women
Echinacea	Antiviral, antibiotic for colds and flu	400–600 mg for 5–14 days Peaks at 5 days	NOT for people with autoimmune disease NOT for pregnant and lactating women
Evening primrose oil	PMS, alcoholism, breast pain, eczema	1–4 g/day	Headache, nausea, skin rash NOT for pregnant and lactating women
Feverfew	Prevention of migraines, arthritis	50–200 mg/day	Chewing leaves can cause mouth sores and loss of taste NOT with prescription headache drugs NOT for pregnant and lactating women
Garlic	Antibiotic, antiviral, antifungal, anticoagulant. infection, hypertension, high blood lipid levels	1–5 cloves/day 1/2–1 teaspoon garlic juice Powder: 600–900 mg/day	Nausea; garlicky scent NOT for people with clotting disorders

(continued)

TABLE 7.3 Common Herbs (*Continued*)

Name	Properties/Use	Form/Dose	Contraindications/Side Effects
Ginger	Nausea and vomiting of various causes, hypertension, high cholesterol; enhances insulin, arthritis, myasthenia gravis	500–1000 mg/day Motion sickness: 1500 mg 30 minutes prior	People taking anticoagulants should use caution
Ginkgo	Attention and memory problems, headaches, tinnitus, intermittent claudication, erectile problems, macular degeneration	80–120 mg/day	Mild gastrointestinal (GI) upset, heart palpitations, dizziness, increases bleeding
Ginseng	Mood swings, improved physical performance, decreases blood glucose, eases cocaine withdrawal	250–500 mg/day	Nervousness, insomnia, euphoria NOT for use when acutely ill with cold or flu NOT for people with hypoglycemia
Glucosamine	Improves pain and movement in osteoarthritis, TMJ discomfort	1000–1500 mg/day	People taking diuretics may need higher doses of glucosamine; increases blood glucose levels; mild GI problems
Goldenseal	Antibiotic, antiseptic, anti-inflammatory for wound healing, colds and flu. Hypertension, uterine bleeding, enhances insulin	465 mg BID or TID for maximum of 3 weeks	Only for short-term use; long-term use may irritate or inflame mucosa NOT during pregnancy—may cause premature uterine contractions
Green tea	Antioxidant, protects against cancer, lowers cholesterol, helps regulate blood sugar and insulin levels; stroke prevention, used in Parkinson's disease	3–4 cups/day	People with anxiety disorder or irregular heartbeat should limit use to no more than 2 cups daily NOT to be used in large quantities during pregnancy
Licorice	Bronchitis, cough, stomach pain, Topically—tendinitis, bursitis, eczema, psoriasis, canker sores	200 mg/day	Increases blood glucose levels. Large doses: hypertension, edema, headache

TABLE 7.3 (Continued)

Name	Properties/Use	Form/Dose	Contraindications/Side Effects
Milk thistle	Antioxidant for liver disorders, psoriasis	420–840 mg/day	May trigger menstruation
Red clover	Isoflavins for menopause, osteoporosis	100–430 mg/day	Breast tenderness, menstrual changes, weight gain NOT for pregnant and lactating women NOT for people with estrogen-responsive tumors
St. John's wort	Mild to moderate depression	240–1800 mg/day Minimum 4–8 weeks	Photosensitivity NOT for use with other antidepressants NOT for children NOT for pregnant and lactating women
SAMe	Analgesic, anti-inflammatory, antidepressant	400–1200 mg/day	Mild GI upset; NOT for people with bipolar disorder NOT to be used with other antidepressants
Saw palmetto	Urinary antiseptic; benign prostatic hyperplasia	640 mg/day	Constipation, diarrhea, headache, urine retention NOT for pregnant and lactating women
Selenium	Antioxidant especially when combined with vitamin E; may prevent some type of tumors; aids in production of antibodies, protects liver	50–140 mcg/day	Metallic taste in mouth, garlicky breath; excessively high levels may lead to liver and kidney impairment
Tea tree oil	Antifungal, antiseptic; acne, minor burns and cuts, athlete's foot, nail infections, herpes, douche for yeast infections	Full strength	Topical use only; do not ingest
Valerian	Insomnia, muscle pain, menstrual and intestinal cramps, benzodiazepine withdrawal	400–900 mg/day	Excitability, uneasiness NOT to be used with alcohol or Antabuse

actions, indications, dosages, side effects, contraindications, drug interactions, and toxicology of at least 300 herbs. The goal is for health care providers in the United States to integrate herbal medicines into treatment plans as their contemporaries have done in other countries.

A small sampling of studies indicate:

- Seven studies met the search criteria for the use of omega-3 fatty acid supplementation in lessening the symptoms of bipolar disorder. Four of the studies using a combination of DHA and EPA demonstrated a statistically significant improvement in symptoms (Turnbull, Cullen-Drill, & Smaldone, 2008).
- A species of South African geranium used in Zulu medicine improves symptoms of respiratory infection (Patrick & Hickner, 2008).
- A double blind, randomized, placebo-controlled study using sugar cane policosanol found that the herb did not lower lipids in persons who had high cholesterol and were resistant to diet changes (Francini-Pesenti, Brocadello, Beltramolli, Nardi, & Caregaro, 2008).
- Hawthorn extract has been studied in 14 randomized, controlled trials. A Cochrane review found that this herb improved cardiac workload, increased exercise tolerance, and reduced shortness of breath and fatigue (Cochrane Library, 2008).
- Saw palmetto is often suggested for men with lower urinary tract symptoms. A randomized clinical, placebo-controlled study followed 225 men taking either 160 mg of saw palmetto or a placebo twice daily for 1 year. Neither group experienced any clinically important adverse effects (Avins et al., 2008).
- Ginkgo has been studied for a variety of conditions. It shows promise for slowing cognitive decline and memory improvement (NCCAM, 2008a).
- It appears that echinacea does not prevent colds and study results are mixed regarding the helpfulness of echinacea in the treatment of upper respiratory infections (NCCAM, 2008b).
- Artichoke leaf extract lowered cholesterol levels in otherwise healthy persons with moderately high serum cholesterol in a randomized double-blind placebo-controlled trial (Bundy, Walker, Middleton, Wallis, & Simpson, 2008).
- A number of studies have found that Saint John's wort and SAMe are effective antidepressants for those with mild to moderate depression. Both products have the potential to induce a manic episode (Andreescu, Mulsant, & Emanuel, 2008; Rahimi, Nikfar, & Abdollahi, 2009; Sarris, Kavanagh, Deed, & Bone, 2009). Although it has been reported that St. John's wort interferes with oral contraceptives, one recent study found there was no interaction with low-dose oral contraceptives (Will-Shahab, Bauer, Kunter, Roots, & Brattstrom, 2009).
- Ginger is effective in treating motion sickness, pregnancy-induced nausea and vomiting, and postoperative nausea and vomiting (White, 2007).

- An herbal mixture, WTTCGE, shortened the length of symptoms for outbreaks of genital herpes with individuals who had recurrent herpes outbreaks for more than 1 year (Hijikata, Yamada, & Yasuhara, 2007).

INTEGRATED NURSING PRACTICE

Because herbs are marketed as "natural" or promoted as foods, consumers may assume incorrectly that herbs are safe and without side effects. It is important to remember that natural remedies be approached with respect. They work because they have strong pharmacological activity. It is important to teach people that although herbs are generally much safer than prescription drugs, if abused or overused they can cause harm.

Although herbs can be quite effective, it is important to caution people about becoming fanatical. If they have a life-threatening illness such as asthma or if they experience chest pain or if they notice more benign symptoms that persist for longer than a few days, they should seek medical attention. While it may be helpful to take echinacea if they feel a cold coming on, any serious ailment should be diagnosed by a health care practitioner before undertaking an herbal cure. Self-diagnosis and self-care are by nature subject to limits. Conventional medicine is best used in crisis situations, and herbs are best used in noncrisis situations. Professionals can save consumers from treating something that does not exist or failing to treat something that does. Further, health practitioners can help individuals evaluate the extent of their progress on the herbal regimen. Consultation is especially important if people are taking other medications; while some herbs can work with prescription drugs, others may not. Some herbs potentiate the effects of drugs, so people may need a lower dose of their regular medication. Suddenly stopping a prescription can be hazardous to one's health. Pregnant and lactating women should always consult their primary care practitioner before taking any herbal medicines.

Nurses must be open to exploring and discussing their clients' use of and questions about herbal medicine. This clinical screening allows evaluation of herbal intake against known and potential adverse interactions with prescription and OTC medications.

As a nurse, you need to educate consumers about potential actions and interactions of herbal remedies. People cannot expect to take an herb for a few days to undo 10 years of poor health habits nor replace a healthy diet with herbal supplements. If people eat a healthy, varied diet that is high in fresh foods, especially fruits, vegetables, and whole grains, they do not need to take other supplements unless they have special needs (Weil, 1998).

Sometimes walking into a health food store or pharmacy is highly confusing. Many people are overwhelmed by the wide assortment of products and brands. As a nurse, you can teach consumers the following basic guidelines in selecting herbal medicines:

- Store clerks are not experts. They do not have an adequate scientific background to counsel people.

- Go with a name brand. Since the industry is unregulated, it is best to choose products made by large, reputable companies that have been in business for a long time. Many excellent products are produced in Germany and France, where they must meet strict production standards.
- Check the label. Look for the word *standardized*, which tells you that the product consistently contains a certain percentage of a specific chemical.
- Check to see if the claims are reasonable. Be wary of promises of instant cures for complicated disorders. If something sounds too good to be true, it probably is.
- Consider the product's form. A liquid, powder, or solid extract is generally best. Bulk herbs can lose their potency quickly. Many herbal tinctures are 50 percent grain alcohol, which may be a problem for people with a history of alcohol abuse or for those who take drugs that can interact with alcohol.
- Be wary of ultra-combination products. If the product has more than six ingredients, it probably contains a small amount of each. The fact that herbs are combined does not make the product necessarily better. If you need ginkgo to boost your memory, it is better to get it full strength than to get a product diluted with ginseng, garlic, and other herbs.
- Take the right dose. Do not take higher doses than the label recommends. Exceeding the recommended dose can lead to toxicity. Most herbal remedies are not to be given to children under the age of 1 unless directed by an experienced practitioner. Children ages 1 to 6 are typically given one-third the adult dose, while children ages 6 to 12 receive one-half the adult dose. People over 65 years may need to reduce the dosage also.
- Watch for side effects. If you have any unusual symptoms, such as allergies, rashes, heart palpitations, or headaches, stop taking the herb immediately and see a health care practitioner.
- Give it time to work. Evaluate how the product makes you feel. After 30 days, ask yourself whether the product has made a difference in your health. If you are not sure, stop taking the herb to gauge the difference.
- Inform your primary health care practitioner about the herbal remedies you are taking.
- If you plan on regularly using herbal remedies, invest in a good herbal reference guide to ensure your access to proper information or consult with the one of the organizations in the resource list. The U.S. Department of Agriculture provides free access to 80,000 records on herb taxonomy and use of herbs worldwide, developed by Dr. James A. Duke.

As a nurse, it is also important that you warn consumers about remedies that can be risky. Chaparral, sold as teas and pills to fight cancer and "purify blood," has been linked to serious liver damage. Dieter's teas, containing such

TRY THIS
Herbal Remedies

Peppermint Tea

Used to soothe an upset stomach, aid digestion, relieve menstrual cramps, soothe sore throats, improve alertness.

How to

Combine 1 to 2 teaspoons of dried peppermint leaf to 8 ounces of water. Steep 3 to 5 minutes. Strain and drink tea.

Chamomile

An excellent home remedy for indigestion, heartburn, and infant colic. It also soothes skin and has mild relaxant and sedative properties.

How to

For an infusion, use 2–3 heaping teaspoons of dried or 1/3 cup of fresh flowers per cup of boiling water. Steep 10–20 minutes. Strain and drink up to 3 cups a day. Diluted infusions may be given to infants for colic.

For a relaxing herbal bath, fill a cloth bag with a few handfuls of dried or fresh flowers and let the water run over it.

For allergic skin rashes, tightly pack a jar of flowerheads, cover with olive oil. Cover and set in a sunny place for 3 weeks. Strain and apply to rashes.

Comfrey

External use only. Promotes the growth of new cells and has a mild anti-inflammatory action. Used in wound and burn treatment.

How to

Mix powdered root with water to make a paste. Apply to injured area and cover with clean bandage. Change daily.

Ginger

Decreases nausea, boosts the immune system, lowers blood pressure.

How to

Use 2 teaspoons of powdered or grated root per cup of boiling water. Steep 20 minutes, strain, add juice from half a lemon and honey to taste. Drink hot up to 3 cups a day. Dilute ginger infusion to treat infant colic. If you buy whole root, refrigerate it.

(continued)

Mint

Relaxes the digestive tract; used to treat colds, coughs, and fevers.

How to

For an infusion, use 1 teaspoon of fresh herb or 2 teaspoons of dried leaves per cup of boiling water. Steep 10 minutes, strain, and drink up to 3 cups a day. Peppermint has a sharper taste than spearmint and feels cooler in the mouth.

For a relaxing herbal bath, fill a cloth bag with a few handfuls of dried or fresh leaves and let the water run over it.

Rosemary

Stimulates circulation and relaxes tired and sore muscles.

How to

For tired, sore feet, make a footbath by adding 10 drops of essential oil to a basin of hot water large enough to hold both feet. Stir the oil into the water with your hand.

---

ingredients as senna, aloe, rhubarb root, buckthorn, cascara, and castor oil, act as laxatives that, when consumed in excessive amounts, can disrupt potassium levels and contribute to cardiac arrhythmias. Ephedra, also called ma huang, is an herb used most often for asthma. It is a cardiac and nervous system stimulant containing ephedrine, which can cause anxiety, psychotic episodes, hypertension, stroke, tachycardia, arrhythmias, and cardiac arrest. Mixing ephedra with caffeine or other substances, as the OTC energy-boosting products do, can increase its dangers. Ephedra should not be combined with theophylline, thyroid hormone, tricyclic antidepressants, methylphenidate, or any other drugs that can cause tachycardia or hypertension. Several states have banned supplements containing ephedrine because of the dangers (Stargrove, Treasure, & McKee, 2007).

The American public is demanding more information about herbal remedies. In the best of all worlds, consumers would have an educated professional—a nurse, a pharmacist, or a doctor—to help guide them through the process of using herbal remedies. That is the situation in Germany, where health care practitioners and pharmacists must be knowledgeable about natural remedies, their approved uses, their potential side effects, and how they should be prescribed. It has not been true in the United States but is sure to change in the near future. Schools of nursing and schools of medicine are including courses on alternative medicine in their curriculum. Pharmacy schools now require their students to take a course in herbal therapy.

As nurse-author Carolyn Kresse Murray (1996) has said, "Part of patient advocacy is making sure you help your patient with all his [her] therapies. Equipping yourself with knowledge about herbal therapies is another way to keep him [her] from harm" (p. 59).

USING RESEARCH TO HEAL

Archer, E. L., & Boyle, D. K. (2008). Herb and supplement use among the retail population of an independent urban herb store. *Journal of Holistic Nursing*, 26(1): 27–35.

What Is This Study About?

The increased use of herbal medicines by Americans is well documented. However, less well-known is the number of users who specifically inform their health care provider of their use of herbs and supplements. Therefore, the purpose of this study was to identify the demographics, beliefs, concurrent pharmaceutical use with herbs and supplements and reporting of use to health care providers by patrons at a herbal specialty retail store.

How Was the Study Done?

This descriptive pilot study used a researcher-developed survey tool to ask customers (N = 35) of an independent, specialty herb store located in the Midwest to anonymously describe their use of herbs and supplements. In addition, participants were requested to name their primary sources of information about herbs and supplements, if they viewed the use of herbs and supplements as "medications," types of insurance and care providers among this group and "reporting practices" of herb, supplements, and pharmaceuticals to their health care provider and herb store staff.

What Were the Results of the Study?

The typical study participant demographics were described as White, female, between 40 to 60 years of age, and highly educated with the majority attaining a bachelor's degree or beyond. Inconsistent with other published studies was that 25.7% of those surveyed were 18 to 28 years old. Ninety-one percent of participants reported the regular use of herbs and supplements for health and wellness while 5.7% indicated they used herbs and supplements only for illness. Thirty-seven percent identified the intake of additional pharmaceuticals on a regular basis. The use of over-the counter-drugs was reported by 63% and another 22% denied the use of over-the counter-drugs. The majority of respondents indicated that the retail staff was their primary source of information about herbs and supplements while the media (including the Internet) was identified as a source of information for 29%. Only 2% acknowledged receiving the majority of their information about herbs and supplements from their doctor, nurse, or pharmacist. The majority (65%) indicated they considered herbs and supplements as medications. Seventy-two percent of those with a "non-traditional" provider considered herbs medications while only 37% of those under the care of a MD or DO considered herbs and supplements medications. The majority of respondents (57%) indicated they were privately insured, 8% reporting government aid for health care benefits and 34% were not insured. The majority of participants (54%) also reported using Western traditional health care for their health problems. Thirty-seven percent identified the consistent reporting of herb and supplement use to all of their health care providers but only 28% consistently reported use specifically to their MD or DO. For participants using a nontraditional care provider, 37% always told of herb and supplement usage.

(continued)

What Additional Questions Might I Have?

Would the results have been significantly different with a larger number, less educated or more culturally diverse study participants? Would the study results be significantly different in various geographic locations within the United States?

How Can I Use This Study?

Nurses need to remain cognizant of the possible use of herbs and supplements by all patients regardless of their age, race, and socioeconomic status. Nurses need to provide an environment that allows individuals to feel comfortable in reporting the use of herbs and supplements and avoid a "don't ask, don't tell" atmosphere. In addition, nurses need to be knowledgeable concerning herb/supplements–pharmaceuticals interaction and provide education to patients about possible reactions that may compromise one's health.

Source: Contributed by Dolores M. Huffman, RN, PhD, Associate Professor of Nursing, Purdue University Calumet.

References

Andreescu, C., Mulsant, B. H., & Emanuel, J. E. (2008). Complementary and alternative medicine in the treatment of bipolar disorder—A review of the evidence. *Affective Disorders*, 110(1–2): 16–26.

Atsumi, T., & Tonosaki, K. (2007). Smelling lavender and rosemary increases free radical scavenging activity and decreases cortisol level in saliva. *Psychiatry Research*, 150(1): 89–96.

Avins, A. L., Bent, S., Staccone, S., Badua, E., Padula, A., Goldberg, H., et al. (2008). A detailed safety assessment of a saw palmetto extract. *Complementary Therapies in Medicine*, 16: 147–154.

Bardia, A., Nisly, N. L., Zimmerman, M. B., Gryzlak, B. M., & Wallace, R. B. (2007). Use of herbs among adults based on evidence-based indications: Findings from the National Health Interview Survey. *Mayo Clinic Proceedings*, 82(5): 561–566.

Bowden, J. (2008). *The Most Effective Natural Cures on Earth*. Beverly, MA: Fair Winds Press.

Bronstein, A. C., Spyker, D. A., Cantilena, L. R., Green, J., Rumack, B. H., & Heard, S. E. (2007). 2006 annual report of the American Association of Poison Control Centers' national poison data system (NPDS). *Clinical Toxicology*, 45(8): 815–917. http://dx.doi.org/10.1080/15563650701754763. Accessed July 28, 2008.

Bundy, R., Walker, A. F., Middleton, R. W., Wallis, C., & Simpson, H. C. (2008). Artichoke leaf extract (Cynara scolymus) reduces plasma cholesterol in otherwise healthy hypercholesterolemic adults. *Phytomedicine*, 15(9): 668–675.

Castleman, M. (2001). *The New Healing Herbs*. Emmaus, PA: Rodale Press.

Cochrane Library. (2008). Issue 1: CD005312.

Cray, D. (1997). Money that grows on trees. *Time*, Fall special issue, 150(19): 21.

Duke, J. A. (2002). *The Green Pharmacy Herbal Handbook*. New York: St. Martin's Press.

Duke, J. A., & Castleman, M. (2001). *The Green Pharmacy Anti-Aging Prescriptions*. Emmaus, PA: Rodale.

Francini-Pesenti, F., Brocadello, F., Beltramolli, D., Nardi, M., & Caregaro, L. (2008). Sugar cane policosanol failed to lower plasma cholesterol in primitive, diet-resistant hypercholesterolaemia. *Complementary Therapies in Medicine*, 16: 61–65.

Hallowell, C. (1997). The plant hunter. *Time*, Fall special issue, 150(19): 17–22.

Hijikata, Y., Yamada, S., & Yasuhara, A. (2007). Herbal mixtures containing the mushroom *ganoderma lucidum* improve recovery time in patients with herpes genitalis and labialis. *The Journal of Alternative and Complementary Medicine*, 13(9): 985–987.

Lynch, N., & Berry, D. (2007). Differences in perceived risks and benefits of herbal, over-the-counter conventional, and prescribed conventional medicines, and the implications of this for the safe and effective use of herbal products. *Complementary Therapies in Medicine*, 15: 84–91.

Murray, C. K. (1996). *Walking the Spiritual Walk*. Virginia Beach, VA: A.R.E. Press.

NCCAM. (2008a). Echinacea. http://nccam.nih.gov/health/Echinacea. Accessed July 26, 2008.

NCCAM. (2008b). Ginkgo. http://nccam.nih.gov/health/ginkgo. Accessed July 26, 2008.

O'Malley, P., Trimble, N., & Browning, M. (2005). Are herbal therapies worth the risks? *Hoslistic Nursing Practice*, 19(1): 44–47.

Patrick, G., & Hickner, J. (2008). This obscure herb works for the common cold. *The Journal of Family Practice*, 57(3): 157–161.

Rahimi, R., Nikfar, S., & Abdollahi, M. (2009). Efficacy and tolerability of hypericum perforatum in major depressive disorder in comparison with selective serotonin reuptake inhibitors: A meta-analysis. *Progress in Neuro-Psychopharmacology & Biological Psychiatry*, 33: 118–127.

Sarris, J., Kavanagh, D. J., Deed, G., & Bone, K. M. (2009). St. John's wort and Kava in treating major depressive disorder with comorbid anxiety: A randomized double-blind placebo-controlled pilot trial. *Human Psychopharmacology*, 24: 41–48.

Stargrove, M. B., Treasure, J., & McKee, D. L. (2007). *Herb, Nutrient, and Drug Interactions: Clinical Implications and Therapeutic Strategies*. St. Louis, MO: Mosby.

Turnbull, T., Cullen-Drill, M., & Smaldone, A. (2008). Efficacy of omega-3 fatty acid supplementation on improvement of bipolar symptoms: A systematic review. *Archives of Psychiatric Nursing*, 22(5): 305–311.

Weil, A. (1998, January–February). Ask the experts. *Natural Health*, pp. 24–28.

White, B. (2007). Ginger: An overview. *American Family Physician*, 75(1): 1689–1691.

Will-Shahab, L., Bauer, S., Kunter, U., Roots, I., & Brattstrom, A. (2009). St. John's wort extract (Ze 117) does not alter the pharmacokinetics of a low-dose oral contraceptive. *European Journal of Clinical Pharmacology*, 65: 287–294.

Resources

American Botanical Council
P.O. Box 144345
Austin, TX 78714-4345
512.926.4900
http://abc.herbalgram.org

American Herbalists Guild
141 Nob Hill Rd.
Cheshire, CT 06410
203.272.6731
www.americanherbalistsguild.com

American Herbal Pharmacopoeia
P.O. Box 66809
Scotts Valley, CA 95067
831.461.6318
http://herbal-ahp.org

British Herbal Medicine Association
Sun House, 26 Church St.
Strand Cloucestershire GL5 1JL, UK
44.(0)20.8398.1036
www.bhma.info

Herb Research Foundation
4140 15th St.
Boulder, CO 80304
800.748.2617
www.herbs.org

NAPRALERT (NAtural PRoducts
ALERT)
College of Pharmacy
University of Illinois at Chicago
833 South Wood St.
Chicago, IL 60612
312.996.9035
www.napralert.org

Ontario Herbalists Association
P.O. Box 123, Station D
Etobicoke, ON, Canada M9A 4X2
877.642.4372
www.herbalists.on.ca

U.S. Food and Drug Administration
Public Health Service
5600 Fishers Lane
Rockville, MD 20857-0001
888.463.6332
www.fda.gov

Wise Woman Apprentice Program
P.O. Box 64
Woodstock, NY 12498
845.246.8081
www.susunweed.com

8

Aromatherapy

Smell is a potent wizard that transports us across thousands of miles and all the years we have lived.

HELEN KELLER

Those who call it quackery assume they know how the universe works, and that is a dangerous assumption.

DAVID E. HOLLOWAY

Aromatherapy is the therapeutic use of essential oils of plants to heal the body, mind, and spirit. It is an offshoot of herbal medicine with the basis of action the same as that of modern pharmacology. The chemicals found in the essential oils are absorbed into the body, resulting in physiological or psychological benefit. Aromatherapy is used to treat symptoms and as such has neither a theory of health and illness nor a system of diagnosis.

Scientists have long known that certain scents have the power to evoke strong physical and emotional reactions but rarely has that knowledge been used in conventional medicine. Healthy humans can smell as many as 10,000 different odors, ranging from the deep fragrance of jasmine to the putrid stench of sewage. Most people, however, do not realize how much the sense of smell affects their daily lives.

Aromatherapy has been forgotten and ignored for many years but is now one of the fastest growing alternative therapies in Europe and the United States. The term *aromatherapy* has become more than a buzzword since the mid-1980s. In the United States, it is now a generic term in the public domain and, as such, cannot be trademarked by an individual or business.

Essential oils come from all over the world—lavender from France, sandalwood and jasmine from India, rose from Turkey and Bulgaria, geranium from the island of Reunion, eucalyptus and tea tree from Australia, and mint from the United States. Today, only 3 percent of essential oils are used in therapy; the remaining 97 percent are used in the perfume and cosmetic industry. With increased popularity, aromatherapy has become a billion-dollar industry.

BACKGROUND

Almost all ancient cultures recognized the value of aromatic plants in maintaining health. Ancient Egyptians used scented oils daily to soften and protect their skin from the harsh, dry climate. They created various fragrances for personal benefit as well as for use in rituals and ceremonies. Fragrances were considered a part of the personal purification necessary to reach a realm of higher spirituality. Oils were dispersed into the air to purify the environment and provide protection from evil spirits. Egyptians were the first to perfect embalming with the use of aromatic plants and oils (Smith & Kyle, 2008).

Priests and physicians used oils thousands of years before the time of Christ. The Ebers Papyrus, discovered in 1817, dates back to 1500 B.C. and mentions more than 800 different formulas of herbal prescriptions and remedies. The Romans diffused oils in their temples and political buildings and bathed in hot tubs scented with oils. Ancient Arabian people studied the chemistry of plants and developed the process of distillation for extraction of essential oils. Throughout Asia perfumes were prized for both medicinal and cosmetic properties. Hundreds of references are made to oils in the Bible such as frankincense, myrrh, and cinnamon. Many were used as protection against disease and for anointing and healing the sick (Cline et al., 2008). Hippocrates, the father of Western medicine, reportedly said, "The way to health is to have an aromatic bath and scented massage every day" (Thomas, 2002, p. 10).

In the twelfth century, trade routes from the Middle East introduced spices, herbs, and exotic scents to Europe, leading to the compilation of many books on therapeutic plant remedies. In the Americas, shamans also used herbs and aromatics in the bathing of patients to transform their energy field. Smoke from plants was often blown over patients as part of healing ceremonies (Schiller & Schiller, 2008).

Although oils were used with great effectiveness in ancient times, they were largely forgotten by the Western world until resurrected in the twentieth century by a French cosmetic chemist, Maurice-Rene Cattefosse. While working in his laboratory in 1920, he had an accident that resulted in a third-degree burn of his hand and forearm. He plunged his arm into a vat of lavender oil, thinking that it was water. To his surprise, the burning stopped within a few moments. With the continual application of lavender oil over the next few weeks, the burn healed completely without a trace of a scar. This incident was the beginning of Cattefosse's fascination with the therapeutic properties of essential oils. He carried out experiments using oils to cure burns, treat wounds, and prevent gangrene and in 1937 coined the term *aromatherapie* (Schiller & Schiller, 2008).

PREPARATION

Since the 1980s, numerous schools of massage and aromatherapy have opened in Britain, France, and Japan. Training in aromatherapy has grown, and courses in it are part of the nursing degree program in some nursing colleges and universities. Aromatherapists practice in a number of settings, including private practices, general medical clinics, and hospitals.

Some people in the United States, after a weekend course, call themselves "aromatherapists." They may know little about plant chemistry and the specific ways in which the oils need to be formulated. Their self-proclaimed title is fine if they use oils only for fragrance and perfume. Using oil formulas for a specific therapeutic action is inappropriate, however, for individuals with this limited knowledge. Jane Buckle, PhD, RN (www.rjbuckle.com) offers a 250 CEU, hands-on clinical aromatherapy program that is only available to licensed health professionals. Those who successfully complete the program are called Certified Clinical Aromatherapy Practitioners (CCAPs). Valerie Cooksley, RN, OCN, FAAIM; and Loraine Kyle, MS, RN, CS, CMT, who founded the Integrative Institute of Aromatherapy, offer a 325 CEU certificate program.

Both these programs have been developed in conjunction with and approved by the American Holistic Nurses Association. In addition, the National Association for Holistic Aromatherapy has established certification guidelines and Standards of Training Levels.

CONCEPTS

Essential Oils

Essential oils are volatile liquids that are distilled or cold pressed from plants. Although chemically they are oils and as such do not mix with water, the term *oil* is somewhat misleading, since they feel like water rather than oil. Varying amounts of essential oil can be extracted from a particular plant, which influences the price of the oil. For example, one ounce of jasmine may cost $150 while the same amount of tea tree oil may cost only a few dollars. The orange tree is a good example of oils extracted from various parts. Neroli oil is from the orange tree blossoms, orange oil from the fruit itself, and petitgrain oil from the leaves of the tree. Other examples are:

Leaves: eucalyptus, peppermint, petitgrain

Flowers: lavender, rose

Blossoms: neroli

Fruits: lemon, mandarin, orange

Grasses: lemongrass

Wood: camphor, sandalwood

Barks: cinnamon

Gum: frankincense

Bulbs: garlic, onion

Dried flower buds: clove

Essential oils are stored in tiny pockets between plant cell walls. As the plant releases the oil, it circulates through the plant and sends messages that help it function efficiently. Oils activate and regulate such activities as cellular metabolism, photosynthesis, and cellular respiration. They may also trigger immune responses to assist in coping with stressful changes in the environment and climate. Some oils protect the plant from predators, especially microorganisms, and in so doing are essentially antibacterial, antiviral, and antifungal. Some oils protect the plant by repelling harmful insects, while others attract insects or animals that are useful for propagation (Clark, 2002).

Plant oils are highly concentrated, and it is important to respect their power. One drop of oil is the medical equivalent of one ounce of the parent plant material used in herbal medicine. Essential oils are chemically diverse and may contain a mixture of more than 100 organic compounds, including esters, alcohols, aldehydes, ketones, phenols, acids, and so on. Each oil may contain more of some compounds than others, which gives the oil its particular therapeutic use. Table 8.1 lists some of the major chemical components and their therapeutic effects.

Hydrosols

Hydrosols, sometimes called plant waters, are extracted from plants during the process of steam distillation. In addition to the essential oil, a condensate water is produced that contains all the components of the plant. In essence, it is equivalent to a homeopathic version of essential oils and is diluted in the same manner (see Chapter 9 for information on dilution). The use of hydrosols in aromatherapy is quite new but growing since they are gentle, safe, and highly effective in extremely low dilutions (Boyraz & Ozcan, 2005).

How Essential Oils Work

The sense of smell is an important part of aromatherapy. Inside the human nose is a small cavity called the *vomero nasal organ* (VMO), which is lined with a cell type that is unlike any other cell in the human body. The VMO is far less prominent in people than in animals, who depend more heavily on smell for guidance. Pheromones are chemical substances produced by one animal that cause a specific reaction in another, usually of the same species, through smell. The VMO appears to specialize in detecting pheromones without people's conscious awareness. In other words, people do not "smell" pheromones in the same way they smell freshly baked apple pies or essential oils. The

TABLE 8.1 Chemical Compounds of Essential Oils and Their Therapeutic Actions

Chemical Compound	Therapeutic Action	Examples of Oils
Hydrocarbons Terpenes	Antiseptic, bactericidal, antiviral. May be expectorant, decongestant, stimulant.	Bay, verbena, pine, juniper, tea tree
Oxygenated hydrocarbons Alcohols	Antiviral, bactericidal, stimulates immune system. Non–skin irritating. Generally safe for children and elderly.	Rose, geranium, citronella, rosewood, coriander, eucalyptus
Esters	Similar to alcohols. Antifungal, anti-inflammatory, antispasmodic. Generally safe, low toxicity.	Ylang-ylang, neroli, bergamot, lavender, clary sage, petitgrain, geranium, citronella
Phenols	Antiseptic, bactericidal, stimulate immune system, stimulate central nervous system. Very potent. Handle with great care since these can irritate the skin and mucous membrane.	Thyme, sage, oregano, clove, cinnamon leaf, ylang-ylang
Aldehydes	Anti-inflammatory, vasodilators, calm central nervous system.	Citronella, melissa, cinnamon bark, lemongrass, lemon, lime, verbena
Ketones	Calming, sedative, analgesic, encourage wound healing. Not for long-time use. Never used in pregnancy.	Caraway, dill, spearmint, peppermint, jasmine, rosemary, sage, fennel
Lactones	Calming. Potentially photocarcinogenic: induce a cancer. Triggered by action of light. Never use before sunbathing.	Bergamot, orange, mandarin, lemon

Sources: Clark, S. (2002). *Essential Chemistry for Safe Aromatherapy*. Edinburgh, UK: Churchill Livingstone; Cooksley, V. G. (2002). *Aromatherapy*. Upper Saddle River, NJ: Prentice Hall; Schiller, C., & Schiller, D. (2008). *The Aromatherapy Encyclopedia*. Laguna Beach, CA: Basic Health Publications.

scent, however, is registered at some brain level, and people respond to it emotionally and/or physically (McGuigan, 2007).

In addition to the VMO, the nose contains 5 million smell-sensing cells that allow people to consciously register smells. Each cell has 6 to 12 hair-like receptors (cilia) that hang down into the stream of air rushing into the nose. These olfactory receptors are the only sensory pathways that open directly to the brain. The cilia detect scents, and the nerve cells relay this information directly to the limbic system, triggering memories and influencing behavior.

The amygdala of the limbic system, which stores and releases emotional memories, is most sensitive to odor or fragrance. Thus, the sense of smell can evoke powerful memories in a split second and change people's perceptions and behaviors. Odors are powerful memory stimulants even when they are not actually present. Just thinking or talking about a particular odor can unleash many memories. Olfactory stimulation can trigger negative responses such as intense fear or panic or can trigger positive feelings with increased release of endorphins and neurotransmitters. Odors stimulate the pituitary gland and hypothalamus and thus impact the production of hormones that control appetite, insulin production, body temperature, metabolism, stress levels, and sex drive. Unlike vision and hearing, the sense of smell is fully functional at birth. Newborns can recognize their mothers by smell, and this sensory response is an important part of bonding. In adult relationships, the sense of smell has a significant role in sensual and sexual attraction (Krautwurst, 2008; La Torre, 2003).

In addition to activating the central nervous system, inhaled oil molecules enter the respiratory system. There the molecules attach to oxygen molecules and circulate through the body, bringing with them the potential for activating self-healing processes. The equivalent in conventional medicine is the use of inhalers in the treatment of asthma. Essential oils can be inhaled directly or mixed with a carrier oil. Electrical and fan-assisted equipment or an aromatherapy light bulb ring may be used to scent a room for therapeutic purposes or to simply make the environment more pleasant. Steam inhalers can be used in the treatment of respiratory infections.

Applied externally, essential oils can calm inflamed or irritated skin, soothe sore muscles, decrease muscular tension, and release muscle spasms. Molecules of essential oils are so tiny they are quickly absorbed through the skin and enter the intercellular fluid and the circulatory system, bringing healing nutrients to the cells. Some oils such as basil, tea tree, and thyme encourage the production of white blood cells, while others such as lavender and eucalyptus fight harmful bacteria, viruses, and fungi. Oils may be applied just about anywhere: neck, face, wrists, over the heart, back, arms, legs, and feet. Massage therapists and acupuncturists often use essential oils in their treatments. Benefits are gained not only from the penetration of the oil through the skin but also from inhalation of the vapor and from direct massage of the skin and muscles. Essential oils do not remain in the body and are excreted in urine, feces, perspiration, and exhalation usually in 3 to 6 hours (Schiller & Schiller, 2008).

A diffuser is a special air pump designed to disburse the oils as an extremely fine vapor into the atmosphere, where they stay suspended for several hours. Diffusing releases oxygenating molecules as well as antiviral, antibacterial, and antiseptic properties. Unlike commercial air fresheners, which mask odors, essential oils clean the air by altering the structure of the molecules that create an unpleasant smell. Essential oils help remove dust particles out of the air and, when diffused in the room, can be an effective air filtration system.

TREATMENT

Essential oils influence health on physical, mental, and emotional levels. They have the ability to penetrate cell walls and transport oxygen and nutrients to the cell. Many have antiviral, antibacterial, antifungal, and antiseptic properties. This property of oils may be significant in the future as microbes continue to mutate and develop resistance to known medications. Aromatherapy can be used for the following purposes:

• Prompt the body and mind to function more efficiently.
• Decrease and manage stress.
• Refresh or recharge oneself.
• Regulate moods—some are energizing and some are sedating.
• Aid restful sleep.
• Act as a first-aid measure.
• Reduce weight.
• Boost the immune system.
• Minimize the discomforts of illness and speed recovery.
• Refresh room environment.

The purity and authenticity of essential oils is critical to their effectiveness. Oils that are diluted, adulterated, or synthetic should not be used for aromatherapy. Those identified as commercial-grade essential oils are likely to be diluted or adulterated in some way. Some are diluted with chemical carriers and passed on to the consumer as "pure essential oils" and are found in bath and cosmetic shops. Those labeled as "infused oils" are also adulterated. "Nature identical" oils are synthetic petrochemical-based products. They have been developed to closely mimic the smell and composition of essential oils. They are not identical, however, and lack many of the healing components of essential oils. Other names for synthetic oils are *aroma-chemicals, perfume oils*, and *fragrance oils*. Manufacturers have no restrictions on how essential oils are labeled. In general, those described with terms such as *genuine, authentic*, or *premium* are more likely to be pure essential oils. Informed consumers read labels carefully and buy from reputable dealers.

Essential oils are quite potent and can irritate the skin, so they should be diluted with a carrier oil before being used on the skin. Carrier oils contain vitamins, proteins, and minerals that provide added nutrients to the body. Some carrier oils can be purchased at supermarkets, while others may be available only at health food stores. Carrier oils include apricot kernel oil, sunflower oil, soy oil, sweet almond oil, grapeseed oil, sesame oil, avocado oil, jojoba, and wheat-germ oil. The fragrance does not have to be intense to be effective. In fact, the more intense the odor, the less pleasant it becomes.

By blending together two or more pure essential oils, a synergy can be created that is more powerful than the individual oils. The interaction of the oils with one another gives an added vibrancy to the blend. Synergistic blends are achieved by combining oils that complement each other. For example, the calming effects of lavender and bergamot or rosemary work well together.

BOX 8.1

Blending Oils According to Effects

Soothing oils: Chamomile

Uplifting oils: Black pepper, coriander, jasmine, juniper, eucalyptus, peppermint, tea tree

Balancing oils: Cypress, lavender

Uplifting and soothing oils: Basil, bergamot, frankincense, ginger, neroli, orange, patchouli, sandalwood

Uplifting and stimulating oils: Cedarwood, lemon, lemongrass, myrrh, pine, rose, rosemary, ylang-ylang

Uplifting and balancing oils: Clary sage, geranium

Examples of Blends

Basil, lavender

Bergamot, cypress, jasmine

Chamomile, lavender

Clary sage, lavender, sandalwood

Eucalyptus, chamomile, lavender, bergamot

Geranium, bergamot, lemon, lavender

Ginger, lavender, orange, neroli

Jasmine, rose, lemon, black pepper

Juniper, bergamot, geranium, frankincense

Lemon, tea tree, ylang-ylang

Pine, eucalyptus, lavender

Patchouli, bergamot, geranium

Peppermint, lavender

Sandalwood, ylang-ylang, black pepper, neroli

Oils with opposite effects, such as a soothing oil and a stimulating oil, should not be blended. It is also important for the blend to have a pleasing scent. See Box 8.1 for categories of oils to consider when formulating blends.

RESEARCH

The research basis for aromatherapy is in its infancy. Much of the research has been performed on animals and isolated tissue cultures. Few trials have been conducted on humans under clinical conditions. Many of the studies are practice based and anecdotal. Little is known at this time about possible interactions with conventional medications or treatments. Nurses are conducting much of the aromatherapy research in conventional health care settings. A number of studies are being done in intensive care settings and in the fields of midwifery, palliative care, and geriatric care.

A small sample of aromatherapy studies have found:

- Young babies bathed by their mothers using lavender-scented bath oil cried less and spent more time in deep sleep after the bath compared to babies bathed without lavender oil. The mothers in the lavender-oil group were more relaxed, smiled, and touched their babies more during the bath compared to the control group (Field et al., 2008).
- A group of 144 healthy volunteers were randomly assigned to ylang-ylang aroma, peppermint aroma, or no aroma (control group). It was found that peppermint increased alertness and enhanced memory and ylang-ylang decreased alertness, impaired memory, but increased a sense of calmness (Moss, Hewitt, Moss, & Wesnes, 2008).
- In a double-blind, placebo-controlled study, senior citizens experiencing knee pain were given six massage sessions with ginger and orange oil (the intervention group) over a 3-week period. The placebo group received the massages using olive oil and the control group had no massages. Knee pain, stiffness, and physical functioning were the measurement parameters. There was significant improvement in the intervention group in the first week following treatment, but by the fourth week this improvement had disappeared (Yip & Tam, 2008).
- In a randomized placebo-controlled trial, 67 female college students who rated their menstrual cramps to be greater than 6 on a 10-point scale were randomized into three groups. The intervention group received abdominal massage using oil infused with lavender, clary sage, and rose. The placebo group received massage using almond oil only and the control group received no treatment. Menstrual cramps were significantly lowered in the aromatherapy group than in the other two groups (Han, Hur, Buckle, Choi, & Lee, 2006)
- 88 individuals with chronic plantar fasciitis were randomized into a double-blind, placebo-controlled trial. The intervention group applied wheatgrass cream daily for 6 weeks, and the control group used a placebo cream. It was found that the wheatgrass cream was no more effective than the placebo cream (Young, Cook, & Webster, 2006).

INTEGRATED NURSING PRACTICE

Nurses are increasingly providing aromatherapy in conventional health care settings, including intensive care areas; renal, burn, and neurologic units; cancer wards; HIV/AIDS units; hospices; geriatric areas; and pediatric units. As a nurse in a conventional health care setting, you can promote the use of aromatherapy in a number of ways. Essential oils can be combined with carrier oils and used for back rubs and foot rubs to help clients relax and decrease their levels of anxiety. Other essential oils can be used as an adjunct to conventional approaches by encouraging the production of white blood cells and for their antibacterial or antiviral action. Acute care and long-term care settings often have unpleasant smells in rooms and hallways. Essential oils, such as rosemary, lemon, tangerine, mandarin, and lemongrass, can be diffused into the air to alter the structure of the molecules creating the odor, thus refreshing the environment. Diffusion of essential oils can also help boost the client's immune system, decrease anxiety and stress, aid restful sleep, and speed recovery. Essential oils can be used to enhance sedation, thereby decreasing the need for night-time medication.

As a nurse, you can teach people a number of things about the use of essential oils. As a general rule, people should purchase essential oils in natural and health food stores rather than stores selling beauty products and perfumes. They should be stored in dark vials, tightly closed and away from heat, light, or dampness. Essential oils should not be ingested, because even modest amounts can be fatal. They must be kept away from children and pets. Pregnant women and persons with epilepsy should consult a knowledgeable health care practitioner or qualified aromatherapist prior to the use of essential oils. Some oils can trigger bronchial spasms, so persons with asthma should consult their primary health care provider before using oils. Oils other than lavender or tea tree oil must always be diluted before applying on the skin. People who have sensitive skin or allergies should take extra care in massaging the oils into the skin or inhaling the essential oil aromas. Caution people not to rub their eyes if they have any essential oil on their hands. Several oils are photosensitive or phototoxic, causing severe sunburn if people are exposed to the sun within 6 hours after application. These oils include clove, bergamot, angelica, verbena, bitter/sweet orange, lemon, lime, and mandarin. Certain oils have high toxicity levels, and their use should be limited to qualified aromatherapists. These oils include boldo leaf, calamus, yellow camphor, horseradish, rue, sassafras, savin, tansy, wintergreen, wormseed, and wormwood.

Professional aromatherapists use up to 50 oils. Most people can meet their home needs with fewer than 30 or even just 10: chamomile, clove, eucalyptus, geranium, lavender, lemon, peppermint, rosemary, tea tree, and thyme. Box 8.2 describes helpful oils you can encourage people to have available at home.

BOX 8.2

Helpful Oils to Have at Home

Oil	Use
Basil	Decrease sinus congestion; soothe GI tract, aid digestion; decrease headache; decrease anxiety; decrease menstrual cramps
Bergamot	Decrease anxiety, decrease depression; urinary antiseptic; acne, disinfectant for wounds, abscesses, boils

Cedarwood	Decrease respiratory congestion and coughs, expectorant; for pain swelling of arthritis; antifungal for skin rashes
Chamomile	Soothe muscle aches, sprains, swollen joints; GI antispasmodic; rub on abdomen for colic, indigestion, gas; decrease anxiety, stress-related headaches; decrease insomnia; can be used with children
Clary sage	Induce sleep; increase sense of well-being; massage or warm compress for menstrual cramps; do not use in pregnancy until onset of labor
Coriander	Improve digestion, decrease colic, decrease diarrhea; decrease muscle aches and stiffness in joints; decrease mental fatigue and increase memory and mental function
Cypress	Massage or cold compress for rheumatic aches; bruising or varicose veins; respiratory antispasmodic (put couple of drops on hanky and inhale deeply), decrease coughs, asthma, bronchitis
Elemi	Boost immune system; cystitis; speed bone healing (massage in prior to casting); increase healing of cuts, sores, wounds; cool inflamed skin; sedative
Eucalyptus	Feels cool to skin and warm to muscles; decrease fever; relieve pain; anti-inflammatory; antiseptic, antiviral, and expectorant to respiratory system in steam inhalation; boost immune system
Frankincense	Bronchodilatory, acts on mucus enabling sputum to be expelled; infected sores; deepen breathing to induce calmness; incense creates a state conducive to prayer
Geranium	Antibacterial; insecticidal; antidepressant; improve yeast infections; first aid on minor cuts and burns
Ginger	Help ward off colds; calm upset stomach, decrease nausea; soothe sprains, muscle spasms
Green apple	Reduce headache severity; decrease anxiety; aid in weight reduction program; reduce symptoms of claustrophobia
Jasmine	Uplifting and stimulating, antidepressant; massage abdomen and lower back for menstrual cramps
Juniper	Calming, decrease stress; diuretic; muscle aches and pains
Lavender	Calming, sedative, for insomnia; massage around temples for headache; inhale to speed recovery from colds, flu; massage chest to decrease congestion; heal burns
Lemongrass	Sedative; skin antiseptic for acne
Marjoram	Insomnia, decrease tension; muscle and joint pain; inhale to clear sinuses and clear congestion; massage abdomen for menstrual cramps
Neroli	Gentle sedative for insomnia, panic attacks; massage abdomen for irritable bowel syndrome
Orange	General tonic; decrease anxiety; GI antispasmodic for colic and indigestion; massage abdomen for constipation; can be used with children

(continued)

Peppermint	Increase alertness; GI antispasmodic for colic and indigestion; massage on temples for headache; decongestant for colds, flu
Petitgrain	Useful for acne and oily skin; decreases muscle spasms; gentle sedative
Rose	Antidepressant; increase alertness; compress for eyestrain, headaches; use in massage for PMS
Rosemary	Stimulating; increase circulation to skin; compress on swollen joints; decrease respiratory congestion; antifungal, antibacterial; deodorize the air
Sandalwood	Calm and cool body; decrease inflammation; drops on handkerchief for sore throat, congestion; in bath water for cystitis; improve chapped dry skin; increase sense of peace in meditation or prayer
Tea Tree	First-aid kit in a bottle; antifungal, good for athlete's foot; soothe insect bites, stings, cuts, wounds; in bath for yeast infection; drops on handkerchief for coughs, congestion
Vetiver	Stimulate production of red blood cells; increase circulation; induce restful sleep; decrease tension
Ylang-ylang	Soothe CNS, decrease depression, increase euphoric mood; decrease BP; regulate respiration; calm heart palpitations

Sources: Cooksley, V. G. (2002). *Aromatherapy*. Upper Saddle River, NJ: Prentice Hall; Devereux, C. (2002). *Aromatherapy*. London: Tuttle; Wilson, R. (2002). *Aromatherapy*. New York: Avery. Schiller, C., & Schiller, D. (2008). *The Aromatherapy Encyclopedia*. Laguna Beach, CA: Basic Health Publications.

TRY THIS

Soothing Potions

Rosewater

Instead of using soap, try splashing your face with rosewater, a simple infusion from rose petals containing some of the flowers' essential oils. Rose oil has mild antiseptic and anti-inflammatory action. It can constrict the tiny blood vessels in your skin to reduce redness, and it is also used in aromatherapy to calm your nerves and elevate your mood. You can buy rosewater in any natural food store, but you can also make your own. Put a handful of fresh rose petals into a small saucepan, add enough water to cover the petals completely, simmer for 15 minutes, then remove the pan from the heat. When it is completely cooled, strain away the petals and transfer your rosewater to a clean glass bottle.

Adult Cold Cure

2 drops eucalyptus

5 drops geranium

3 drops peppermint

5 drops rosemary

Mix oils together. Use in any of the following ways:

- Put several drops in a diffuser.
- Put 2 drops on a tissue and breathe in the aroma.
- Put 4 drops in a bath.
- Add 8 drops to 2 tablespoons of carrier oil and massage the chest, back, neck, forehead, nose, and cheekbones.

Natural Sleep Aid

- Put 2 drops of lavender on your pillowcase.
- Combine 3 drops chamomile, 4 drops lavender, 3 drops orange, and 5 ounces of water. Using a spray bottle, spray linens and room air before sleeping.

Source: Fitzsimmons J., & Bousquet, P. M. (1998). *Aromatherapy Through the Seasons.* Berkeley, CA: Conari Press; Hoffman, R., & Fox, B. (2006). *Alternative Cures That Really Work.* New York: Rodale; Schiller, C., & Schiller, D. (2008). *The Aromatherapy Encyclopedia.* Laguna Beach, CA: Basic Health Publications.

USING RESEARCH TO HEAL

Han, S. H., Hur, M. H., Buckle, J., Choi, J., & Lee, M. S. (2006). Effect of aromatherapy on symptoms of dysmenorrhea in college students: A randomized placebo-controlled clinical trial. *Journal of Alternative and Complementary Medicine*, 12(6), 535–541.

What Is This Study About?

Many women experience menstrual cramps and symptoms of dysmenorrhea. Complementary and alternative medicine may be a remedy for the reduction of these symptoms. The purpose of this research was to investigate the effectiveness of aromatherapy, specifically a combination of lavender, clary sage, and rose applied topically in decreasing menstrual cramps and symptoms associated with dysmenorrhea.

How Was the Study Done?

Fifty-seven college women attending Korean universities were recruited for this double-blind, three group experimental pre-test/post-test design study. Sample participants were randomly assigned to one of the three groups. The students assigned to the experimental group (n = 25) received aromatherapy in almond oil massage, the placebo group (n = 20) received massage with almond oil only, and the control group (n = 22) did not receive treatment. Institutional Review Board approval was granted for this study. Subjects in the aromatherapy group and placebo group had no knowledge as to

(continued)

whether they were receiving real or sham aromatherapy. The participants in the experimental group received aromatherapy (lavender, clary sage, and rose in a 2:1:1 ratio) for 15 minutes in the form of a prescribed abdominal massage in a specific treatment room every day beginning one week before the start of menses and continuing until the first day of menstruation. Treatment room beds were warmed by heating pads. Participants in the placebo group received the same treatment but only with almond oil. The control group was instructed to continue with their normal daily routine. Severity of cramps data were collected on the first and second days of menses after the experimental treatment and designated as post-test data. Measurement of menstrual cramps was measured with a 10-point Visual Analog Scale and the severity of dysmenorrhea was measured by a verbal multidimensional scoring system.

What Were the Results of the Study?

Severity of cramps was significantly lower in the aromatherapy group than in the other two groups. Findings revealed that the levels of the menstrual cramps and change in the severity of dysmenorrhea during the first few days of menstruation were decreased in the experimental group more significantly as compared with the placebo and control groups.

What Additional Questions Might I Have?

Would a larger sample size significantly influence the results of this study? Were the women receiving any other treatment modality for menstrual cramps and dysmenorrhea?

How Can I Use This Study?

Nurses can suggest that women use aromatherapy as an alternative treatment to decrease menstrual cramps and dysmenorrheal symptoms and enhance quality of life.

Source: Contributed by Dolores M. Huffman, RN, PhD, Associate Professor of Nursing, Purdue University Calumet.

References

Boyraz, N., & Ozcan, M. (2005). Antifungal effect of some spice hydrosols. *Fitoterapia*, 76(7–8): 661–665.

Clark, S. (2002). *Essential Chemistry for Safe Aromatherapy*. Edinburgh: Churchill Livingstone.

Cline, M., Taylor, J. E., Flores, J., Bracken, S., McCall, S., & Ceremuga, T. E. (2008). Investigation of the anxiolytic effects of linalool, a lavender extract, in the male Sprague-Dawley rat. *American Association of Nurse Anesthetists Journal*, 76(1): 47–52.

Field, T., Field, T., Cullen, C., Largie, S., Diego, M., Schanberg, S., et al. (2008). Lavender bath oil reduces stress and crying and enhances sleep in very young infants. *Early Human Development*, 84(6): 399–401.

Han, S. H., Hur, M. H., Buckle, J., Choi, J., & Lee, M. S. (2006). Effect of aromatherapy on symptoms of dysmenorrheal in college students. *Journal of Alternative and Complementary Medicine*, 12(6): 535–541.

Krautwurst, D. (2008). Human olfactory receptor families and their odorants. *Chemistry & Biodiversity*, 5(6): 842–852.

La Torre, M. A. (2003). Aromatherapy and the use of scents in psychotherapy.

Perspectives in Psychiatric Care, 39(1): 35–37.

McGuigan, M. (2007). Hypothesis: Do homeopathic medicines exert their action in humans and animals via the vomeronasal system? *Homeopathy*, 96(2): 113–119.

Moss, M., Hewitt, S., Moss, L., & Wesnes, K. (2008). Modulation of cognitive performance and mood by aromas of peppermint and ylang-ylang. *The International Journal of Neuroscience*, 118(1): 59–77.

Schiller, C., & Schiller, D. (2008). *The Aromatherapy Encyclopedia*. Laguna Beach, CA: Basic Health Publications.

Smith, M. C., & Kyle, L. (2008). Holistic foundations of aromatherapy for nursing. *Holistic Nursing Practice*, 22(6): 3–9.

Thomas, D. V. (2002). Aromatherapy: Mythical, magical, or medicinal? *Holistic Nursing Practice*, 17(1): 8–16.

Yip, Y. B., & Tam, A. C. Y. (2008). An experimental study on the effectiveness of massage with aromatic ginger and orange essential oil for moderate-to-severe knee pain among elderly in Hong Kong. *Complementary Therapies in Medicine*, 16: 131–138.

Young, M. A., Cook, J. L., & Webster, K. E. (2006).The effect of topical wheatgrass cream on chronic plantar fasciitis. *Complementary Therapies in Medicine*, 14: 3–9.

Resources

Aromatherapy Registration Council
  5940 SW Hood Ave.
  Portland, OR 97039
  503.244.0726
  www.aromatherapycouncil.co.uk

Institute of Integrative Aromatherapy
  P.O. Box 19241
  Boulder, CO 80308
  303.545.2002
  www.aroma-rn.com

International Federation of
    Aromatherapists
  Suite 70, Walpole Court, Ealing Green
  London W5 5ED UK
  020.8567.1923
  www.ifaroma.org

National Association for Holistic
    Aromatherapy (NAHA)
  3327 W. Indian Trail Rd. PMB 144
  Spokane, WA 99208
  509.325.3419
  www.naha.org

Smell and Taste Treatment and Research
    Foundation
  845 North Michigan Ave., Suite 990W
  Chicago, IL 60611
  312.938.1047

9

Homeopathy

*People take different roads seeking
fulfillment and happiness. Just because
they're not on your road doesn't mean
they've gotten lost.*

H. Jackson Browne

*Miracles do not happen in contradiction
of nature, but in contradiction to what we
know about nature.*

Saint Augustine

The term **homeopathy** is derived from the Greek words
omoios, meaning "similar," and *pathos*, meaning "feeling." It
is a self-healing system, assisted by small doses of remedies
or medicines, that is useful in a variety of acute and chronic disorders. The practice of homeopathy in the United States has increased tremendously since the 1980s, corresponding to the
increase in other forms of alternative medicine. Homeopathic
medicine is practiced worldwide, especially in Europe, Latin
America, and Asia.

In the United States, the homeopathic drug market has
grown into a multimillion-dollar industry. Most of these remedies
are not regulated by the FDA and are available as over-the-
counter medications.

BACKGROUND

Homeopathy, as a therapeutic system, is approximately 200 years
old. It was developed by Samuel Hahnemann (1755–1843), a
German physician and chemist. Homeopathy came to most of
Europe, the United States, Russia, and Latin America in the 1830s.

During epidemics of cholera, typhus, and scarlet fever, homeopathy was significantly more effective than the conventional medical approaches of the times. In 1869, the American Institute of Homeopathy opened free dispensaries for the poor and voted to admit female physicians, unheard of in conventional medicine. By the 1890s, 15 percent of American physicians used some homeopathic remedies in their practice, learned in the 22 homeopathic medical schools and practiced in more than 100 homeopathic hospitals (Feingold, 2008).

During and after the Civil War, the practice of medicine began to change with technical achievements such as anesthesia, antisepsis, surgery, microbiology, vaccines, and antibiotics. State legislatures began to license physicians and accredit medical schools. The American Medical Association (AMA) invited homeopaths to become members in exchange for licensing, seeking to create a monopoly against lay healers, midwives, and herbalists. When the homeopaths chose not to join forces, the AMA began to persecute homeopathy and, in 1914, proposed uniform standards of medical education and assumed the power of accreditation, using it to phase out homeopathic colleges. Between the 1920s and 1970s, homeopathic education in the United States was almost nonexistent (Wauters, 2007).

PREPARATION

About half of the homeopaths in the United States are physicians. The others are licensed health care practitioners such as nurse practitioners, dentists, naturopathic physicians, chiropractors, acupuncturists, and veterinarians. The Council for Homeopathic Certification administers the certification process, which involves a specified number of hours of training, three years of clinical practice, and written and oral examinations. Certification earns the right to place the designation *DHt* after one's name.

CONCEPTS

Law of Similars

Hahnemann proposed the use of the **law of similars,** which claims that a natural substance that produces a given symptom in a healthy person cures it in a sick person. The substance whose symptom-picture most closely resembles the illness being treated is the one most likely to initiate a curative response for that person. Hence the name *homeopathy*—"similar feeling."

If taken in large amounts, these natural compounds will produce symptoms of disease. In the doses used by homeopaths, however, these remedies stimulate a person's self-healing capacity. As Andrew Weil states, "The difference between a poison and a medicine is the dose" (Frye, 1997, p. 846). An example is seen in the use of Ipecac, which in large doses causes severe nausea and vomiting. Women who are experiencing the nausea and vomiting of pregnancy, however, can use small doses of Ipecac to cure those same symptoms (Wauters, 2007).

Law of Infinitesimals

Natural healing compounds are specially prepared for homeopathic use through a process of serial dilution. The compound is first dissolved in a water–alcohol mixture called the "mother tincture." One drop of the tincture is then mixed with 10 drops of water–alcohol, and this process is repeated hundreds or thousands of times depending on the potency being prepared. At each step of the dilution, the vial is vigorously shaken, called **succussion,** which seems to be an essential step. The homeopathic belief is that the more the substance is diluted, the more potent it becomes as a remedy.

The remedies are diluted beyond the point at which any molecules of the substance can theoretically still be found in the solution. This paradox, that the remedy becomes more potent through dilution, is the reason many biomedical scientists reject homeopathic medicine. Just as biomedical pharmacologists do not understand the mechanisms of many conventional drugs, it is not presently understood how homeopathic remedies work. A number of theories are proposed. A remedy may be like a hologram. No matter how many times a substance is diluted, a smaller but complete essence of the substance remains. Modern chaos theory supports the observation that major changes occur in living organisms when bodily substances are activated only slightly. The basic assumption of chaos theory is that minute changes can have huge effects. Advances in quantum physics have led some scientists to suggest that the imprinting of electromagnetic energy in the remedies interacts with the body on some level. Gas discharge visualization technology may provide an electromagnetic probe into the properties of homeopathic remedies in the future. Researchers in physical chemistry have proposed the memory of water theory in which the structure of the water–alcohol solution is altered during the process of dilution and retains its new structure even after the substance is no longer present. It seems likely that remedies work through a bioenergetic or subatomic mechanism that we are not as yet capable of understanding. The situation may be likened to any number of advances in the understanding of energy such as radio, television, microwave ovens, and cordless telephones that previously were virtually unimaginable (Novella et al., 2008; Smith, 2008; Witt et al., 2007).

In the 1920s and 1930s, Dr. Bach, a conventional physician, a homeopathic physician, and an intuitive healer, discovered **flower essences.** He believed that emotions such as anger, hate, or fear negatively impact the immune system leading to stress, pain, and illness. He experimented with a number of flowers, eventually creating a treatment system involving 38 different types of wildflowers. Flowers are placed in a clear glass bowl filled with purified water and placed in direct sunlight, which transfers the energy of the blossom into the water—a process called **infusion.** Bach's flower essences are diluted but not as much as homeopathic remedies. The remedies are placed under the tongue or in a glass of liquid four times a day. They are usually safe for even infants and the elderly and are thought to contribute to physical, emotional, mental, and spiritual healing. The best known remedy is the Bach

Rescue Remedy®, which is used to calm people (and pets) in any stressful situation (Sekhar et al., 2008; Wauters, 2007).

VIEW OF HEALTH AND ILLNESS

Homeopathy is a method for treating the sick rather than a set of hypotheses about the nature of health and illness. The assumption is, however, that a vital force—known as qi or prana in other traditions—exists. It is necessary to have adequate nutrition, exercise, rest, good hygiene, and a healthy environment to adapt and maintain homeostasis. In other words, health is the ability of people to adapt their equilibrium in response to internal and external change. Illness is primarily a disturbance of the vital force manifesting as symptoms of distress. Vital force or life energy is the ultimate origin of health and illness, alike, ending only with the death of the person (Griffith, 2006).

Symptoms of illness represent people's attempts to heal themselves. Thus, homeopathy views symptoms as an *adaptive reaction* that is the best possible response that can be made in the present circumstances. For example, a cough is the body's attempt to clear the bronchi; inflammation is the body's effort to wall off and burn out invading foreign bodies; and fever is the body's way of creating an internal environment that is less conducive to bacterial or viral growth. Given this perspective, the therapeutic approach is to aid the body's efforts to adapt to stress or infection. Thus, for someone with a high fever, homeopaths may recommend belladonna, which increases the natural healing response of body heat. The law of similars is a stimulation of immune and defense responses leading to spontaneous resolution of symptoms as the illness is conquered. In like manner, two of the few conventional therapies that seek to stimulate the body's own healing reaction, immunization and allergy treatment, have the homeopathic law of similars as their basis. Other applications in conventional medicine include the use of radiation in the treatment of cancer and Ritalin in the treatment of hyperactive children. The majority of interventions in biomedicine, however, attempt to oppose symptoms by exerting a greater and opposite force. Medicines are designed to "cure" by suppressing symptoms such as the use of aspirin in an effort to control or limit people's fevers. The danger is that, over time, suppressive treatments may actually strengthen disease processes instead of resolving them (Research Report, 2008).

DIAGNOSTIC METHODS

Homeopathic diagnosis is holistic and detailed. The initial assessment may last several hours. Practitioners assess the whole person, looking at every aspect of physical, emotional, and mental life. A multitude of factors are considered, such as nutritional status, emotional imbalance, and environmental stress. It is believed that no part can be isolated from the whole person. The homeopathic interview itself is a powerful healing experience because clients are encouraged to tell their story in its entirety. They are encouraged to speak for as long a time as possible. This process of sharing pain and suffering begins the healing process. During the interview, the practitioner observes everything about the person, including posture, dress, facial expression, tone of voice, rate of speech, and so forth. The physical exam is a head-to-toe assessment with the inclusion of laboratory work as needed to establish a diagnosis. Answers to questions are elicited in an attempt to fully understand the significance of the symptoms:

- Subjective symptoms such as pain, vertigo, fatigue, or anger
- Localization of symptoms such as one sided, wandering, radiating, or diffuse
- Factors that modify the symptoms, making them better or worse, such as time of day, hot or cold, weather, diet, or emotional state
- Quality of symptoms such as burning, aching, throbbing
- Rate of onset or resolution of the symptoms such as sudden or gradual
- Symptoms that appear simultaneously or in sequence

Symptoms are classified into three categories—the general physical symptoms, the local symptoms, and the mental and emotional symptoms. *General physical symptoms* include such things as sleep, appetite, energy, temperature, or generalized body pain. *Local symptoms* occur in particular parts of the body such as swelling in the right elbow or pain in the left leg. Included in local symptoms are those related to a specific organ function such as shortness of breath or palpitations. *Mental and emotional symptoms* include anxiety, irritability, anger, tearfulness, isolation, or suspiciousness. This composite picture of the person is far more important than any isolated laboratory findings or abstract disease category in formulating the diagnosis. Homeopathic practitioners do not hesitate to refer to biomedical specialists for conventional drugs or surgery.

TREATMENT

Homeopathy is not a complete system of medicine in itself and should be used in conjunction with biomedicine. As in other complementary practices, the initial question is always "Who is the person?" rather than "What is the disease?" This focus ensures an individualized approach to treatment. Each person with the same presenting complaint may be treated with different remedies depending on the totality of physical, mental, and emotional symptoms. A person with a sore throat may be prescribed one of six or seven common remedies for sore throats, depending on whether the pain is worse on the right or left side, what time of day it is worse, how thirst and appetite are affected, and the individual's emotional state (Feingold, 2008).

The science and the art of homeopathy is to find the remedy with the ability to mimic most closely the sick person's pattern of symptoms. Practitioners use only one remedy at a time, since administering different remedies for different symptoms makes it difficult to know which remedy was effective. Not only are the smallest possible doses used, typically only one dose is given, which allows time for the remedy to complete its action without further interference. If necessary, a dose may be repeated or another remedy may be tried. A temporary worsening of the symptoms may occur after receiving the remedy, which is usually mild and short lived and may be an indication that the correct remedy was chosen (Feingold, 2008).

Homeopathy is used to treat both acute and chronic health problems as well as for health promotion. It cannot cure conditions resulting from structural, long-term, organic changes such as cirrhosis, diabetes, chronic obstructive lung disease, advanced neurological diseases, or cancer. In some of these cases, homeopathy can palliate the symptoms and increase the client's comfort level. Traumatic injuries affect nearly everyone in similar ways and thus the remedies are fairly standard. Epidemic infectious diseases also tend to affect most victims in the same way and individuals are usually treated with the same remedy. Common infectious illnesses such as urinary tract infections, respiratory infections, or ear infections demonstrate more individual symptoms and require more individualization in selecting the remedy. Chronic illness such as ulcerative colitis, rheumatoid arthritis, asthma, and skin disorders are considered to be constitutional. Thus, these disorders require the most skillful assessment, individualized prescription, and follow-up (Schneider, Schneider, Hanisch, & van Haselen, 2008; Wauters, 2007).

The Homeopathic Pharmacopoeia of the United States (Borneman & Foxman, 1989), listing more than 2,000 remedies, is the official standard for preparation and prescription. Most remedies come from plants used in traditional herbal medicine. A few remedies come from animal sources and others from naturally occurring chemical compounds. Box 9.1 lists examples of remedies. Some, such as mercury and belladonna, would be poisonous in large doses but are safe in the superdilute homeopathic doses. These remedies rank among the safest medicines available (Research Report, 2008; Wauters, 2007). Homeopathic medicines found in most health food stores are called *combination medicines* or *formulas*, because they have between three and eight different homeopathic medicines mixed together. The various manufacturers choose the medicines most commonly prescribed for specific symptoms and assume that one of them will help cure the ailment that the consumer has. Professional homeopaths believe that the remedy individually chosen for the person tends to work more often and more effectively than these combinations.

RESEARCH

As in other areas of medical research, the two questions are "How does it work?" and "How well does it work?" Many researchers are studying the physics of how homeopathic remedies work. At this time, it seems likely that remedies work through a bioenergetic or subatomic mechanism that is not yet understood or measurable. Research in the areas of quantum physics,

BOX 9.1

Examples of Homeopathic Remedies

Plant	Mineral	Animal
Herbs: comfrey, eyebright, mullein, yellow dock	**Metals:** copper, gold, lead, tin, zinc	**Venoms:** jellyfish, insects, spiders, mollusks, crustaceans, fish, snakes, amphibians
Foods and spices: cayenne, garlic, mustard, onion	**Salts:** calcium sulfate, sodium chloride, potassium carbonate	**Secretions:** ambergris, musk, cuttlefish ink
Fragrances, resins, residues: amber, petroleum, charcoal, creosote	**Acids:** hydrochloric, nitric, phosphoric, sulfuric	**Milks**
Mushrooms, lichens, mosses	**Elemental substances:** carbon, hydrogen, iodine, phosphorus, sulfur	**Hormones**
	Constituents of earth's crust: silica, aluminum oxide, ores, rocks, lavas, mineral waters	**Glandular and tissue extracts**
		Disease products: vaccines, abscesses, tuberculosis, gonorrhea, syphilis

physical chemistry, and biochemistry may someday be able to answer the question of how the remedies work.

One of the difficulties in using the standard randomized, placebo-controlled paradigm for homeopathic remedies is the individualization of the treatment. Unlike biomedicine, each person with the illness is likely to be prescribed a different remedy based on holistic assessment.

A small sampling of studies include the following:

- Three randomized, placebo-controlled, double-blind clinical trials investigated the effectiveness of arnica on postoperative swelling and pain after knee surgery for cruciate ligament reconstruction (CLR), artificial knee joint implantation (AKJ), and arthroscopy (ART). All three trials demonstrated a trend toward less swelling for the patients receiving arnica. The only significant difference was found in the CLR group (Brinkhaus et al., 2006).

- A multicenter cohort study investigated homeopathic versus conventional treatment for children with eczema. Over a period of one year, both groups demonstrated similar improvement (Keil et al., 2008).
- A new Cochrane review has found some evidence that cranberry juice can prevent recurrent urinary tract infections in women (Cochrane Library, 2008).

INTEGRATED NURSING PRACTICE

Nurses, like homeopathic practitioners, emphasize listening to clients' stories of their lives. It is within the context of people's lives that we identify patterns of response to illnesses and disorders and formulate nursing diagnoses. Nursing diagnoses and outcome criteria focus our attention on adaptations that may help people live healthier lifestyles. The study of mental health nursing in our basic educational program teaches us the value of listening and attending to people's pain as an intervention to help them begin the process of healing. These principles are common to both nursing and homeopathy, illustrating, once again, the broad base of nursing practice. Some nurse practitioners, valuing the contributions of homeopathy to well-being, continue their education and achieve licensure to practice homeopathic medicine. As nurses educated in Western approaches, we are more likely to suppress symptoms in an attempt to "cure" the disease. In many situations, it may be more beneficial to follow the homeopathic approach and view symptoms as the body's attempt to heal itself. We may find clients improve more quickly when non-life-threatening symptoms are supported rather than suppressed, such as low- to moderate-grade fevers or productive coughs.

People who are interested in homeopathic remedies can find low-potency remedies in health food stores. Higher potency remedies are obtained from homeopathic pharmaceutical companies under the direction of experienced homeopathic prescribers. Because remedies are inactivated by direct sunlight and heat, teach people to store the preparations in a dark, dry place, away from other strong-smelling substances. When taking a remedy, patients should have nothing by mouth for at least 30 minutes before and after the dose. Many homeopaths discourage the use of coffee, mint, camphor, and other strongly aromatic substances while undergoing treatment, since such substances may reverse the effects of the remedy. Camphor is a component in chest rubs as well as in many cosmetics, skin creams, and lip balms. If the remedy is in the form of a pellet, it should be held under the tongue and allowed to dissolve slowly. If the remedy is a liquid, it is held in the mouth for one to two minutes before swallowing.

Prescription medications, especially those given for potentially life-threatening disorders such as asthma, should not be stopped abruptly when beginning homeopathic care. As the person improves, however, a downward titration of the biomedical prescription may be needed. Acupuncture and chiropractic medicine should not be started at the same time as homeopathic remedies, but if already instituted, may be continued (Griffith, 2006).

A number of homeopathic remedies can be used to speed recovery and prevent recurrences of acute conditions such as colds, stomachaches, coughs, and headaches. Although many remedies are used for conditions that subside on their own, they can dramatically speed recovery and often prevent recurrences. Because homeopathic medicines are considerably safer than conventional drugs, it often makes sense to use them as the first resort and to consider using conventional drugs if the homeopathic remedies work too slowly or not at all. People should read all the information on the label to select the right remedy. If it says, for example, that the remedy is best used when the symptoms appear suddenly, then that remedy is not likely to be effective for a condition that emerged almost unnoticed over several days. You can teach clients the following three guidelines for the use of homeopathic remedies:

1. *The more the better.* The more the symptoms match that of the remedy, the more likely it will work.
2. *The less the better.* The more dilute the remedy, the more powerful it is.
3. *It's working if you feel better within 24 hours.* If not, you may have the wrong remedy and may need a different remedy or may need to see a health care practitioner.

Many people keep homeopathic remedies on hand and ready to use. See *Try This: Top Ten Remedies* for the most popular remedies that help with the majority of common physical problems and emotional difficulties.

TRY THIS

Top Ten Remedies

Bryonia (wild hops): Used for coughs that are worsened by simple breathing; headaches that are increased by bending over, walking, or even moving the eyes; constipation with dry, hard stools.

Allium cepa (onion): Used for colds or respiratory allergies where symptoms resemble the reaction of a person exposed to the mist of an onion: watery eyes, clear nasal discharge, and sneezes, all of which are aggravated by exposure to heat.

Pulsatilla (windflower): Need is based on the type of person, rather than a specific ailment. Helpful for people who are highly emotional, weepy, impressionable, easily influenced, fearful of abandonment, and worried about what others think of them. May also be used for digestive disorders, allergies, earaches, headaches, insomnia, and premenstrual syndrome.

Ignatia (St. Ignatius bean): Used by people who experience anxiety or grief.

Arsenicum album (arsenic): Used for many conditions, especially when symptoms are worse after midnight, when burning symptoms are predominant, when great thirst occurs, or when the person is high-strung and restless.

Belladonna (deadly nightshade): Used for fever or inflammation that begins rapidly, with a red or flushed appearance; the person is hypersensitive to touch or light.

Gelsemium (yellow jessamine): Used for classic flu symptoms accompanied by lack of thirst. Helpful for headaches in the back part of the head.

Nux vomica (poison nut): Useful after overdosing with food or drink, indigestion, constipation, and headaches that are worse at night and on waking.

Aconitum (monkshood): Used for colds, flu, coughs, and sore throats with rapid onset.

Rhus toxicodendron (poison ivy): Helpful for arthritis syndromes, flu, sprains and strains, and sore throats; used by people who feel pain on initial motion that eases with continued motion and who have symptoms that worse in cold or wet weather.

Sources: Feingold, E. (2008). *Homeopathy, Herbal Remedies, & Nutritional Supplements*. Albany, NY: Whitston Publishing; Griffith, C. (2006). *The Practical Handbook of Homeopathy*. London: Watkins Publishing; Wauters, A. (2007). *The Homeopathy Bible*. New York: Sterling Publishing Company.

TRY THIS

Pet Remedies

Mercurius solubilis: Inflamed gums; swollen nasal bones and a greenish thick discharge

Podophyllum: Diarrhea with gushy feces containing mucus

Baryta carb: Diarrhea in puppies and young dogs

Arsenicum album or allium cepa: Respiratory symptoms where the nasal and ocular discharge is thin and watery

Sulphur: Red and itchy skin

Lycopodium or thallium acetas: Hair loss secondary to skin disorders

Source: Hunter, F. E. (2004). *Everyday Homeopathy for Animals*. Beaconsfield, UK: Beaconsfield Publishers; Messonnier, S. (2003). Is homeopathy right for your dog? *Dog World*, 87(2): 42–47; Juta, C. (2005). *Animal Homeopathy*. Charleston, SC: BookSurge Publishing.

References

Borneman, J. P. & Foxman, E. L. (1989). *Homeopathic Pharmacopoeia of the United States*. Southeastern, PA: Homeopathic Pharmacopoeia.

Brinkhaus, B., Wilkens, J. M., Ludtke, R., Hunger, J., Witt, C. M., & Willich, S. N. (2006). Homeopathic arnica therapy in patients receiving knee surgery: Results of three randomized double-blind trials. *Complementary Therapies in Medicine*, 14: 237–246.

Cochrane Library. (2008). Issue 1, CD001321.

Feingold, E. (2008). *Homeopathy, Herbal Remedies, & Nutritional Supplements*. Albany, NY: Whitston Publishing.

Frye, J. (1997). Homeopathy in office practice. *Primary Care*, 24(4): 845–864.

Griffith, C. (2006). *The Practical Handbook of Homeopathy*. London: Watkins Publishing.

Keil, T., Witt, C. M., Roll, S., Vance, W., Weber, K., Wegscheider, K., et al. (2008). Homeopathic versus conventional treatment of children with eczema: A comparative cohort study. *Complementary Therapies in Medicine*, 16: 15–21.

Novella, S., Roy, R., Marcus, D., Bell, I. R., Davidovitch, N., & Saine, A. (2008). A debate: Homeopathy—quackery or a key to the future of medicine? *Journal of Alternative and Complementary Medicine*, 14(1): 9–15.

Research Report. (2008). Questions and answers about homeopathy. *National Center for Complementary and Alternative Medicine*. http://nccam.nih.gov/health/homeopathy/. Accessed July 26, 2008.

Schneider, C., Schneider, B, Hanisch, J., & van Haselen. (2008). The role of a homeopathic preparation compared with conventional therapy in the treatment of injuries: An observational cohort study. *Complementary Therapies in Medicine*, 16: 22–27.

Sekhar, M. S., Aneesh, T. P., Varghese, K. J., Vasudaven, D. T., Deepa, R., & Revikumar, K. G. (2008). Herbalism: A phenomenon of new age in medicine. *Internet Journal of Pharmacology*, 15312976, 6(1): 1–10. Accessed January 11, 2008, from ContentSelect Research Navigator.

Smith, K. (2008). *Awakening the Energy Body*. Rochester, VT: Bear & Company.

Wauters, A. (2007). *The Homeopathy Bible*. New York: Sterling Publishing Company.

Witt, C. M., Bluth, M., Albrecht, H., Weishuhn, T.E. R., Baumgartner, S., & Willich, S. N. (2007). The in vitro evidence for an effect of high homeopathic potencies—A systematic review of the literature. *Complementary Therapies in Medicine*, 15, 128–138.

Resources

American Institute of Homeopathy
801 N. Fairfax St., Suite 306
Alexandria, VA 22314
888.445.9988
www.homeopathyusa.org

European Council for Classical Homeopathy
School House, Market Place
Kenninghall, Norfolk NR16 2AH, UK
44.1953.888163
www.homeopathy-ecch.org

Hahnemann Center for Heilkunst
13 Mill St.
Manotick ON, Canada, K4M 1A3
613.692.1700
www.homeopathy.com

Homeopathic Educational Services
2124B Kittredge St.
Berkeley, CA 94704
501.649.0294
www.homeopathic.com

The Academy of Veterinary Homeopathy
P.O. Box 9280
Wilmington, DE 19809
866.652.1590
www.theavh.org

10

Naturopathy

It is more important to know what sort of person has a disease than to know what sort of disease a person has.

HIPPOCRATES

If you are distressed by anything external, the pain is not due to the thing itself but to your own estimate of it; and this you have the power to revoke at any moment.

MARCUS AURELIUS

Naturopathic medicine is not only a system of medicine but also a way of life with emphasis on client responsibility, client education, health maintenance, and disease prevention. It may be the model health system of the future with the movement toward healthy lifestyles, healthy diets, and preventive health care.

BACKGROUND

The basic precepts of naturopathy are similar to those in ancient medical systems throughout the world. Naturopathy can trace its philosophical roots to the Hippocratic school of medicine around 400 B.C. Hippocrates had a holistic approach to clients and instructed his students to prescribe only wholesome treatments and avoid causing harm or hurt. Furthermore, Hippocrates thought that the entire universe followed natural laws, and the role of the physician was to understand and support nature's own cures (Backgrounder, 2008).

Naturopathic medicine grew out of the nineteenth-century medical systems of America and Europe. Dr. John Scheel of New

York City coined the term itself in 1895, although it was Benedict Lust who formalized **naturopathy** in 1902 as both a system of medicine and a way of life. By the early 1900s, more than 20 naturopathic schools of medicine were operating in the United States. In the 1920s and 1930s, naturopathic journals encouraged a diet high in fiber and low in red meat, the same type of diet promoted by the National Institutes of Health and the National Cancer Institute in the 1990s. With the development of antibiotics and vaccines in the 1940s and 1950s, the popularity of naturopathy began to decline as people began to rely on these medical breakthroughs. The 1970s saw a renewal in the importance of nutrition, healthy lifestyles, and environmental cleanup programs. This interest continued to grow into what is now the American interest in alternative medicine (Backgrounder, 2008).

PREPARATION

In order for naturopathic medicine to establish itself as a legitimate health care system, it needed to establish accredited schools and conduct credible research. Currently five schools exist in the United States and Canada: Bastyr University in Kenmore, Washington; National College of Naturopathic Medicine in Portland, Oregon; the Southwest College of Naturopathic Medicine and Health Science in Tempe, Arizona; University of Bridgeport College of Naturopathic Medicine in Bridgeport, Connecticut; and the Canadian College of Naturopathic Medicine in North York, Ontario. Two candidate programs awaiting accreditation are Boucher Institute of Naturopathic Medicine in New Westminster, British Columbia, and National University of Health Sciences in Lombard, Illinois. The Council on Naturopathic Medical Education is the accrediting agency for programs in the United States and Canada.

State law determines the scope of naturopathic practice since there is no national licensure for naturopathy. The laws typically allow standard diagnostic procedures, a range of therapies, vaccinations, and limited prescriptive rights. Some states allow the practice of natural childbirth. In states that do not license naturopathic doctors, anyone can call herself/himself a naturopathic doctor after completing some correspondence courses. These individuals may give seminars and advise people on healthy lifestyles, but they are not permitted to diagnose illness or to prescribe treatment. When seeking a naturopathic doctor as a primary care physician, people must ask for verification of graduation from an accredited naturopathic medical school.

The education of naturopathic physicians is extensive and similar to conventional medical education. Four years of medical school follow a college degree in a biological science. The first two years of medical school include courses in anatomy, cell biology, nutrition, physiology, pathology, neurosciences, histology, pharmacology, biostatistics, epidemiology, and public health as well as alternative therapies. Some differences are significant. For example, conventional medical students may have only 4 course hours in nutritional education, while naturopathic medical students have 138 course hours in nutrition. The third and fourth years of medical school are oriented toward clinical experience in diagnosis and treatment. Today's naturopathic doctor is an extensively educated, primary care physician able to utilize a broad range of conventional and alternative therapies.

CONCEPTS

Naturopathic medicine holds the same view of human physiology, bodily functions, and disease processes as conventional medicine. Although many alternative health care professions are defined by the therapies used, naturopathy is defined more by basic concepts.

Healing Power of Nature

It is believed that the body innately knows how to maintain health and heal itself. Natural laws of life operate inside and outside the body, and the physician's job is to support and restore them by using techniques and medicines that are in harmony with the natural processes. These natural methods are geared to strengthen the body's own healing ability. Faith, hope, and beliefs may be the most significant aspects of any treatment. Many studies have documented the ability of the mind to affect the process of disease, either positively or negatively. Physicians consider issues such as "What does it mean, for this person, to be in balance?" and "What are the healing powers available for this person?"

First Do No Harm

Iatrogenic illness, the creation of additional problems from medical treatment, is a major health problem in the United States. Adverse drug reactions appear to be between the fourth and sixth leading cause of death in the United States (Davies, Green, Mottram, & Pirmohamed, 2007). Hospital-acquired infections have become a major problem in the United States.

As Hippocrates said, "Above all else, do no harm." Naturopathic physicians prefer noninvasive treatments that minimize the risk of harmful side effects. Issues considered are "Will a delay in treatment be of benefit?" and "What is the potential for harm with this particular treatment plan?"

Find the Cause

Naturopathic physicians look for the underlying causes of disease and try to help patients eliminate them. These causes are often found in people's lifestyles, habits, and/or diets. Physical, mental, emotional, and spiritual factors are important in determining cause. Issues considered are "What are the causative factors contributing to 'disease' in this person? Of these causative factors, which are avoidable or preventable? What are the limiting factors in this person's life?"

Physician as Teacher

The word *doctor* comes from the Latin *docere*, meaning "to teach." Unlike many conventional medical physicians who have little time to teach, the primary focus of naturopathic physicians is teaching people how to achieve health and avoid disease. The emphasis is on people learning to assume responsibility for themselves and their well-being. A growing awareness among consumers views good health as dependent to a great extent on treating the body properly. Consumers are looking for health care practitioners who can teach them how to treat all aspects in a healthy manner, and naturopathic physicians are an appropriate choice for many. Issues to be considered include "What type of patient education is the physician providing?" and "In what ways does the physician encourage and support patient responsibility?"

VIEW OF HEALTH AND ILLNESS

Naturopathy views health as more than the absence of disease. Health is a dynamic process that allows people to thrive despite various internal and external stresses. Health arises from a complex interaction of physical, mental, emotional, spiritual, dietary, genetic, environmental, lifestyle, and other components. Health is characterized by positive emotions, thoughts, and actions. Healthy people are energetic and creative as they live goal-directed lives. Health does not come from doctors, pills, or surgery, but rather from people's own efforts to take appropriate care of themselves.

Naturopathic physicians recognize the role of bacteria and viruses in illness but view these as secondary factors. They believe that most disease is the direct result of ignoring natural laws. These violations include eating processed foods, having little exercise and rest, living a fast-paced lifestyle, focusing on negative thoughts and emotions, and being exposed to environmental toxins. Disease-promoting habits lead people away from optimal function toward progressively greater dysfunction in body, mind, and spirit. Naturopathy recognizes that death is inevitable, but believes progressive disability is often avoidable.

DIAGNOSTIC METHODS

Naturopathic physicians practice as primary care providers. They see people of all ages suffering from all types of disorders and diseases. They make conventional medical diagnoses using standard diagnostic procedures such as physical examinations, laboratory tests, and radiology. They also perform a detailed assessment of lifestyle, looking for physical, emotional, dietary, genetic, environmental, and family dynamics contributing to a disorder. Since health or disease is a complex interaction of factors, naturopathic physicians treat the whole person, taking all these elements into account. Careful attention to each person's individuality and susceptibility to disease is critical to accurate diagnosis. When necessary, naturopathic physicians, like family practice physicians, refer patients to other health care professionals for hospitalization, surgery, or other specialized care.

TREATMENT

Naturopathic physicians do not provide emergency care, nor do they do major surgery. They rarely prescribe drugs and they treat clients in private practice and outpatient clinics, not in hospitals. Some physicians practice natural childbirth at home or in a clinic.

The therapeutic approach of the naturopathic doctor is to help people heal themselves and to use opportunities to guide and educate people in developing healthier lifestyles. The goal of treatment is the restoration of health and normal body function, rather than the application of a particular therapy. Virtually every natural medical therapy is utilized, most of which are described in this text. Physicians mix and match different approaches, customizing treatment for each person. The least invasive intervention to support the body's natural healing processes is a primary consideration. These interventions include dietetics, therapeutic nutrition, herbs (European, Native American, and Chinese), physical therapy, spinal manipulation, acupuncture, lifestyle counseling, stress management, exercise therapy, homeopathy, and hydrotherapy.

Counseling is an important intervention because mental, emotional, and spiritual factors are part of the holistic approach. Lifestyle modification is crucial to the success of naturopathy. While it is relatively easy to tell a person to stop smoking, get more exercise, and reduce stress, such lifestyle changes are often difficult for people to make. The naturopathic physician is educated to assist people in making the needed changes. This process involves helping people acknowledge the need to change habits; identifying reinforcers for unhealthy habits; setting realistic and progressive goals; establishing a support group of family, friends, and others with similar difficulties; and giving people positive recognition for their gains (Backgrounder, 2008).

RESEARCH

The American Association of Naturopathic Physicians publishes the *Journal of Naturopathic Medicine*, which includes articles on original research, research reviews, and news and review articles relating to naturopathic medicine. Naturopathic schools of medicine have active research departments investigating a number of healing therapies. Because treatment programs are individually designed, it is nearly impossible to compare naturopathic medicine with conventional medicine; simply too many variables are involved. Scientific research in particular therapies has been conducted in China, India, Germany, France, and England. In the United States, substantial scientific information is readily available on the effectiveness of diet and lifestyle in modifying the risk of severe illness such as heart disease and cancer. Hundreds of scientific papers address diet, nutritional supplements, herbs, exercise, and acupuncture. Some of the other natural healing therapies have not been fully investigated from the Western scientific perspective. The National Institutes of Health is conducting 12 clinical trials involving naturopathic medicine. It may be many years before science is sophisticated enough to understand some of these therapies.

INTEGRATED NURSING PRACTICE

Interestingly, the bond between nursing and naturopathy is demonstrated by the enrollment in U.S. naturopathic colleges of medicine; one third of the students are nurses who have chosen this path to continue their post-baccalaureate education. The profession of nursing, like naturopathy, has traditionally embraced the concept of the healing power of nature and the belief that the locus of restoring health is within each person and cannot be "given" to a client by health care practitioners. Drugs, herbs, procedures, surgeries, or mind–body techniques may be helpful or necessary, but by themselves do not cure disease. People must, and do, rebalance and repair themselves. The profession of nursing was founded on this philosophy and view of life as noted by Florence Nightingale's (1969) basic premise that healing is a function of nature that comes from within the individual. She saw the role of the nurse as putting the "patient in the best condition for nature to act on him."

Nursing has always focused on education of those who have been entrusted to our care. We believe that through education we empower others by providing the knowledge, skills, and support to tap into their inner wisdom and make healthy decisions for themselves. This concept is basic to the practice of nursing and is evidenced in the American Nurses Association's Standard of Nursing Practice where health teaching is one of the standards. The goal of nursing, as in naturopathy, is one of healing and, if possible, the restoration of health.

Because nurses spend so much more time with clients than do physicians, we are often in position to prevent or respond quickly to iatrogenic illnesses. To this end, it is critically important that we monitor closely the impact of medications on the recipients. We must know the physiological action, expected effects, side effects, and adverse effects of every medication we administer. We must assess and reassess clients who are receiving medications. Likewise, we must understand procedures and their potential problems for all clients in our care. It is up to each one of us to maintain clinical skills through self-study and continuing education.

TRY THIS

Visualization

Visualization is one of the many interventions used by nurses. This visualization is called "Winched up the Hill." Next time you are faced with a hill to ascend, imagine a winch at the top and a chord from it to your solar plexus. Invite the winch to draw you upward, easily and effortlessly. At first it may make little difference, but keep practicing the visualization at every opportunity until you train yourself to tune into this extra source of energy.

Source: Rutherford, L. (1996). *Principles of Shamanism.* San Francisco: Thorsons.

References

Backgrounder. (2008). An introduction to naturopathy. http://nccam.nih.gov/health/naturopathy. Accessed July 26, 2008.

Davies, E. C., Green, C. F., Mottram, D. R., & Pirmohamed, M. (2007). Adverse drug reactions in hospitals. *Current Drug Safety*, 2(1): 79–87.

Nightingale, F. (1969). *Notes on Nursing*. New York: Dover Press.

Rutherford, L. (1996). *Principles of Shamanism*. San Francisco: Thorsons.

Resources

American Association of Naturopathic
   Physicians
4435 Wisconsin Ave., NW, Suite 403
Washington, DC 20016
866.538.2267
www.naturopathic.org

British Naturopathic and Osteopathic
   Association
3 Park Terrace
Manor Rd.
Luton, Bedfordshire LU1 3HN, UK
01582.488.455
www.osteopathy.org

Manual Healing Methods

The time will come when, after harnessing the winds, the tides, and gravitation, we shall harness for God the energies of Love. And on that day, for the second time in the history of the world, man (humankind) will have discovered fire.

TEILHARD DE CHARDIN

11

Chiropractic

All things are connected.
Whatever befalls the earth
befalls the sons of the earth.
Man did not weave the
web of life.
He is merely a strand in it.
Whatever he does to the web
He does to himself.

CHIEF SEATTLE, upon surrendering
his tribal lands in 1856

The word **chiropractic** comes from two Greek words, *cheir* (hand) and *praktikos* (practical), which were combined to mean "done by hand." Chiropractic, by numbers of practitioners, is the third largest independent health profession in the United States, following conventional medicine and dentistry. It is also the most frequently used form of alternative medicine. Chiropractors are primary health care providers, licensed both for diagnosis and treatment. The practice is limited by procedure (manipulation of the spine) and excludes surgery and prescription medications.

BACKGROUND

Manipulation, as a healing technique, was practiced long before chiropractic. Chinese artifacts as early as 2700 B.C. describe manipulation of the spine. In 1500 B.C., the Greeks gave written instructions on how to manipulate the lumbar spine for back care. Hippocrates, born about 460 B.C. and called the "father of medicine," used spinal manipulation to reposition vertebrae and cure a variety of dysfunctions. Galen, born about A.D. 130, a Greek physician, anatomist, and physiologist, also used manipulation and reported the cure of a patient's hand weakness and numbness through manipulation of the seventh cervical vertebra. Hippocrates and Galen helped form the foundation of Renaissance medicine, during which manipulative healers were known as "bone-setters." The "father of surgery," Ambroise Pare, born about A.D. 1517, incorporated manipulation into his treatment of patients. In the centuries that followed, manipulative techniques were passed down from generation to generation, often within families (Lenarz, 2003).

Daniel David Palmer, a self-educated American healer, founded chiropractic in 1895. Palmer administered the first chiropractic adjustment to Harvey Lillard, a janitor who had gone deaf 17 years earlier while stooping in a mine. Palmer found what he called a misaligned vertebra, which he manipulated, allowing Lillard to stand up straight, free of back pain, and with his hearing restored. Within two years of this discovery, Palmer founded his Chiropractic School and Cure while at the same time developing the underlying concepts. In 1906, a split in the profession occurred that still exists today. Several faculty members, including John Howard, left Palmer College because of significant differences with Palmer's son, B. J. Palmer. B. J. Palmer believed that spinal subluxation or misalignment of the spinal vertebrae was the cause of all disease, whereas Howard believed that additional causes were generally present. Howard opened his National School of Chiropractic around a broad-based and scientific educational curriculum. To this day, those who follow Palmer's path are called "straight" chiropractors, while those who follow the Howard model are called "mixer" chiropractors (Theberge, 2008).

PREPARATION

Chiropractors are licensed in all states of the United States as well as in many other countries. The 15 American chiropractic colleges graduate more than 2,800 chiropractors each year. Colleges also exist in Canada, Australia, England, France, and Japan. Chiropractic education requires at least 90 undergraduate credit hours, including many in the basic sciences. Chiropractic college is a five-year program that includes courses in anatomy, physiology, pathology, and diagnosis, as well as spinal adjusting, nutrition, physical therapy, and rehabilitation. Programs for a doctor of chiropractic (DC) degree require 4,820 hours of education compared with 4,670 hours for doctor of medicine (MD) degree programs. Educational standards in the United States are supervised by a government-recognized accrediting agency, the Council of Chiropractic Education (NCCAM, 2008).

Chiropractors practice in more than 60 countries and function almost entirely in free-standing private practices. Some continue their education with postdoctoral training in specialty areas such as radiology, orthopedics, neurology, behavioral medicine, family practice, occupational health, and sports medicine. The majority of states have mandated health insurance coverage for chiropractic treatment.

CONCEPTS

Anatomy

The **craniosacral system** is composed of the brain and spinal cord, the cerebrospinal fluid, the meninges, and the bones of the spine and skull. The adult vertebral column is composed of seven cervical, twelve thoracic, five lumbar, one sacral, and one coccygeal vertebrae. The vertebrae provide attachment for various muscles and protection for the spinal cord and are separated by intervertebral disks. Several curves in the vertebral column increase its strength. The spinal cord, housed in the vertebral canal, conducts sensory and motor impulses to and from the brain and controls many reflexes. Thirty-one pairs of spinal nerves originate from the cord: eight cervical, twelve thoracic, five lumbar, five sacral, and one coccygeal.

The vertebrae, with the exception of the first and second cervical, are much alike and are composed of a body, an arch, and seven projections called *processes* (see Figure 11.1). The two processes at the top are the superior articular processes, and the two at the bottom are the interior articular processes; these four processes are of particular interest to the chiropractic physician. At the end of each of these processes is a facet, which, like the facet of a diamond, is smooth and capped with cartilage to allow for friction-free movement. The two superior articular processes from each vertebra join with the two inferior articular processes of the vertebra above. The resulting structure is called a *facet joint*, which is encased in a strong, fibrous joint capsule that prevents the joint from coming apart. The other anatomical feature that is of concern to chiropractic is the sacroiliac joint, which is formed where the sacrum attaches to the ilia.

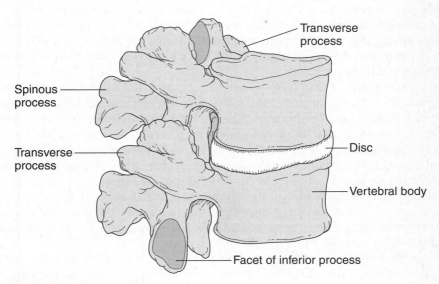

FIGURE 11.1 The Vertebrae

Assumptions

Chiropractic practitioners believe that the body possesses a unique internal wisdom that continually strives to maintain a state of health within the body. This body wisdom means that every person has an innate healing potential. Accessing this internal healing system is the goal of the healing arts. In addition, it is believed that a balanced, natural diet and regular exercise are essential to proper bodily function and good health. The assumptions of chiropractic are as follows (Lenarz, 2003):

- Structure and function exist in intimate relation with one another.
- Structural distortions can cause functional abnormalities.
- The vertebral subluxation is a significant form of structural distortion and leads to a variety of functional abnormalities.
- The nervous system plays a prominent role in the restoration and maintenance of proper bodily function.
- Subluxation influences bodily function primarily through neurologic means.
- Chiropractic adjustment is a specific and definitive method for the correction of vertebral subluxation.

Chiropractic addresses the application of this knowledge to diagnose and treat structural dysfunctions that affect the nervous system. Since the nervous system is highly developed in humans, it influences all other systems in the body, thereby playing a significant role in health and disease.

VIEW OF HEALTH AND ILLNESS

Chiropractic practitioners believe that health is a state of balance, especially of the nervous and musculoskeletal systems. When the spine is fully aligned, nerve energy flows freely to every cell and organ in the body. This free flow of energy nurtures the innate ability of the body to work effectively and coordinate normal body functions.

Traditionally, chiropractic viewed illness and disease as caused by misalignment of the spinal vertebrae, referred to as **vertebral subluxation,** leading to irritation and dysfunction of nerves and blood vessels. The disrupted flow of impulses was thought to interfere with normal muscle function, respiration, heartbeat, arterial tone, digestion, and resistance to disease. A more recent theory is that of **intervertebral motion dysfunction.** This motion theory contends that loss of mobility in the facet joints (see Figure 11.2), rather than misalignment, is the key factor in the concept of subluxation. Subluxation can be caused by just about anything—falls, injuries, genetic spinal weaknesses, improper sleeping habits, poor posture, obesity, stress, and occupational hazards ((NCCAM, 2008; Upledger, 2008).

Although this "one cause" philosophy has been a central concept in chiropractic history, few chiropractors today would endorse this simplistic formulation of illness. They recognize the existence of bacteria and viruses in

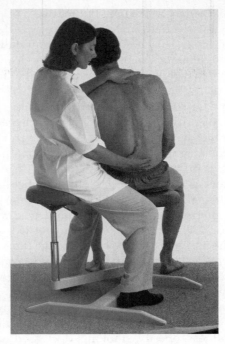

FIGURE 11.2 Practitioner uses her hands to discover which spinal joints are moving freely and which joints are stiff.

Source: Dorling Kindersley Media Library/Andy Crawford

creating disease, especially in a susceptible person. Susceptibility depends on many factors, one of which is spinal misalignment. Although it now embraces a multifactoral explanation of disease, the chiropractic treatment of choice is spinal adjustment. The biomechanical explanation states that range of motion is improved when fibrous adhesions within joints are broken or small tags from the joint capsule are released through manipulation. The neurophysiologic explanation proposes that mechanoreceptors in the joint are stimulated through manipulation, resulting in a relaxation of the paraspinal muscles (Upledger, 2008).

DIAGNOSTIC METHODS

Ninety percent of those seeking chiropractic services have neuromusculoskeletal symptoms or disorders, primarily back pain, neck pain, and headaches. The central focus of chiropractic diagnosis is the determination of when and where **spinal manual therapy** (SMT) is appropriate. The diagnostic process also determines what type of adjustment would be most appropriate. Unlike conventional medicine, which typically assumes that the site of a pain is the site of its cause, chiropractors evaluate the site of pain in a regional and whole-body context. Joint pain in the upper extremities, for example, can be caused by injury or pathology in the joint but may also originate from cervical spine dysfunction. Similarly, the source of joint pain in the lower extremities can be in the lumbar spine. The chiropractic assumption is that the source of the pain should be sought along the path of the nerves leading to and from the site of the symptoms. This whole-body approach is a hallmark of chiropractic (Theberge, 2008).

The process for assessing a client is much the same as that followed by any other physician or nurse practitioner. The chiropractor may spend as much as 60 to 90 minutes with a new client, examining, explaining the results of the examination, the diagnosis, and the proposed treatment plan. The quality of the relationship is primary to chiropractic.

A detailed history is the first step in chiropractic diagnosis. The chiropractor asks about the pattern and quality of the pain and its chronology. Is the pain constant or intermittent? Is the pain a dull ache, a nagging sensation, or a burning sensation? What causes the pain to get worse? What causes the pain to get better? The answers to these types of questions are key to the diagnostic process. The physical examination includes postural assessment, range-of-motion studies, inspection and palpation of affected areas, muscle strength testing, and neurological screening.

A number of back pain risk factors are critical to diagnosis and are consistently assessed by the physician. *Individual factors* contributing to back pain include older age, tallness, obesity, smoking, decreased muscle strength, decreased flexibility, lack of physical conditioning, and multiple pregnancies. Other health conditions are considered, such as osteoporosis, multiple myeloma, osteoarthritis, scoliosis, and ruptured disk. *Psychological factors* include the person's levels of anxiety, stress, and pain tolerance. *Occupational risk factors* for back pain include heavy physical work; frequent bending, twisting, lifting, pushing, pulling; repetitive strain; and injury or accidents. *Recreational risk factors* include hockey, football, gymnastics, golf, racquetball, bowling, squash, handball, tennis, backpacking, wrestling, skiing, and other high-impact sports. All applicable risk factors are noted during the history (Upledger, 2008).

The chiropractic physician relies heavily on hands-on procedures using palpation to determine both structural and functional problems. These hands-on procedures are complemented by a neurological physical examination. It is the same neurological assessment done by a conventional physician. Following the neurological evaluation is the motion palpation exam in which the chiropractor physically examines the spine, noting how it feels as well as how the client says it feels. The client is gently moved into and out of various postures during this part of the exam. Some postures are done standing while others are done lying down. This process often informs the chiropractor what movements or positions reproduce or aggravate the pain. X-rays to confirm diagnostic findings may or may not be done.

Hypermobility of spinal joints is diagnosed by the sound of a repeated click when a joint is moved through its normal range of motion. This unstable type of subluxation is related to flaccid ligaments and is more problematic than the fixated type of subluxation. Hypermobile joints should not be forcibly manipulated since manipulation can move the joint beyond the safe range of motion and increase the degree of hypermobility. Rather, nearby joints that have become fixated to compensate for the unstable joint can be manipulated, and muscle strength and tone can be increased with exercise (Upledger, 2008).

The chiropractor rules out pathologies that are contraindicative to SMT. For example, advanced, degenerative joint disease would rule out all forms of SMT that use significant force on the joint. Chiropractic treatment is not appropriate in the case of spinal infections, fractures, or tumors, which fortunately are fairly rare. In addition, SMT is not done on a woman in late pregnancy or on people whose pain is increased with manipulation. Diagnosis determines appropriate chiropractic treatment, referral for appropriate conventional medical care, or concurrent care.

TREATMENT

Three primary clinical goals guide chiropractic intervention. The *first clinical goal* is to reduce or eliminate people's pain. Typically this goal is the client's primary—and often only—goal. The *second clinical goal* is to correct the subluxation, thereby restoring biomechanical balance to reestablish shock absorption, leverage, and range of motion. In addition, muscles and ligaments are strengthened by spinal rehabilitative exercises to increase resistance to further injury. The *third clinical goal* is preventive maintenance to ensure the problem does not recur. This goal is comparable to the idea of having teeth cleaned periodically to prevent decay. Maintenance intervals vary from person to person depending on lifestyle.

Back pain is a leading cause of disability and the second most common reason (after the common cold) people visit a doctor. Chiropractors have two times the number of visits for back pain as conventional physicians. Most chiropractors also treat peripheral joints—elbows, knees, and shoulders. In 1994, a panel for the Agency for Health Care Policy and Research of the U.S. Department of Health and Human Services concluded that spinal manual therapy speeds recovery from acute low back pain and recommended it either in combination with or as a replacement for nonsteroidal anti-inflammatory drugs. At the same time, the panel rejected many methods used for years by conventional medicine such as bed rest, traction, and various other physical therapy modalities and cautioned against spinal surgery except in the most severe cases (Theberge, 2008). **Spinal manipulation** is an assisted (chiropractor) passive (client) motion applied to the spinal facet joints or the sacroiliac joints. Chiropractors use their hands to apply pressure in specific location and direction. The skill lies in the ability to be specific about which joint is being manipulated, which is especially important in the presence of any unstable joints. A chiropractor has 10 to 20 different ways of manipulating every movable joint in the body. Chiropractors also practice soft-tissue manipulation to stretch contracted muscles and decrease muscle spasms.

High-velocity, low-amplitude (HVLA) thrust adjustment is the most common form of manipulation. It is performed by manually moving a joint to the end point of its normal range of motion, isolating it by local pressure on bony prominences, and then giving a swift, specific, low-amplitude thrust. Often a series of these thrusts are applied to the back and neck. When the facet joints are forced apart, a small vacuum is created and then released, which creates a popping sound much like people cracking their knuckles. This manipulation does not cause pain, though people may feel a little discomfort the next day due to rebalancing of the contracted muscles. This sensation can be compared to muscular soreness at the beginning of a weight training program. HVLA is *absolutely contraindicated* in malignancies, bone and joint infections, acute myelopathy, acute fractures and dislocations, acute rheumatoid or rheumatoid-like joint pathology, and unstable joints. Adverse effects with cervical adjustment may be more serious such as disk injury, vertebrobasilar infarction, or vertebral fracture. Other adjusting methods include low-velocity thrust adjustment with mechanically assisted drop-piece tables, various light touch techniques, ultrasound, and electrical muscle stimulation (Lenarz, 2003).

Network chiropractic spinal analysis blends chiropractic and energy field principles. This approach assesses two types of subluxations: structural, involving the joint facets, and soft tissue involving tension in the muscles and other soft tissue connected to the spine. Network chiropractors treat the soft-tissue subluxations with energy techniques before the structural subluxations are corrected with manipulation. Similar to network chiropractic is **Bio-Energic Synchronization Technique** (BEST). Chiropractors using BEST look at the part of the body responsible for misalignment of the spine and use energy balancing to treat the malfunction (Morter Health System, 2008).

Craniosacral therapy involves manipulation of the sutures in the skull, resulting in decreased cerebrospinal fluid pressure and increased mobility of the cranial bones. Stimulating nerve endings in the scalp triggers the nervous system to turn off stress signals. The goal of craniosacral therapy is to reestablish structural stability and improve neurologic function. It is used to treat problems of the brain and spinal cord such as chronic pain, headache, temporomandibular joint (TMJ) syndrome, stroke, epilepsy, cerebral palsy, dizziness, and tinnitus. Craniosacral therapy is rapidly gaining acceptance in Western medicine. In addition to chiropractors, nurses, physicians, dentists, and physical therapists are incorporating craniosacral techniques into their practice (Mann et al., 2008).

As holistic practitioners, chiropractors work with many facets of clients' lifestyles. Nutrition education is provided, exercise programs are designed, rehabilitation measures are planned, correct posture and lifting techniques are explained, and activities of daily living are assessed and improved. Conditions commonly seen by a chiropractor include the following:

- Lower back syndromes
- Mid-back conditions

- Neck syndromes
- Headaches
- Carpal tunnel syndrome
- Sciatica
- Muscle spasms
- Sports-related injuries
- Whiplash and accident-related injuries
- Arthritic conditions
- Shoulder conditions
- Torticolis
- Extremity trauma

RESEARCH

Procedures have been researched since the early days of chiropractic, though researchers frequently had difficulty in finding a source for publication. Today the *Journal of Manipulative and Physiological Therapeutics* and *Spine* publish much of the chiropractic-related research, and increasingly more chiropractic studies are reported each year in conventional medical journals. The most significant research in the 1980s and 1990s was done outside the United States. The quality and quantity of chiropractic research in the United States is beginning to change, however, as chiropractors become more accepted by biomedical physicians. Professional groups such as the American Back Society, the North American Spine Society, the International Society for the Study of the Lumbar Spine, and the American Public Health Association all accept chiropractic physicians as full members.

The National Institutes of Health has funded 84 clinical trials for chiropractic. These include studies on balance, posture, back pain, knee pain, neck pain, headaches, arthritis, insomnia, and tobacco use cessation (www.clinicaltrials.gov). A sampling of studies has demonstrated the short-term and long-term benefits of chiropractic:

- In a double-blind, placebo-controlled study, 25 individuals with Stage 1 hypertension who received manipulation of the Atlas vertebra (C1) had a significant reduction in both their systolic and diastolic readings (Bakris et al., 2007).
- A randomized, controlled trial compared pain clinic management with chiropractic treatment for individuals with chronic low-back pain. The chiropractic group demonstrated highly significant improvements in disability scores (Wilkey, Gregory, Byfield, & McCarthy, 2008).
- A systematic review of the entire clinical encounter of chiropractic care found that it benefited clients with asthma, cervicogenic vertigo, and infantile colic. Promising benefit was evidenced in children with otitis media and elderly people with pneumonia (Hawk, Khorsan, Lisi, Ferrance, & Evans, 2007).

- A systematic review of psychological response in spinal manipulation found that there was some evidence that spinal manipulation improved psychological outcomes compared with verbal interventions (Williams et al., 2007).

Chiropractic researchers are now looking at the effectiveness in organic or somatovisceral disorders. With the atmosphere of growing medical–chiropractic cooperation and new federal funding of studies comes the anticipation of more widely disseminated research findings.

INTEGRATED NURSING PRACTICE

Observing a client's posture and gait is a key component of basic nursing assessment. Normally, people's posture should be erect and at ease with the shoulders level and straight. Movements should be smooth and relaxed. A normal walk is rhythmic, in a straight, upright position with the arms swinging naturally at each side. General nursing assessment data provided by the client includes the following:

- Description of current mobility, mobility 2 months ago, and mobility 2 years ago
- Description of changes in the ability to walk, sit, or stand
- History of injuries and treatments
- Description of daily exercise routine
- List of sport activities
- Description of repetitive movements related to work or other activities

During a nursing assessment, clients are asked to walk across the room and back as you observe for any difficulties with gait or posture that require further evaluation. An older client's gait may include short, shuffling, uncertain, and sometimes unsteady steps with a decreased arm swing. As people age, they often develop slumped shoulders and a more stooped body posture. Pregnant women often experience changes in body posture and gait as their pregnancy advances. The pelvis tips forward, increasing the lumbosacral curve, creating a gradual lordosis—an exaggerated lumbar curve in the spine. The enlarging breasts may pull the shoulders forward, contributing to a stooped body posture. As the pelvic joints relax and the weight and size of the fetus increase, the woman's center of gravity, stance, and gait are altered, contributing to the common complaint of backaches.

As a nurse, you can intervene to help with minor difficulties of gait and posture. Teach people to warm up and stretch before exercising and cool down and stretch upon completion. Many people can participate in low-impact aerobic activity that does not stress muscles and joints, such as walking, swimming, dancing, weight training, and bicycling. Other activities you can encourage are yoga, t'ai chi, and qigong, which are presented in other chapters in this text. Help people become aware of problems they are experiencing in posture, and encourage them to walk and sit "straight, tall, and relaxed." Good standing posture is with one's feet facing forward, knees slightly flexed, chest up, shoulders back, and chin parallel to the floor. Good sitting posture includes feet flat on the floor with knees, ankles, and hips at right angles, and chin parallel to the floor.

Nursing practice and chiropractic medicine support the belief that prevention of injuries is preferred over treatment of injuries. Many nursing activities such as lifting, transferring, or positioning clients require muscle exertion by the nurse. To reduce the risk of injury to your clients and yourself, practice proper body mechanics. The coordinated motion of the body depends on the integrated functioning of bones, joints, muscles, and the nervous system. You achieve better body balance from a wide base of support created by separating your feet to a comfortable distance. Bending your knees and flexing your hips, thus bringing the center of gravity closer to your support base, will also improve your balance. When you are lifting an object or person, use your legs to lift and your arms to support. Facing the direction of movement and pivoting with your feet prevents abnormal twisting of the spine. Balancing activity between arms and legs protects the back from strain.

A referral to chiropractic evaluation and treatment is appropriate for the conditions listed earlier in the chapter. Chiropractors view themselves as contributing members of the health care team and refer to conventional physicians for problems outside their scope of practice. Although chiropractors have clear guidelines for referring to conventional practitioners, biomedical professionals have not developed formal guidelines for referring to chiropractors. It is time for communication and cooperation to be broadened between conventional practitioners and chiropractors in an effort to create the most effective health care system for the greatest number of people.

TRY THIS

Energy Boosters

Poor posture robs your body of energy. You may spend many hours of your day walking incorrectly or slumped in a chair, which interrupts the flow of energy and oxygen through your body and spinal cord. Take a moment to sit up or stand straight. Imagine that a cord is attached to the top of your head, pulling it gently toward the sky. This image helps readjust your posture. Feel your head, neck, shoulders, and spine relax as they realign from a constricting position. This imagery, practiced either sitting or standing, will revive you.

Take your shoes off; sit on the floor with your legs stretched out in front of you and your palms facing down at your sides. Point your toes as hard as you can and hold for 5 seconds, then flex your feet as hard as you can and hold for 5 seconds. Repeat 10 times.

References

Bakris, G., Dickholtz, M., Sr., Meyer, P. M., Kravitz, G., Avery, E., Miller, M., et al. (2007). Atlas vertebra realignment and achievement of arterial pressure goal in hypertensive patients. *Journal of Human Hypertension*, 21(5): 347–352.

Hawk, C., Khorsan, R., Lisi, A. J., Ferrance, R. J., & Evans, M. W. (2007). Chiropractic care for nonmusculoskeletal conditions: A systematic review with implications for whole systems research. *Journal of Alternative and Complementary Medicine*, 13(5): 491–512.

Lenarz, M. (2003). *The Chiropractic Way*. New York: Bantam Books.

Mann, J. D., Faurot, K. R., Wilkinson, L., Curtis, P., Coeytaux, R. R., Suchindran, C., et al. (2008). Craniosacral therapy for migraine: Protocol development for an exploratory controlled clinical trial. *BMC Complementary and Alternative Medicine*, 8: 8–28.

Morter Health System. www.morter.com/morter.php. Accessed September 14, 2008.

National Center for Complementary and Alternative Medicine. (2008). An introduction to chiropractic. http://nccam.nih.gov/health/chiropractic/. Accessed July 26, 2008.

Theberge, N. (2008). The integration of chiropractors into health care teams. *Sociology of Health and Illness*, 30(1): 19–34.

Upledger, J. E. (2008). *Cranio Sacral Therapy*. Berkeley, CA: North Atlantic Books.

Wilkey, A., Gregory, M., Byfield, D., & McCarthy, P. W. (2008). A comparison between chiropractic management and pain clinic management for chronic low-back pain in a National Health Service outpatient clinic. *The Journal of Alternative and Complementary Medicine*, 14(5): 465–473.

Williams, N. H., Hendry, M., Lewis, R., Russell, I., Westmoreland, A., & Wilkinson, C. (2007). Psychological response in spinal manipulation (PRISM): A systematic review of psychological outcomes in randomized controlled trials. *Complementary Therapies in Medicine*, 15: 271–283. www.clinicaltrials.gov. Accessed on September 14, 2008.

Resources

American Chiropractic Association
1701 Clarendon Blvd.
Arlington, VA 22209
703.276.8800
www.acatoday.org

British Chiropractic Association
59 Castle St.
Reading, Berkshire Rg1 7SN, UK
0118.950.5950
www.chiropractic-uk.co.uk

Canadian Chiropractic Association
600-30 St. Patrick St.
Toronto, ON, Canada, M5T 3A3
877.222.9303
www.ccachiro.org

Chiropractors' Association of Australia
2/36 Woodriff St., Penrith NSW 2750
P.O. Box 335
Penrith N 2751
1800.075.003
http://chiropractors.asn.au

Federation of Chiropractic Licensing Boards
5401 West 10th St., Suite 101
Greeley, CO 80634-4400
970.356.3500
www.fclb.org

World Chiropractic Alliance
2950 N. Dobson, Suite 3
Chandler, AZ 85224
800.347.1011

12

Massage

What a desire! To live in peace with that world: Myself.

Sylvia Ashton-Warner

Few men (women) during their lifetime come anywhere near exhausting the resources dwelling within them. There are deep wells of strength that are never used.

Richard E. Byrd

Massage therapy, the scientific manipulation of the soft tissues of the body, is a healing art, an act of physical caring, and a way of communicating without words. Massage, a hands-on touch therapy, has reached out to an ever-widening U.S. audience. Massage is the most prevalent complementary therapy offered in hospitals in the United States. The goal of massage therapy is to achieve or increase health and well-being and to help the body heal itself. Although massage therapists may hold general views of health and well-being, massage therapy has no specific theoretical framework or diagnostic system of disease.

Compared with members of other cultures, people in the United States are generally touch-phobic and touch-deprived. Cross-cultural studies have revealed that people in the United States have one of the lowest rates of casual touch in the world. When psychologist Sidney Jourard observed rates of casual touch among couples in cafes, he reported the highest rates in Puerto Rico (180 times per hour) and Paris (110 times per hour) and one of the lowest rates in the United States (2 times per hour). French parents and children touch each other three times more frequently than their U.S. counterparts. French teens demonstrate significantly more casual touching of friends than U.S. adolescents, who are more likely to fiddle with their rings, crack their knuckles, and demonstrate other forms of self-stimulation. Other studies have found that cultures that are more physically affectionate toward infants and children tend to have lower rates of adult violence. In spite of advertising pleas to "reach out and touch someone," the majority of North Americans have precious little physical contact with family members, friends, and co-workers (Field, 1999, 2001).

Concerns have escalated about "inappropriate" touch, sexual abuse, and sexual harassment in schools and workplaces in the United States. Touch, unfortunately, has become associated with sex. Some schools have instituted "teach, but don't touch" policies. It is rare to see teachers put their hands on the shoulder of a child who is crying. Sadly, to protect themselves from being accused of inappropriate touch, many people are not touching at all. While concern for protecting children from those who would touch inappropriately is valid, the implications of a "hands-off" barrier have significant negative effects on growth, development, and emotional well-being.

BACKGROUND

The idea that touch can heal is an old one. Cave paintings in the Pyrenees show that 15,000 years ago people treated injuries with what looks like massage. References to massage are found in 4,000-year-old Chinese medical texts. Hippocrates, in the fourth century B.C. wrote, "The physician must be acquainted with many things and assuredly with rubbing" (the ancient Greek and Roman term for massage). Some of the greatest physicians in history advocated massage, including Celsus (25 B.C.–A.D. 50), Galen (130–200), and Avicenna (980–1037). Ambroise Pare (1517–1590), the "father of surgery"; William Harvey (1578–1657), who demonstrated the circulation of blood; and Herman Boerhaave (1668–1738), who introduced the clinical method of teaching medicine, all utilized massage as a healing technique. Roman gladiators were massaged before entering the arenas, and eighteenth-century Swedish cavalrymen were rubbed down between battles. In the Middle Ages, Christians viewed massage as the work of the devil, and many therapists were burned at the stake as witches. Remnants of this attitude have continued into the twentieth century as massage is sometimes assumed to be a front for prostitution (Hughes, Ladas, Rooney, & Kelly, 2008).

The thirteenth-century German emperor Frederick II was curious to know what language children would speak if they were raised without hearing any words at all. Stealing a number of newborns from their parents, he gave them to nurses who physically cared for the infants but were forbidden to cuddle or talk to them. All the children died before they could talk. The discovery that was made was important: Tactile stimulation can be a matter of life and death. Most recently a similar situation occurred in the early 1990s in Romania when thousands of infants were stockpiled into orphanages. Some were virtually left alone in their cribs for 2 years and were discovered to be severely impaired as a result of this isolation (Colt, 1997).

Two New York physicians who were trained in Sweden introduced massage into the United States in the mid-nineteenth century. The first massage therapy clinics were opened by Swedish physicians after the Civil War and had among their clients members of Congress and Presidents Harrison and Grant. At first physicians performed massage, but they eventually delegated the technique to nurses and physical therapists and by the mid-twentieth century, massage therapy was virtually abandoned by most health care professionals except nurses. For many years, during the time of relatively little technology, it was standard nursing practice to give back rubs after bathing clients, and back rubs were also a routine part of Hour of Sleep Care. Advanced medical technology, sophisticated equipment, and nurses assuming more of a management role left little time for hands-on nursing care. An upsurge of interest in the field began in the 1970s with Dr. Dolores Kreiger and Dr. Martha Rogers, two nurse pioneers who advocated the art and caring form of touch in nursing practice. Nurses are now returning to their tradition in providing comfort and care through the use of touch and massage. Most communities of Catholic sisters have at least one sister trained in massage therapy, and massage is routinely offered at spiritual retreats. These sisters have come to recognize the power for spiritual renewal from physical contact in their healing ministries. If clients choose, they also pray with them. Going beyond what most massage therapists do, they often set aside time after the massage if the client wants to talk about a problem or issue.

In the United States, some insurance companies will pay for massage that has been ordered by a primary health care provider, but it is still considered an alternative or complementary treatment. In many areas of the world massage is an integral part of health systems. In the former Soviet Union, Germany, China, and Japan, massage therapists work along with physicians in the hospital setting as important members of the health care team.

PREPARATION

Therapists who have 500 or more hours of education from a recognized school are eligible to take the National Certification Examination offered by the National Certification Board of Therapeutic Massage and Bodywork. The International Association of Infant Massage further certifies instructors who take four days of training, read course material, and pass a take-home exam.

CONCEPTS

Skin

In many ways, human beings are wired for touch. The skin is the body's largest organ, covering almost 20 square feet and accounting for nearly one-quarter of the body's total weight. As many as five million touch receptors in the skin—3,000 in a fingertip—send messages via the spinal cord to the brain. The skin has four main functions: protection from mechanical and radiation injuries and from invasion by foreign substances; as a sense organ; as a temperature regulator; and as a metabolic organ. Of all the sensory organs, the skin is the most important. People can survive without the senses of sight, sound, smell, and taste, but would find it difficult to survive without the functions performed by the skin.

Touch

Touch is a primal need, as necessary for growth and development as food, clothing, or shelter. The sense of touch is the earliest to develop in the human embryo and at less than six weeks of gestation, a light stroking of the face will cause bending of the neck and trunk away from the source of stimulation. Touch continues to function even after seeing and hearing begin to fade as we age. Touch can be thought of as a nutrient transmitted through the skin in many different ways: holding, cuddling, nuzzling, caressing, and massage. From the bonding of parent and newborn to holding the hand of a dying loved one, touch is the most intimate and powerful form of communication between people. It can be aggressive as in the spanking of a child or a punch in the face. It can be tender as in the hug that comforts a crying friend or the touch of a lover. Even casual touch has an effect. Waitresses who touched their customers on the hand or shoulder as they returned change, for example, received larger tips than those who did not. Politicians act on this knowledge when they reach out to touch potential voters (Moore, 2005).

The importance of the sense of touch is evident in many English expressions. Some people have to be "handled" carefully because they are "thin-skinned" while others are "thick-skinned." "Touchy" people are overly sensitive or easily angered. Some people are "soft touches" and other have "the human touch." Some people "rub" others the wrong way. "Feeling" for another person is a description of empathy. A "touching" experience is something that is deeply felt. As biomedicine continues to make incredible advances in technology, it leaves behind one of the most valuable senses of a human being—that of touch. This sense of isolation may explain, in part, the increasing interest in healing practices, most of which include the experience of touch.

Trigger Points

When a person is injured or bodily systems are malfunctioning, trigger points or pain reflexes appear throughout the body. A trigger point is a "knot" of tensed muscles, which, when stimulated, triggers a referred pain response in other parts of the body. Some of the trigger points are in the area of the injury or problem, while others are at a distance. Rubbing and exerting pressure on these points have been found to have a positive effect on the healing process (Kaye et al., 2008).

Fascia and Fascial Restrictions

The fascia is the tough connective tissue that exists in the body almost like a three-dimensional web from head to foot. If somehow every structure of the body were removed except the fascia, the body would retain its shape. Every muscle, bone, organ, nerve, and blood vessel of the body is covered with fascia like a continuous saran wrapping. It varies in thickness and density and in the amount of collagenous fiber, elastic fiber, and tissue fluid it contains. The function of the fascia is to support cells, muscles, groups of muscles, and organs and act as a shock absorber. At the cellular level, fascia creates the interstitial spaces and is important in cellular respiration, elimination, metabolism, fluid, and lymphatic flow.

Each time a person experiences a trauma, undergoes an inflammatory process, or suffers from poor posture over time, the fascial system becomes restricted and the person loses flexibility and spontaneity of motion. As the fascia continues to slowly tighten, an abnormal pressure develops on the nerves, muscles, bones, or organs, resulting in poor cellular efficiency, necrosis, pain, and dysfunction throughout the body (Kaye et al., 2008).

VIEW OF HEALTH AND ILLNESS

It is believed that massage aids the ability of the body to heal itself and is aimed at achieving or increasing health and well-being. Only now is science beginning to catch up with people when it comes to appreciating the importance—and the power—of touch. The Touch Research Institutes (TRIs) at the University of Miami School of Medicine bring together researchers from Duke, Harvard, Maryland, and other universities to study touch and how it might be used to promote health and treat disease.

Stronger, sustained touch in massage can have an even greater effect than other forms of touch. A skilled massage therapist not only stretches and loosens muscle and connective tissue, but also greatly improves blood flow and the movement of lymph fluid throughout the body. Massage speeds the removal of metabolic waste products resulting from exercise or inactivity, allowing more oxygen and nutrients to reach the cells and tissues. The release of muscular tension also helps to unblock and balance the overall flow of life energy throughout the body known as qi, ki, prana, or subtle energy. In addition, massage can stimulate the release of endorphins, serotonin, dopamine, and oxytocin. The benefits of massage are described in Box 12.1.

As an adjunct to medical treatment, massage may be helpful in relieving backaches, headaches, muscle spasm and pain, hypertension, swelling and pain from injuries or after surgery, grand mal epileptic seizures, insomnia, anxiety, and depression. It can be a palliative treatment for the comfort of those with terminal conditions and can help maintain circulation and muscle tone for bedridden people. Even people in deep comas may show improved heart rates when their hands are held. Most comprehensive cancer treatment programs offer massage as a standard component of care. Massage can reduce agitation in people with Alzheimer's disease, and it has been used to relieve stress at disaster sites.

Massage has been used with individuals who have psychiatric disabilities as an adjunct to conventional psychiatric interventions. Clients are given a chair massage, done with the client fully dressed and seated on a massage

BOX 12.1

The Benefits of Massage

Physical Level

- Relieves muscle tension and stiffness
- Reduces muscle spasm and tension
- Provides relief from pain
- Speeds recovery from exertion
- Improves joint flexibility and range of motion
- Increases ease and efficiency of movement
- Improves posture
- Stimulates lymphatic circulation, which decreases edema
- Improves local circulation, which increases healing of injured tissues
- Lowers blood pressure, slows heart rate
- Promotes deeper, easier breathing
- Eases tension headaches
- Improves the health of the skin

Mental Level

- Induces a relaxed state of alertness
- Reduces mental stress, thus clearing the mind
- Increases capacity for clearer thinking

Emotional Level

- Satisfies the need for caring and nurturing touch
- Increases feelings of well-being, decreases mild depression
- Enhances self-image
- Reduces levels of anxiety
- Increases awareness of mind–body connection

chair. The head, neck, back, arms, and legs are massaged for 10 to 20 minutes per session. Hilliard's (1995) study found that massage was an effective stress reducer for inpatient and outpatient clients who sought safe touch and relaxation resulting in a sense of emotional well-being.

TREATMENT

Touch is the fundamental medium of massage therapy. It is, however, more than just mechanical manipulation. Touch is a form of communication; thus one of its most significant benefits is the comfort of human care conveyed by the therapist. Massage communicates gentleness and connection, trust and receiving, and peace and alertness.

The first massage therapy appointment begins with questions about one's physical condition, medical history, and current aches and pains. The therapist determines what a client hopes to gain from the massage. The client undresses in private and uses a sheet or blanket for draping. The individual decides whether underwear is on or off. The client lies on a cushioned table and the therapist uncovers only that part of the body that is being massaged, using oil or lotion to help the hands move smoothly. It is recommended that clients not eat just before a massage and drink extra water afterward to clear the body of toxins released from deep tissues. At home, clients are encouraged to enjoy a salt bath as another aid in detoxifying the body. One-half cup each of sea salt, Epsom salts, and baking soda is added to a tub of warm water for the salt bath.

From hour-long massages in therapists' offices to ten-minute massages at the workplace, a massage is available for practically every body and budget. Massage therapists offer their services in a wide variety of settings such as private practice clinics, health clubs and fitness centers, chiropractic offices, nursing homes and hospitals, salons and resorts, on site in the workplace, and even in clients' homes. There are almost as many styles of massage as there are practitioners. Most therapists combine a variety of methods in their work, which allows them to tailor each session to the specific needs of the client.

There are minimal side effects when being treated by a massage therapist. In one study of 91 participants, only 10% said that they experienced some minor discomfort, swelling, or bruising after the massage. Twenty three percent experienced unexpected positive changes such as improvement in mood and emotional well-being, digestive function, and respiration (Cambron, Dexheimer, Coe, & Swenson, 2007).

There are, however, some situations in which massage is *contraindicated*:

- Phlebitis/thrombosis
- Severe varicose veins
- Any acute inflammation of the skin, soft tissue, or joints
- Burns
- Areas of hemorrhage or heavy tissue damage
- Unregulated blood pressure
- Febrile state
- Herniated disk
- Recent fractures or sprains
- Advanced osteoporosis
- A bleeding disorder or taking blood-thinning drugs
- Some types of cancer

Swedish Massage

Peter Ling of Sweden, who integrated ancient Asian massage with a Western understanding of anatomy and physiology, developed **Swedish massage** about 150 years ago. It is the most common form of massage in the United

States. Swedish massage uses a system of long gliding strokes, as well as kneading and friction techniques on the more superficial layers of the muscles, combined with active and passive movements of the joints. It is used primarily for a full-body massage to promote general relaxation, improve circulation and range of motion, and relieve muscle tension.

Swedish massage uses five basic strokes. *Effleurage*, French for "touching," is the introductory stroke. The therapist uses the whole hand providing long, gliding strokes relaxing the central nervous system and preparing the local area for the other strokes. *Petrissage* involves grasping muscle groups and lifting them, stretching them away from the bones and then kneading or rolling them. This technique is the closest in imitating exercise because it makes the muscles contract. This stroke is used mostly on flaccid muscles that need to have their contractile ability increased. Petrissage also stimulates the central nervous system and therefore, is not used with clients who have cerebral vascular dysfunctions. *Friction* involves using the fingers and thumbs to press on small areas and move in a circular motion around the area. *Vibration* involves placing the hands on a muscle group and moving them back and forth quickly in a shaking motion. *Tapotement* or *percussion* involves striking the skin with the outside edges of the hands, fingers, or cupped palms to stimulate circulation (Stewart, 2006).

Shiatsu Massage

In Japanese, *shi* means "finger" and *atsu* means "pressure." **Shiatsu massage** is the Japanese adaptation of acupressure. Like Chinese acupuncture and acupressure, shiatsu is based on the idea that life energy, *ki*, flows along invisible pathways called meridians. Health is related to a free flow of energy, and illness is caused by blockages to the flow. Blocked energy can cause physical discomforts, so the aim is to release the blocks associated with the discomfort or disease and rebalance the energy flow. Therapists use their hands, elbows, and even their feet to press for about 30 seconds on each point. Depending on the way it is done, shiatsu can be gentle or quite forceful. Done on a floor mat rather than a massage table, a typical shiatsu session lasts about an hour (Hughes et al., 2008).

Sports Massage

Sports massage uses techniques of Swedish massage and shiatsu massage but focuses on parts of the body that are likely to be stressed by a particular sport. It takes less time than Swedish or Shiatsu and is usually more vigorous. For example, runners might need to have their hamstrings worked extensively. This technique also concentrates on reducing or eliminating factors that interfere with human performance such as muscle spasms, tendonitis, and muscle fatigue.

Prior to the athletic event, massage loosens, warms, and readies the muscle for intensive use, especially when combined with stretching. Besides helping prevent injury, it can improve performance and endurance.

Post-event massage relieves pain, prevents stiffness, and returns the muscles to their normal state more rapidly. The use of massage in sports health care is increasing rapidly in both training and competition. Recreational athletes have also discovered the benefits of sports massage as a regular part of their workouts.

Trigger Point Massage

Trigger point massage is a type of deep massage in which the fingers are used to release knots and tender spots in muscles. Rubbing and exerting pressure on these points has been found to have a positive effect on the healing process by interrupting the cycle of spasm and pain. Techniques are similar to those used in shiatsu but are based on Western anatomy and physiology. Trigger point massage is typically a technique incorporated into Swedish or sports massage.

Myofascial Release

Myofascial release is a whole-body therapy preceded by a comprehensive evaluation and diagnostic workup. The therapist evaluates the fascial system through visual analysis and palpation of tissue and fascial layers. Normal tissue is soft and mobile in all directions. Abnormal tissue may feel hot, hard, sensitive, or somewhat stringy or crunchy. When the therapist has determined where the fascial restrictions lie, gentle pressure is applied in the direction of the restriction, which is designed to break up the collagen of the fascia. Myofascial release is effective in strains and sprains, headaches, chronic pain, temporomandibular joint (TMJ) pain, and adhesions. Myofascial release is contraindicated in malignancy, open wounds, cellulitis, febrile state, hematoma, infection, advanced degenerative changes, acute circulatory conditions, and acute rheumatoid arthritis (Hughes et al., 2008; Riggs, 2007).

Rolfing

Developed by the late biochemist Ida P. Rolf, **Rolfing**® (also known as structural integration) is a system of whole-body manipulation in which the Rolfer uses the fingers, knuckles, and elbows to stretch the fascia, which tends to bind up because of injury, bad posture, emotional problems, or genetic weaknesses. The fascia is stretched to release patterns of tension and rigidity and return the body to a state of correct alignment. Other massage therapists work by applying smooth strokes over muscles; Rolfers press deeply into muscle tissue and fascia to release them. Clients are asked to breathe deeply during the session and visualize the muscle lengthening. The current Rolfing method is more gentle and far less painful than the original style of treatment. Practitioners use a broad range of touch and pressure from feather-light to deep massage. When performed with the right sensitivity, even deep and heavy pressure may not be painful.

Thai Massage

Some people call **Thai massage** "passive yoga," because the receiver is fully clothed, lies on a futon, and is deeply stretched, compressed, and gently rocked. The whole body of the therapist is used to treat the whole body of the receiver. The experience feels like a combination of yoga, shiatsu, and meditation. Point pressure and kneading of the tissues is similar to massage techniques. Yoga techniques involve positioning the client in numerous stretches similar to yoga poses, then gently rocking the person to deepen the stretch and open the joints. The gentle rocking creates an energy flow through the different stretches. Thai massage gives the person the flexibility, inner organ massage, oxygenation of the blood, and quieting of the mind that comes with yoga, but because the receiver is passive, the session becomes meditative. Sometimes the therapist stands on the recipient and gently rolls one foot on and off the body. This compression can be gentle to deep and can energize or relax the recipient.

Chinese Massage

Tui Na is one of the four main branches of Traditional Chinese Medicine, the others being herbs, acupuncture, and qigong. Tui Na is the forerunner of all forms of massage that exist today. It differs from other types of massage in that it is used to treat specific illnesses as well as musculoskeletal problems. A practitioner of Tui Na must be a Traditional Chinese Medicine physician in order to make an accurate diagnosis before instituting treatment. Tui Na is often combined with qigong exercises for building up general health and strength. See Chapter 23 for information on qigong.

Chair Massage

Chair massage is done with the client fully dressed, seated on a portable massage chair. A doughnut-shaped pillow that allows for easy breathing supports the person's face. The sessions, which last 10 to 20 minutes, involve massage of the head, neck, back, arms, and hands. This type of massage is often provided in the workplace, shopping malls, or in airports. The purpose of the massage is to decrease tension, reduce stress, and enhance people's adaptive capabilities.

Pregnancy Massage

Massage is contraindicated until after the first trimester of pregnancy, because of the danger of miscarriage during that time. During the second and third trimesters, massage can ease pain and provide comfort to the pregnant woman. Massage relaxes the woman and reduces the flow of stress hormones to the baby. It also nurtures the woman, which helps her nurture her baby after birth. Pregnancy massage is usually done in a side-lying position with plenty of pillows or cushions for support (see Figure 12.1). The

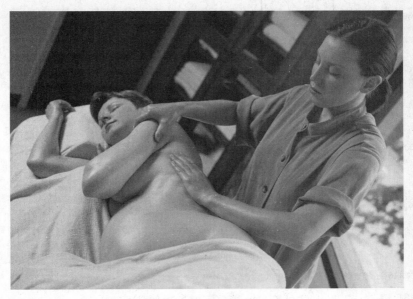

FIGURE 12.1   Pregnant Woman Getting a Massage

Source: Getty Images, Inc.-Photodisc/Steve Mason

massage usually is done to the neck, arms/hands, back, pelvis, and legs/feet. Since not all massage therapists are trained in pregnancy massage, consumers must ask about the experience and/or credentials of a particular therapist.

Infant Massage

Infant massage is gaining in popularity in the United States (see Figure 12.2). Researchers have found that infant massage produces weight gains in premature infants, reduces complications in cocaine babies, and helps depressed mothers soothe their babies. In healthy babies, it improves parent–infant bonding, eases painful procedures such as inoculations, reduces pain from teething and constipation, reduces colic, induces sleep, and makes parents feel good (Moore, 2005).

Self-Massage

Self-massage is a wonderful way for people to better acquaint themselves with their entire bodies. It is a process in which they learn to be aware of and release tensions and inhibitions, to reclaim parts of themselves that have been neglected, and to accept themselves as they are. Self-massage increases one's ability to listen to the body and enhance one's healing journey. Getting to know and appreciate one's body through touch is an important part of self-acceptance. The more in touch people are with themselves, the more they

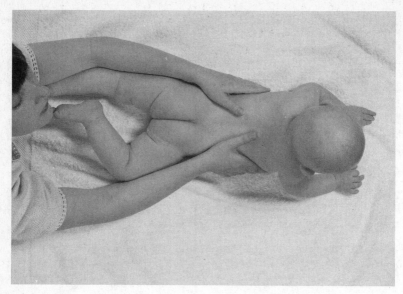

FIGURE 12.2   Baby Boy Having His Back and Side Massaged
Source: Alamy Images/BananaStock

come in touch with the reality and experience of the world around them. Heightened awareness of the unity of body, mind, and spirit often leads to an increased perception of the unity of all nature. As it builds self-confidence and self-acceptance, this awareness enables people to respond with more compassion and caring to others.

Self-massage is done in a warm, comfortable, and quiet environment. Breath work and relaxation techniques are utilized to ground and center before the experience. Self-massage often begins with gazing at oneself naked in a mirror, withholding judgment and criticism. The next step is to stretch like a cat and pay attention to how the body feels. If there is an area that is stiff or tender, the person slowly moves, gently holds, or massages that part. Then the person finds a position that is relaxing and comfortable. Without a set route or sequence, individual senses guide self-massage. At times the whole body may be explored and massaged and at other times people may feel like spending the time on one part, such as the face and head. Self-massage is done slowly and rhythmically with the eyes closed so that all one's attention can be focused on the sensation (Tulku, 2003).

RESEARCH

During the past half-century, numerous reports on clinical trials have been published in health care literature. These reports have documented the benefits of massage therapy for the treatment of pain, inflammation, lymphedema, nausea, muscle spasm, various soft-tissue dysfunctions, grand mal seizures, anxiety, depression, and insomnia. Randomized, controlled trials are somewhat difficult since therapists individualize treatment approaches for each client. Russell, Sumler, Beinhorn, and Frenkel (2008) searched for randomized trials of massage in people with cancer. The six reports that fit the criteria were unable to retain enough subjects to have a statistically adequate sample size. These six reports studied pain relief, anxiety relief, improvements in nausea, or a lessening of depression. A Cochrane Database Systematic Review looked at eight studies of massage therapy. Four trials found a reduction in anxiety and one trial reported a significant improvement in depression (Hughes et al., 2008).

The following is a small sample of the current research:

- Mothers scoring high on the Edinburgh Postnatal Depression Scale at 4 weeks postpartum were randomly assigned to attend baby massage classes or a support group. They completed questionnaires and were filmed interacting with their babies before and after six intervention sessions and at one year. Both intervention groups showed reductions in depression across the study period, but the massage group showed significantly better interactions with their infants (O'Higgins, St James Roberts, & Glover, 2008).
- A study involving 263 volunteers experiencing moderate to severe muscle spasm/muscle strain looked at the effect of deep-tissue massage on blood pressure and heart rate. It was found that following a 45- or 60-minute massage, the average systolic pressure had a reduction of 10.4 mm Hg, a diastolic pressure reduction of 5.3 mm Hg, a mean arterial pressure reduction of 7.0 mm Hg, and an average heart rate reduction of 10.8 beats per minute (Kaye et al., 2008).
- A systematic review of 10 randomized, controlled trials of massage therapy for adults with a diagnosis of cancer found that massage might lessen anxiety, pain, and nausea, but lack of rigorous evidence does not support definitive conclusions (Wilkinson, Barnes, & Storey, 2008).
- A randomized, controlled trial of women undergoing chemotherapy for breast cancer found that massage treatment (20 minutes of massage on five occasions) significantly reduced nausea compared with control treatment (five 20-minute visits) (Billhult, Bergbom, & Stener-Victorin, 2007).
- A randomized study of the effects of massage on well-being and stress perception among older adults found that there was significant improvement in the massage group (50-minute massages twice a week for 4 weeks) compared to the control group (guided relaxation sessions for the same frequency). The massage group demonstrated improvement in anxiety, depression, vitality, general health, and positive well-being on the General Well-being Schedule and the Perceived Stress Scale (Sharpe, Williams, Granner, & Hussey, 2007).

INTEGRATED NURSING PRACTICE

Massage provides a valuable tactile approach, which, when combined with verbal approaches, communicates nurses' care and compassion. Back rubs, lasting 3 to 5 minutes, offer physiological and mechanical benefits to clients in a variety of settings. A back rub is usually given after the bath, but you may also find that one given in the evening will help clients to relax and fall asleep. Massage the back in a slow, rhythmical, and relaxed manner. Tightness through the shoulder and neck muscles from an uncomfortable resting position can be relieved with friction or petrissage. Gently rubbing the skin over bony areas increases circulation and helps prevent skin breakdown. If you are caring for someone who is in bed a great deal of the time, offer massage each time the person's position is changed. Observe for areas of redness, especially over the sacrum and the back of the heels, elbows, and knees. Stroking toward the pressure areas encourages capillary dilatation.

Some people, self-conscious about full-body or even back massage, may accept and benefit from hand and foot massage. Figure 12.3 illustrates the procedure for a hand massage. These same steps can be adapted for a foot massage. By stimulating the circulation, massage eases stiffness and pain in persons with arthritis and helps drain lymph and decrease fluid retention in persons with dependent edema.

Childbirth nurses and *nurse midwives* have long advocated massage during pregnancy. A light, natural oil such as tangerine, almond, or safflower is used, avoiding the addition of any essential oils, which may have ill effects on the fetus. The benefits of massage during pregnancy (Walters, 2002) are as follows:

- *Relaxes.* Massage helps reduce tension in the neck and shoulders and, in the later stages of pregnancy, in the lower back.
- *Uplifts.* Massage minimizes fatigue and improves the flow of energy and induces a general feeling of well-being.
- *Improves circulation.* Massage may help prevent varicose veins that may accompany pregnancy.
- *Stimulates lymphatic drainage.* Massage helps reduce fluid retention in the ankles and feet that often occurs during the later stages of pregnancy.
- *Tones muscles.* Massage helps relieve the pain of distended ligaments and decreases the tendency to cramp that may occur toward the fifth month of pregnancy.
- *Maintains skin tone.* Massage increases the skin's suppleness and elasticity and may help prevent stretch marks.

Midwives and *maternal child nurses* incorporate massage during labor and delivery. During contractions, deep massage of the lower back and hips provides counterpressure that many women find helpful. In between contractions, you can massage the shoulders, back, hands, and feet to increase comfort and relaxation. If contractions are lagging, a light massage of the breasts may stimulate activity. After delivery, gentle heat may be applied to

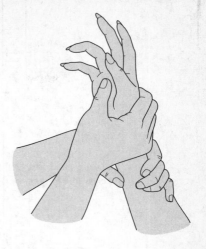

While holding the client's hand, place massage oil or lotion on the hand. Gently bend the hand backward and forward to limber the wrist. Grasp each finger and do range-of-motion exercises.

A

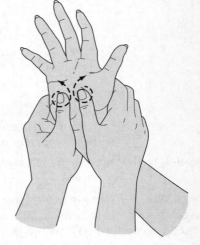

With the client's elbow resting on the table, hold the hand upright and massage the palm of the hand with the cushions of your thumbs, using circular movements in opposite directions.

B

FIGURE 12.3   Procedure for Hand Massage

the breasts followed by a firm massage around the breast toward the nipple to assist in milk letdown.

If you practice nursing in *newborn nurseries* and neonatal intensive care units, you should advocate infant massage and incorporate it as a basic nursing intervention. Most premature and drug-exposed infants given three massages a day are more alert, active, and responsive than nonmassaged infants. Massaged infants are also able to calm themselves, sleep more deeply, and have fewer episodes of apnea.

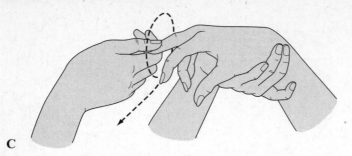

C

Massage each finger from the base to the tip, along all surfaces of the finger.

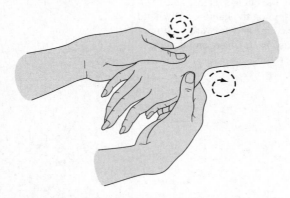

D

Use your thumbs to massage the wrist and top of the hand, using circular movements. Repeat three times. Repeat the entire procedure on the other hand.

FIGURE 12.3 Procedure for Hand Massage (*continued*)

Whether you are massaging a newborn or teaching parents infant massage, the process lasts for as little as a few minutes or as long as a half hour but should be performed only when a baby is willing. If a baby is crying, hiccuping, or turning his head to the side, the massage should be discontinued and tried another time. The oil for infant massage should be a light textured, unscented oil such as almond, coconut, or safflower oil. Infants should not be massaged with synthetic, petroleum-based products because they have no nutritional value and are not absorbed into the skin. The following are some gentle massage strokes for infants:

- *Foot.* Press all over the bottom of the foot using the thumbs.
- *Leg.* Hold the leg like a baseball bat and move the hands up the leg squeezing slightly and turning in opposite directions.
- *Stomach.* Make scooping strokes, one hand following the other.
- *Chest.* Begin with both hands at the center and gently push out to the sides along the rib cage.

- *Back.* With fingers spread apart, "comb" the back from the neck to the buttocks.
- *Hand.* Roll each finger between one's finger and thumb; press gently all over the palm, using the thumbs.
- *Face.* Make small circles around the jaw using the fingertips.

In the *psychiatric* setting, you may integrate executive massages for those clients who wish to use massage as a stress reducer. Debbie Hilliard (1995), a clinical nurse specialist and a certified massage practitioner, has utilized massage for several years with people experiencing persistent mental illness. She found that, while massage was not suitable for all clients, the majority who sought the treatment reported subjective relief from tension, anxiety, and muscle pain. Massage also provides an appropriate way to meet people's basic need for touch.

If you are a *hospice* nurse, an important part of your care might be massage, which often helps manage pain and symptom distress. As well as integrating it into your routine nursing care, it can be taught easily to family members. Touch is a primal need, even during the process of dying. Being able to communicate caring through massage makes the process a little easier for all concerned.

You may wish to expand your expertise in massage by becoming a massage therapist and combining that practice with your practice of nursing. Contact the National Association of Nurse Massage Therapists (see this chapter's Resource section) for appropriate programs.

TRY THIS

Massage

One-Minute Massage

Revive your hair and your spirits with a simple scalp massage you can do anytime and almost anywhere. With your fingertips, rub entire scalp using small circular motions. Massage stimulates the scalp oils that bring out the natural shine in hair. It is also an all-over energy booster.

Two-Minute Massage

Mix a tablespoon each of wheat germ, olive oil, and sunflower oil. Rub on your shoulders and neckline. After two minutes, rinse and pat dry. Lavish damp skin with lotion.

Partner Massage

- Set the mood with scented candles and soft music in a dimly lit room.
- Lay folded quilts on the floor rather than using your bed so you can easily move around your partner.

(continued)

- Remove jewelry to avoid catching hairs as you work.
- Comfort your partner by covering her/him with a sheet and placing a pillow under the knees when lying on the back and under the ankles when lying on the front.
- Massage works best when strokes are lubricated. Any vegetable oil will work, but scented massage oils can add to the sense of relaxation and sensuality.
- Begin with both of you doing slow deep breathing to center and ground.
- Warm up the oil by rubbing it between your hands before applying it.
- Begin with light strokes and proceed to deeper pressure only after the muscles in the area have relaxed and warmed up.
- Your partner should tell you if any strokes feel uncomfortable: too light, too deep, or on a tender spot.
- Take your time: ideally 2 to 3 minutes per foot, 10 minutes per leg, 15 to 20 minutes for the back, and 15 minutes for the front including 5 minutes on the face.
- Stroke toward the heart instead of against the flow of blood returning to the heart.
- Never press directly on the spinal column, just on the muscles on either side of it.
- The best massage comes from using your whole body, not just your arms.

Sources: Cassar, M. P. (2002). *Massage Made Easy.* New York: MetroBooks; Coughlin, P. (2002). *Principles and Practice of Manual Therapeutics.* New York: Churchill Livingstone; and Walters, L. (2002). *Kind Touch Massage.* New York: Sterling.

USING RESEARCH TO HEAL

Billhult, A., Bergbom, I., & Stener-Victorin, E. (2007). Massage relieves nausea in women with breast cancer who are undergoing chemotherapy. *The Journal of Alternative and Complementary Medicine*, 13(1): 53–57.

What Is This Study About?

Breast cancer is one of the most common malignancies in women in the United States. Frequently, women undergoing chemotherapy treatment for this cancer complain of side effects such as nausea, anxiety, and depression. The purpose of this study was to explore the effect of skin massage (effleurage) on nausea, anxiety, and depression in women diagnosed with breast cancer and undergoing chemotherapy.

How Was the Study Done?

The design of the study was a prospective, randomized, controlled trial. Thirty-nine Swedish women (mean age = 51.8, ranging in age from 33–69 years) diagnosed with breast cancer and receiving chemotherapy were randomly assigned to a massage group (n = 19, 20 minutes on five occasions) or a control group (n = 20, five 20-minute visits by hospital staff without a massage). Nausea and anxiety were measured on the Visual Analog Scale before and after each intervention. Depression was measured by the Hospital Anxiety and Depression Scale. The Ethical Committee approved this study. Participants in the intervention group were given five massage treatment sessions choosing between lower leg/foot massage and lower arm/hand massage. A cold-pressed vegetable oil was used for the massage followed by immediately wrapping the massaged limb in a towel.

What Were the Results of the Study?

Differences in reports of nausea were statistically significant between the two groups. Complaints of nausea were significantly decreased in the women experiencing a massage of a limb. No statistical significance was found for differences in anxiety and depression between the groups.

What Additional Questions Might I Have?

Were the participants using any other treatments for the symptoms (nausea, anxiety, and depresion) during the course of the study? Would a different type of massage (whole body, Swedish, Shiatsu, Sports, Trigger Point, etc.) have influenced participant's experience of nausea, anxiety, and depression? Would the results have been significantly different with a larger number of participants? Would massage be effective for persons experiencing nausea as a side effect of other treatments or health problems?

How Can I Use This Study?

Nurses caring for women undergoing chemotherapy need to support decisions to use massage as a treatment option. Nurses should realize the importance of massage as an intervention that may enhance the quality of life for persons living with a diagnosis of breast cancer.

Source: Contributed by Dolores M. Huffman, PhD, RN, Associate Professor of Nursing, Purdue University Calumet.

References

Billhult, A., Bergbom, I., & Stener-Vicorin, E. (2007). Massage relieves nausea in women with breast cancer who are undergoing chemotherapy. *The Journal of Alternative and Complementary Medicine*, 13(1): 53–57.

Cambron, J. A., Dexheimer, J., Coe, P., & Swenson, R. (2007). Side-effects of massage therapy. *The Journal of Alternative and Complementary Medicine*, 13(8): 793–796.

Cassar, M. P. (2002). *Massage Made Easy*. New York: MetroBooks.

Colt, G. H. (1997). The magic of touch. *Life*, 52–62.

Coughlin, P. (2002). *Principles and Practice of Manual Therapeutics*. New York: Churchill Livingstone.

Field, T. M. (1999). American adolescents touch each other less and are more aggressive toward their peers as compared with French adolescents. *Adolescence*, 34: 753–758.

Field, T. M. (2001). *Touch*. Cambridge, MA: The MIT Press.

Field, T. M., Diego, M., Cullen, C., Hernandez-Reif, M., Sunshine, W., & Douglas, S. (2002). Fibromyalgia pain and substance P decrease and sleep improves after massage therapy. *Journal of Clinical Rheumatology*, 8: 72–76.

Hilliard, D. (1995). Massage for the seriously mentally ill. *Journal of Psychosocial Nursing*, 33(7): 29–30.

Hughes, D., Ladas, E., Rooney, D., & Kelly, K. (2008). Massage therapy as a supportive intervention for children with cancer. *Oncology Nursing Forum*, 35(3): 431–442.

Kaye, A. D., Kaye, A. J., Swinford, J., Baluch, A., Bawcom, B. A., Lambert, T. J., et al. (2008). The effect of deep-tissue massage therapy on blood pressure and heart rate. *The Journal of Alternative and Complementary Medicine*, 14(2): 125–128.

Moore, R. (2005). The joy of giving infant massage. *International Journal of Childbirth Education*, 20(4): 34–37.

O'Higgins, M., St. James Roberts, I., & Glover, V. (2008). Postnatal depression and mother and infant outcomes after infant massage. *Journal of Affective Disorders*, 109(1–2): 189–192.

Riggs, A. (2007). *Deep Tissue Massage*. Berkeley, CA: North Atlantic Books.

Russell, N. C., Sumler, S. S., Beinhorn, C. M., & Frenkel, M. A. (2008). Role of massage therapy in cancer care. *The Journal of Alternative and Complementary Medicine*, 14(2): 209–214.

Sharpe, P. A., Williams, H. G., Granner, M. L., & Hussey, J. R. (2007). A randomized study of the effects of massage therapy compared to guided relaxation on well-being and stress perception among older adults. *Complementary Therapies in Medicine*, 15: 157–163.

Stewart, N. (2006). *The Complete Body Massage Course*. London: Collins & Brown.

Tulku, T. (2003). *Tibetan Relaxation*. London: Duncan Baird Publishers.

Walters, L. (2002). *Kind Touch Massage*. New York: Sterling.

Wilkinson, S., Barnes, K., & Storey, L. (2008). Massage for symptom relief in patients with cancer: Systematic review. *Journal of Advanced Nursing*, 63(5): 430–439.

Resources

American Massage Therapy Association
500 Davis St., Suite 900
Evanston, IL 60201-4695
877.905.2700
www.amtamassage.org

American Oriental Bodywork Therapy
Association
1010 Haddonfield-Berlin Rd.,
Suite 408
Voorhees, NJ 08043-3514
856.782.1616
www.aobta.org

British Federation of Massage
Practitioners
78 Meadow St.
Preston, Lancashire PR1 1TS, UK
01772.881063

International Association of Infant
Massage
26 Chigwell Rd.
South Woodford, London, E18 1LS, UK
020.8989.9597
www.iaim.org.uk

National Association of Nurse Massage
Therapists
28 Lowry Drive
P.O. Box 232
West Milton, OH 45383
800.262.4017
www.nanmt.org

National Certification Board of
Therapeutic Massage and Bodywork
1901 South Meyers Rd., Suite 240
Oakbrook Terrace, IL 60181
630.627.8000
www.ncbtmb.com

Rolf Institute of Structural Integration
5055 Chaparral Ct., Suite 103
Boulder, CO 80301
800.530.8875
www.rolf.org

Touch Research Institutes
University of Miami School of Medicine
P.O. Box 016820
Miami, FL 33101
305.243.6781
www.miami.edu/touch-research

13

Pressure Point Therapies

Let parents then bequeath to their children not riches but the spirit of reverence.

PLATO

It is in my caring for the otherness of the other that determines my humanity, and my spirituality.

ELIE WIESEL

Acupuncture, acupressure, Jin Shin Jyutsu™, Jin Shin Do™, and reflexology are different forms of the same practice of stimulating points on the body to balance the body's life energy. Jin Shin Jyutsu, Jin Shin Do, and reflexology are forms of acupressure and in this chapter, the term *acupressure* includes all the forms. **Acupuncture** and **acupressure** are based on the theory that applying pressure or stimulation to specific points on the body, known as acupuncture points, can relieve pain, cure certain illnesses, and promote wellness. Acupuncture uses needles, whereas acupressure uses finger pressure. Although the older of the two techniques, acupressure is not as powerful and could be considered the over-the-counter version of acupuncture. Acupressure is easy to learn and convenient for self-care, whereas acupuncture requires training to use the needles. Frequently, these practices are part of a holistic approach to wellness and are combined with diet, herbs, massage, mind–body techniques, and spiritual therapies. Used with great success on humans for thousands of years, acupuncture and acupressure are now available for cats, dogs, and horses through veterinarians trained in Traditional Chinese Medicine.

BACKGROUND

Acupuncture and acupressure started in China several thousand years ago. The practice spread to Korea around 300 A.D. and to Japan and Europe in the seventeenth century. In the late nineteenth century, a Canadian physician, Sir William Osler, became interested in acupressure techniques, but they remained largely unknown in North America until the 1970s. Accompanying President Richard Nixon on his trip to China in 1972, James Reston, a reporter for the *New York Times*, wrote about his experience with acupuncture for relief of pain following abdominal surgery in China. This article began the upsurge of interest in these therapies in the United States. At the present time, acupuncture and acupressure are practiced widely in Asia, the former Soviet Union, and Europe and are gaining in popularity in North America (Lin, 2006).

Jin Shin Jyutsu (pronounced "jin-shin, jit-soo") and **Jin Shin Do** are Japanese phrases meaning "The Way of the Compassionate Spirit." They are ancient practices that fell into relative obscurity until they were dramatically revived in the early 1900s by Master Jiro Murai in Japan. Dying from a terminal illness, he turned in desperation to Jin Shin Jyutsu and meditation. Within a week, he was completely well. He spent the remaining 50 years of his life researching and sharing his knowledge of this healing art, which he referred to as the art of happiness, the art of longevity, and the art of benevolence. After World War II, a Japanese American, Mary Burmeister, studied with Master Murai for many years and eventually returned to the United States with the "gift" of Jin Shin Jyutsu and Jin Shin Do. Today, thousands of students throughout the United States and around the world study and practice Jin Shin Jyutsu and Jin Shin Do (Cross, 2002).

Reflexology, an associated ancient practice, limits the use of acupressure points, or reflexes, to the feet, hands, and ears. William Fitzgerald, an American physician, introduced reflexology to the West in 1913. He noted that postoperative pain was less when pressure was applied to people's feet and hands just before surgery. In spite of Fitzgerald's work, it was the efforts of Eunice Ingham, a physical therapist, who expanded and refined Fitzgerald's observations and found that reflexology not only reduced pain but provided other health benefits as well. Ingham mapped the specific reflex zones on the feet, hands, and ears that reflexologists use today. This work gave her the distinction of being the founder of modern reflexology in the West (Keet, 2009).

PREPARATION

The United States has 53 schools and colleges of acupuncture approved by the Council of Colleges of Acupuncture and Oriental Medicine. In most states the National Commission for the Certification of Acupuncture and Oriental Medicine (NCCAOM) exam is required to become licensed. To take the exam, candidates must have completed a formal education program at an accredited school or have 4,000 hours of training with a documented preceptor. More than 10,000 practitioners have been certified to date.

An estimated 7,000 to 8,000 American doctors now include acupuncture in their practices. Most are family physicians, anesthesiologists, orthopedists, and pain specialists. Few physicians are NCCAOM certified, but most are certified by the American Academy of Medical Acupuncture instead. Even though acupuncture is used in China to treat many conditions, in the United States, conventional physicians have taken the technique out of context, basing it more on a biomedical model of diagnosis and treatment. Nationally, an estimated 15,000 nonmedical professionals practice acupuncture, including nurses, naturopathic physicians, and chiropractors (Shan, 2007).

Professionals using acupressure are usually physical therapists or massage therapists with special training in this field. Some nurses are trained in acupressure and use it to help clients sleep and to reduce levels of anxiety. Midwives may use acupressure techniques to promote relaxation during labor and reduce breast engorgement after delivery. No specific license or certification is needed to practice any of the forms of acupressure, although practitioners of reflexology have the option to become certified by the American Reflexology Certification Board.

CONCEPTS

Meridians

Acupuncture, acupressure, Jin Shin Jyutsu, Jin Shin Do, and reflexology are treatments rooted in the traditional Eastern philosophy that *qi*, or life energy, flows through the body along pathways known as **meridians.** Like major power lines, the meridians connect all parts of the body. As vital energy flows through the meridians, it forms tiny whirlpools close to the skin's surface at places called *hsueh*, which means "cave" or "hollow." In Traditional Chinese Medicine, these are acupuncture points; in India, *marma* points. These pressure points function somewhat like gates to moderate the flow of qi. Acupuncture needles inserted into these points or pressure on these points releases blocked energy and improves the circulation of qi in the body (Dale, 2009).

The body has 14 major meridians and 360 to 365 classic points through which qi can be accessed. Most practitioners, however, focus on 150 points. The points themselves are metaphors for a person's journey through life with names such as "Spirit Gate," "Great Esteem," "Joining the Valleys," and "Inner Frontier Gate." Each meridian is also associated with an internal organ after which it is named: stomach, spleen, heart, small intestine, bladder, kidney, circulation—sex, gallbladder, liver, lung, and large intestine. The triple-warmer meridian is associated with the thyroid and adrenal glands, the governing meridian with the spine, and the central meridian with the brain. Chapters 2 and 4 present more detailed information regarding energy and meridians.

Microsystems

At many points in the body the meridians converge. These points are reflexes to distant parts of the body and are called **microsystems.** Microsystems are areas of the body that are small, local representations of the whole body and are located on the feet, hands, and ears. In other words, each individual part of the body has an associated reflex on the ear, the hand, and the foot. The reflexes are symmetrical in that organs on the right side of the body are in the right foot, and the left organs on the left foot. The reflexes also correspond in descending order: the brain reflexes are in the tips of the toes, the eyes and ears under the toes, the shoulders and lungs on the ball of the foot, the stomach and pancreas on the instep, the intestines and colon toward the heel, and the hips on the heel. See Figures 13.1(A), (B), and (C) for reflexology maps.

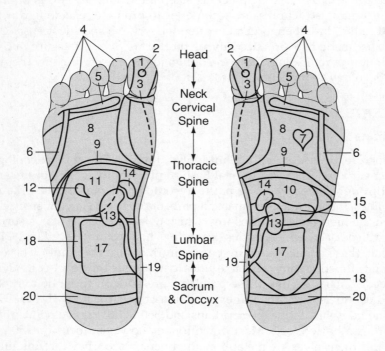

1. Head and brain	11. Liver
2. Pituitary and pineal glands	12. Gallbladder
3. Throat and thyroid gland	13. Kidney
4. Sinus	14. Adrenal gland
5. Eyes and ears	15. Spleen
6. Shoulder	16. Pancreas
7. Heart	17. Small intestine
8. Lungs and thymus gland	18. Large intestine
9. Diaphragm and solar plexus	19. Bladder
10. Stomach	20. Sacrum and sciatic nerve

FIGURE 13.1A   Foot Reflexology Points

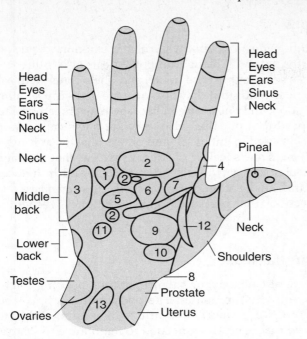

1. Heart (left hand) and thymus gland
2. Lungs
3. Liver (right hand) and shoulders
4. Solar plexus
5. Pancreas
6. Kidneys and adrenals
7. Stomach
8. Large intestine
9. Small intestine
10. Bladder
11. Appendix
12. Thyroid
13. Sacrum and pelvis

FIGURE 13.1B   Hand Reflexology Points

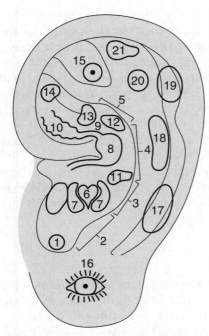

1. Endocrine glands and hormones
2. Head and brain
3. Neck
4. Upper and middle back
5. Lower back
6. Heart and thymus gland
7. Lungs
8. Stomach
9. Small intestine
10. Large intestine
11. Spleen
12. Liver
13. Kidney
14. Bladder
15. Nervous system and spirit
16. Eyes and face
17. Shoulders
18. Arm and elbow
19. Hand
20. Leg and knee
21. Foot

FIGURE 13.1C   Ear Reflexology Points

Mind–Body Connections

In the pressure point tradition, the mind, body, spirit, and emotions are never separated. Thus, the heart is not just a blood pump; the heart also influences one's capacity for joy, one's sense of purpose in life, and one's connectedness with others. The kidneys filter fluids, but they also manage one's capacity for fear, one's will and motivation, and one's faith in life. The lungs breathe in air and breathe out waste products, but they also regulate one's capacity to grieve, as well as one's acknowledgment of self and others. The liver cleanses the body, and it also influences one's feeling of anger as well as that of vision and creativity. The stomach has a part in digestion of food and influences one's ability to be thoughtful, kind, and nurturing as well. These are just a few of the mind–body connections that pressure point practitioners recognize (Smith, 2008).

VIEW OF HEALTH AND ILLNESS

Health is viewed as a state of harmony, or balance, of the opposing forces of nature, both internal and environmental. The body requires balanced yin and yang energy to function properly and utilize its natural ability to resist disease. It is believed that everything needed to maintain and restore health already exists in nature and that pressure point therapies free up energy and restore balance, thus enabling individuals to maintain or regain their health.

Symptoms are caused by an imbalance of yin and yang in some part of the body leading to excesses or deficiencies of life energy throughout the body. When the flow of energy becomes blocked or congested, people experience discomfort or pain on a physical level, may feel frustrated or irritable on an emotional level, and may experience a sense of vulnerability or lack of purpose in life on a spiritual level. When the flow of energy is interrupted, the area cannot nourish or cleanse. If not corrected, these blocks and imbalances in energy channels can result in disease and eventually illness.

The goal of care is to recognize and manage the disruption before illness or disease occurs. Qi can be thrown out of balance in a number of ways, including genetic vulnerability, accident or trauma, diet, lifestyle, emotional upset, spiritual distress, climate, or noxious agents. Pressure point practitioners bring balance to the body's energies, which promotes optimal health and well-being and facilitates people's own healing capacities.

DIAGNOSTIC METHODS

The initial consultation involves a holistic assessment, because no part of the self is considered a neutral bystander when the body is in a state of imbalance. A detailed medical history is an important part of the diagnostic process. Special attention is paid to the connection between body, mind, emotions, and spirit.

If pressure point therapies are done within the context of Traditional Chinese Medicine, palpation is the major diagnostic method. Reading the pulses provides a remarkable amount of information about the person's condition. Imbalances in the body can be detected through palpating microsystems on the feet, hands, and ears. If something feels different in the microsystems, the corresponding organ is examined in more detail. Chapter 4 discusses the diagnostic process of Traditional Chinese Medicine in greater detail.

TREATMENT

Pressure point therapies consider symptoms to be an expression of the condition of the person as a whole. Thus, sessions focus not only on relieving pain and discomfort, but also on responding to disruptions before they develop into illnesses.

Acupuncture

To restore the flow of energy, acupuncturists insert sterile, hair-thin needles at points along the meridians. The needles are rotated, twirled, or accompanied by a weak electrical current, and are often left in several minutes or longer. Acupuncturists also may apply heat or use finger pressure to alter the flow of qi. Clients feel little, if any, pain. Some people experience sensations of warmth, tingling, heaviness, or a dull ache.

Evidence now indicates that, in addition to restoring the flow of energy within the meridians, acupuncture reduces pain by triggering the release of endogenous opioids. Many of the analgesic effects of acupuncture can be partially or completely blocked by the use of opioid antagonists such as naloxone. Acupuncture also stimulates the nervous system to release ACTH, a chemical that aids in fighting inflammation; prostaglandins, which help wounds heal more quickly; and other substances that may promote nerve regeneration. The antiemetic effects apparently stem from the increase in endorphins and ACTH, which inhibits the chemoreceptor trigger zone and the vomiting center in the brain. Acupuncture also calms the upper gastrointestinal tract. Research has found that acupuncture is effective for nausea from morning sickness, motion sickness, postoperative nausea, and chemotherapy-induced nausea. Unlike drugs and surgery, acupuncture has virtually no side effects (Samuels, Gropp, Singer, & Oberbaum, 2008; Spira, 2008).

Jin Shin Jyutsu and Jin Shin Do

Jin Shin Jyutsu and Jin Shin Do can be applied as self-help and also by a trained practitioner. It is practiced by placing the fingertips over clothing on designated pressure points, to harmonize and restore the energy flow. Rather than doing something to the body, Jin Shin encourages the body to "let go," which is seen as the path to awakening one's awareness of harmony within the self and the universe.

A session generally lasts about an hour with the client lying on a table fully clothed. The practitioner's hands act as "jumper cables" to "kick start" the correct flow of energy. A spot on the shoulder may be held at the same time as a spot on the knee. The practitioner uses special sequences of hand positions to stimulate the circulation of energy. The touch is gentle, steady, and never involves force. It is generally pain free; any tenderness in a particular area is caused by a blockage and tends to dissipate as the area is held. Some people may feel hot or cold or feel a sensation in another part of the body than the one where the practitioner is working. Most people experience a sense of deep relaxation with Jin Shin Jyutsu and Jin Shin Do (Andry, 2008).

Reflexology

Reflexologists manipulate the reflex zones most commonly on the feet, but the hands or ears may also be manipulated. A session usually lasts about 45 minutes with the client sitting comfortably in a chair and the practitioner using thumb and fingers in small, creeping movements over the sole of the foot. This manipulation prompts the nervous system to speed up the body's response to an afflicted area by stimulating the flushing of toxins from the area.

Uses

Pressure point therapies are widely used around the world to treat many conditions, including addiction, allergies, bronchitis, cerebral palsy, depression, diabetes, hemorrhoids, hepatitis, herpes, infertility, irritable bowel syndrome, nausea, premenstrual syndrome, stroke, and ulcers. In the United States, reduction of pain is a major therapeutic use including pain from dental work, temporomandibular joint (TMJ) syndrome, migraine headaches, osteoarthritis, low back pain, sciatica, carpal tunnel syndrome, and sports injuries. Acupuncture can provide symptomatic relief from the pain of bursitis and is much safer than anti-inflammatory drugs and injections of steroids (Bonafede, Dick, Noyes, Klein, & Brown, 2008; Park et al., 2008).

Contraindications

Pressure point therapy is not appropriate for every ailment. It is not indicated for an acute or infectious illness or fever or if surgery is needed. Foot injuries need to heal before reflexology is used on the foot. If someone has a pacemaker, practitioners avoid stimulating the left chest zone. If someone has gallstones or kidney stones, the gallbladder and kidney points are avoided. If the person is pregnant, uterine points are avoided.

USING RESEARCH TO HEAL

Courbasson, C. M. A., de Sorkin, A. A., Dullerud, R., & Van Wyk, L. (2007). Acupuncture treatment for women with concurrent substance use and anxiety/depression: An effective therapy? *Family & Community Health*, 30(2): 112–120.

What Is This Study About?

Relapse following treatment for alcohol and substance abuse is well documented. This relapse is due to many factors including physiological effects of the substance itself or anxiety and depression. To prevent relapse following addiction treatment, an effective program must be found and frequently includes a combination of treatment modalities. The purpose of this study was to evaluate the benefits of adding auricular acupuncture for women living with alcohol/drug addiction and participating in a 21-day outpatient structured treatment program.

How Was the Study Done?

This was an exploratory study using a sequential comparative research design. The women were recruited for the study from a 21-day residential/day treatment center in Toronto, Canada. The participants ranged in age from 15 to 71, majority was not married, and most were seeking treatment for alcohol addiction. Trained acupuncturists provided acupuncture three mornings per week for 45 minutes per session for the 204 women voluntarily enrolled in the study. Women (n = 101) attending the center but not wishing to take part in the acupuncture served as a comparison group. In addition, both groups of women were seated together in a meeting room and were instructed to view the 45 minutes acupuncture treatment period as a "quiet time" for themselves. (Women who were enrolled in the treatment as usual without acupuncture were also requested to participate in the same 45 minutes of quiet time but without acupuncture intervention.) Additionally, both groups were asked to write down their thoughts of self-reflection at a later time. Both groups completed four brief self-report measures. The measures used were the Beck Depression Inventory, Beck Anxiety Inventory, Reflective Activity Scale, and the Drug-Taking Confidence Questionnaire. All measures were completed at four specific times during the program. Women who agreed to take part in the study after discharge from the center were provided questionnaires via the mail service.

What Were the Results of the Study?

At the completion of treatment, the women in acupuncture group reported significantly less depression, less anxiety, and were better able to reflect on and resolve difficulties than the women in the comparison group. Women in the acupuncture group had stronger feelings about their ability to cope and enhanced confidence in their ability to refrain from substance use when encountering stressful situations as compared to the group not experiencing acupuncture. Responses to questions about acupuncture included "calming effect," "reduced cravings for substances (including nicotine)," and "less anger" and "irritability". Eighty-six percent said they would recommend acupuncture to others in a recovery program for alcohol and substance abuse. Additionally, significant differences were reported between the two groups in alcohol and drug coping self-efficacy at 1 month and

(continued)

3 months. However, statistically significant differences (may be due to small number of women returning questionnaires) on levels of depression and anxiety were not found at follow-up.

What Additional Questions Might I Have?

Would results have been significantly different if a randomized control clinical trial design was implemented to address the research question? How would the findings have been affected if more women responded to the follow-up questionnaires? What would be the findings if a longitudinal design requiring follow-up at 1 year, 2 years, and so forth was implemented? What is the effect of acupuncture for other addictions such as eating, gambling, etc.? Would the results be similar for men living with substance abuse addiction?

How Can I Use This Study?

This study has considerable clinical value for nurses caring for persons living with a dependence on alcohol and drugs. Nurses should value and promote the use of acupuncture as an adjunct treatment for addiction. Acupuncture can be considered an effective and perhaps cost-effective intervention in promoting an enhanced quality of life for those individual desiring to improve their addiction behavior.

Source: Contributed by Dolores M. Huffman, PhD, RN, Associate Professor of Nursing, Purdue University Calumet.

RESEARCH

In 1997, the National Institutes of Health (NIH) assembled a panel of experts in a scientific court known officially as a consensus conference. A panel of 12 experts was drawn from a variety of backgrounds, including biomedical research scientists, physicians, and others. The panel's task was to listen to as much evidence as the acupuncture/pressure point research community could present in the first half of the 3-day conference. The panel's judgment included the following statement: "There is sufficient evidence of acupuncture's value to expand its use into conventional medicine and to encourage further studies of its physiology and clinical value" (NIH, 1998). The panel determined that acupuncture was clearly effective for nausea and vomiting from pregnancy, motion sickness, chemotherapy, and anesthesia and for postoperative pain from dental surgery. The panel also noted "other situations such as addiction, stroke rehabilitation, headache, menstrual cramps, tennis elbow, fibromyalgia, myofascial pain, osteoarthritis, low back pain, carpal tunnel syndrome, and asthma where acupuncture may be useful as an adjunct treatment or an acceptable alternative or be included in a comprehensive management program" (NIH, 1998). This panel focused only on data collected by means of randomized controlled clinical trials and, as such, did not review data on technique, cost benefit, patient preference, or practitioner education.

The following is a small sample of recent research results. It is anticipated that further research in pressure point therapies will be available in the not-too-distant future.

- In conducting a review of the evidence, Rooney (2008) concluded that a number of studies reported inconsistent evidence of the efficacy of acupuncture for the treatment of nonspecific acute low back pain. She further stated that since some people respond to acupuncture, the decision should be made case-by-case.
- A systematic review, including seven trials with 1366 women, found that women undergoing in vitro fertilization had an increased chance of pregnancy when receiving acupuncture within one day of embryo transfer (Manheimer et al., 2008).
- A group of people with mild-to-moderate dementia were divided into two groups. The first group had 4 weeks of weekly reflexology treatment followed by a control condition of friendly visits. The other group has 4 weeks of friendly visits followed by 4 weeks of reflexology. It was found that the subjects demonstrated significant reduction in pain and stress when receiving reflexology as compared to friendly visits (Hodgson & Andersen, 2008).
- A systematic review found that acupuncture and moxibustion demonstrated a statistically significant correction in breech presentation of the fetus (van den Berg et al., 2008).
- A study of 30 individuals with chronic obstructive pulmonary disease (COPD) were either treated with conservative treatment with medication or received acupuncture as well as conservative treatment with medication. After 10 weeks, there was a significant difference in the improvement of dyspnea with exercise in the acupuncture group (Suzuki et al., 2008).

INTEGRATED NURSING PRACTICE

If you are interested in incorporating pressure point therapies into your nursing practice, you may want to attend a weekend or weeklong program on reflexology, Jin Shin Jyutsu, or Jin Shin Do. Even without further education, you can incorporate hand, foot, or ear massages into your practice. This type of massage is easy to learn and nonintrusive. The procedure for a hand massage is shown in Figure 12.3 in the chapter on massage therapy. These procedures can be modified for an ear massage. The hands, feet, and ears are fairly small. If you simply massage them, focusing on any tender spots you find, you are bound to send qi or energy to all parts of the body. Few people object to this type of massage. Even if the recipient has no particular physical complaints, this type of massage is wonderfully relaxing.

You can teach clients about a number of pressure points as you advocate self-help. Box 13.1 describes this process for headaches, hiccups, and carpal tunnel syndrome. To ease tension and restore energy, try this pressure point:

BOX 13.1

Self-Help: Pressure Points

The following are several examples of how people can use pressure points to relieve discomfort or pain. Once you think you have located one of the appropriate points, probe the area with a fingertip or pencil eraser in a tight circular motion in the general location. Points often feel tender, sore, or tingling. Press the point for 1 minute, then stop for a few seconds, and press again. Work the point for 5 to 20 minutes. If you are experiencing a headache, hiccups, or symptoms of carpal tunnel syndrome, experiment for yourself and find which points work best for you. Remember, only some of the points need to be worked to achieve relief.

Headache

Point 1.   Hold your hand open, palm down, and find the point in the center of the fleshy webbing between the thumb and index finger.

Point 2.   Find the point on the top of the foot in the valley between the big toe and second toe.

Point 3.   This point is at the base of the back of the skull in the hollow above the two large vertical neck muscles.

Point 4.   This point is in the hollow above the inner eyes, where the bridge of the nose meets the ridge of the eyebrows.

Point 5.   Find the point between the eyebrows in the indentation where the bridge of the nose meets the forehead.

Point 6.   This point is two finger-widths above the webbing of the fourth and fifth toes in the groove between the bones.

Hiccups

Point 1.   Find the point in the indentation behind each earlobe.

Point 2.   This point is located at the base of the throat in the center of the collarbone.

Point 3.   Find this point on the center of the breastbone three thumb-widths up from the base of the bone.

Point 4.   This point is located three finger-widths below the base of the breastbone in the pit of the abdomen. If you are healthy, do not press this point for more than 2 minutes. If you are not healthy, do not press this point at all.

Carpal Tunnel Syndrome

Point 1.   Find the point in the middle of the inner side of the forearm, two and a half finger-widths below the wrist crease.

Point 2.   This point is located in the middle of the inside of the wrist crease.

Point 3.   Find the point on the outside of the forearm, midway between the radius and ulna, two and a half finger-widths below the wrist crease.

Sources: Forem, J., & Shimer, S. (1999). *Healing with Pressure Point Therapy*. Upper Saddle River, NJ: Prentice Hall; Keet, L. (2009). *Hand Reflexology*. New York: Hamlyn; Wills, P. (2009). *Easy Reflexology*. Courtenay, BC: Connections.

Hold your left palm in front of you, fingers together. The fleshy spot between your thumb and index finger is a key pressure point. Using your right thumb, massage this spot in a circular motion for a slow count of 15. Then switch hands and repeat the process. You can also teach clients several finger holds to improve their general level of well-being. Explain that they should gently hold the appropriate finger on either hand while imagining the negative emotions melting away and physical symptoms easing.

- *Thumb.* Corresponds to worrying, depression, anxiety. Physical symptoms may include stomachaches, headaches, skin problems, and nervousness.
- *Index finger.* Corresponds to fear, mental confusion, frustration. Physical symptoms are digestive problems and muscle problems such as backaches.
- *Middle finger.* Corresponds with anger, irritability, indecisiveness. Physical symptoms are eye or vision problems, fatigue, and circulation problems.
- *Ring finger.* Corresponds with sadness, fear of rejection, grief, negativity. Physical symptoms are digestive, breathing, or serious skin problems.
- *Little finger.* Corresponds with insecurity, effort, overdoing it, nervousness. Physical symptoms are sore throat and bone or nerve problems.

Clients can be taught acupressure for relief of nausea from a variety of causes. The pericardium 6 point is located in the midline of the inner wrist between 2 and 3 finger-widths up from the crease where the hand joins the wrist. People can stimulate this point using their own finger or apply an acupressure wristband to the point.

TRY THIS

Foot Massage

When your feet ache, your whole body suffers. Here are instructions for a 10- to 15-minute foot massage to relax and soothe your feet and perhaps your entire body.

- Sit in a comfortable, quiet place where you will not be disturbed. You may want to have soothing music in the background.

(continued)

- Pour a small amount of nongreasy lotion or massage oil into your hands and rub them together.
- Begin massaging one foot, stroking each toe in an up-and-down motion. Then massage the entire foot using kneading, wringing motions until the lotion is absorbed.
- Holding your foot firmly in one hand, press the thumb of the other hand (slightly bent) on the sole of the foot near the heel. Apply even pressure with the thumb and "walk it" forward, little by little. Press one spot, move forward, press again, move forward, and so on.
- When you get to the toes, go back to the heel and trace another line from heel to toe. Continue this process until the entire sole of the foot has been worked.
- Repeat the entire process with the other foot.

Sources: Cross, J. R. (2002). *Acupressure and Reflexology in the Treatment of Medical Conditions.* St. Louis, MO: Butterworth-Heinemann; Mackereth, P. A., & Tiran, D. (2002). *Clinical Reflexology.* New York: Churchill Livingstone; Rose, M. (2009). *Comfort Touch: Massage for the Elderly and the Ill.* Hagerstown, MD: Lippincott Williams & Wilkins.

References

Andry, J. B. (2008). *A Touching Good-Bye: The Gentle Use of Jin Shin Jyutsu Acupressure at Time of Critical Illness and Death.* Santa Barbara, CA: Ampersand, Inc.

Bonafede, M., Dick, A., Noyes, K., Klein, J. D., & Brown, T. (2008). The effect of acupuncture utilization on healthcare utilization. *Medical Care, 46*(1): 41–48.

Cross, J. R. (2002). *Acupressure & Reflexology in the Treatment of Medical Conditions.* St. Louis, MO: Butterworth-Heinemann.

Dale, C. (2009). *The Subtle Body.* Louisville, CO: Sounds True, Inc.

Hodgson, N. A., & Andersen, S. (2008). The clinical efficacy of reflexology in nursing home residents with dementia. *The Journal of Alternative and Complementary Medicine, 14*(3): 269–275.

Keet, L. (2009). *The Reflexology Bible: The Definitive Guide to Pressure Point Healing.* New York: Sterling.

Lin, Y. C. (2006). Preoperative usage of acupuncture. *Pediatric Anesthesia, 16:* 231–235.

Manheimer, E., Zhang, G., Udoff, L., Haramati, A., Langenberg, P., Berman, B. M., et al. (2008). Effects of acupuncture on rates of pregnancy and live birth among women undergoing in vitro fertilization: Systematic review and meta-analysis. *British Medical Journal, 336*(7643): 545–549.

National Institutes of Health. (1998). NIH consensus conference: Acupuncture. *Journal of the American Medical Association, 280:* 1518–1524.

Park, J., Linde, K., Manheimer, E., Molsberger, A., Sherman, K., Smith, C., et al. (2008). The status and future of acupuncture clinical research. *Journal of Alternative and Complementary Medicine, 14*(7): 871–881.

Rooney, L. (2008). Acupuncture in the treatment of non-specific low back pain in an adult population: A review of the evidence. *Internet Journal of Advanced Nursing Practice, 9*(2): 1–8. Accessed October 21, 2008, at Academic Search Premier.

Samuels, N., Gropp, C., Singer, S. R., & Oberbaum, M. (2008). Acupuncture for psychiatric illness: A literature review. *Behavioral Medicine, 34:* 55–62.

Shan, Y. (2007). Using acupuncture to manage pain. *Primary Health Care,* 17(7): 25–29.

Smith, K. (2008). *Awakening the Energy Body.* Rochester, VT: Bear & Company.

Spira, A. (2008). Acupuncture: A useful tool for health care in an operational medicine environment. *Military Medicine,* 173(7): 629–634.

Suzuki, M., Namura, K., Ohno, Y., Tanaka, H., Egawa, M., Yokoyama, Y., et al. (2008). The effect of acupuncture in the treatment of chronic obstructive pulmonary disease. *Journal of Alternative and Complementary Medicine,* 14(9): 1097–1105.

van den Berg, I., Bosch, J. L., Jacobs, B., Bouman, I., Duvekot, J. J., & Hunink, M. G. (2008). Effectiveness of acupuncture-type interventions versus expectant management to correct breech presentation: A systematic review. *Complementary Therapies in Medicine,* 16: 92–100.

Resources

American Association of Acupuncture and Oriental Medicine
P.O. Box 162340
Sacramento, CA 95816
866.455.7999
www.aaaom.edu

American Academy of Medical Acupuncture
1970 E. Grand Ave., Suite 330
El Segundo, CA 90245
310.364.0193
www.medicalacupuncture.org

American Reflexology Certification Board
P.O. Box 5147
Gulfport, FL 33737
www.arcb.net

British Acupuncture Council
63 Jeddo Rd.
London W12 9HQ, UK
020.8735.0400
www.acupuncture.org.uk

Canadian Acupressure Institute Inc.
256 Linden Ave.
Victoria, BC, Canada V8W 4E5
877.909.2244
www.acupressureshiatsuschool.com

Jin Shin Foundation for Bodymind Acupressure
P.O. Box 416
Idyllwild, CA 92549
951.659.5707
www.jinshindo.org

National Commission for the Certification of Acupuncture and Oriental Medicine
76 South Laura St., Suite 1290
Jacksonville, FL 32202
904.598.1005
www.nccaom.org

14

Hand-Mediated Biofield Therapies

> *Often hands will solve a mystery that the intellect has struggled with in vain.*
>
> C. G. JUNG

> *Happiness, grief, gaiety, sadness are by nature contagious. Bring your health and your strength to the weak and sickly, and so you will be of use to them. Give them, not your weakness, but your energy, so you will revive and lift them up.*
>
> HENRI-FREDERIC AMIEL

A wide variety of alternative, complementary, and integrative healing practices are emerging in popularity and are designed to balance the body's **biofield,** or energy field, and increase the flow of energy. The National Center for Complementary and Alternative Medicine (NCCAM, 2007) classifies energy medicine as a domain in complementary and alternative medicine with two types of energy fields: veritable (can be measured) or putative (have yet to be measured). Examples of veritable energy medicine include magnetic therapy, millimeter wave therapy, sound energy therapy, and light therapy. Putative energy fields are also called biofields and are based on the concept that human beings are infused with a subtle form of energy. More detailed discussion of the concept of body energy is found in Chapter 2.

Practices related to biofield therapies have been utilized cross-culturally for millenia, but it is only recently that programs of related research have emerged. In the 1980s, scientists in the emerging field of psychoneuroimmunology (PNI), or mind–body medicine, began to study energy medicine. Among them were Herbert Benson, MD, and Joan Borysenko, PhD, who discovered and studied the body's innate "relaxation response" as it relates to self-healing. Many of the PNI researchers were influenced by Eastern traditions that view the mind, body, spirit, and health as one and energy as something that people can deliberately nurture within themselves. Today, the field of mind–body medicine is well established and recognized with scientific breakthroughs occurring regularly.

The three most prominent therapies using the hands to alter the biofield and impact the healing process are *Therapeutic Touch* (TT), *Healing Touch* (HT), and *Reiki*. All three approaches could be simply defined as the use of the hands on or near the body with the intention to support and facilitate self-healing in a heart-centered and intentional way in order to rebalance the energy field. Actually, the word *touch* is a misnomer in TT and HT, because the practitioner need not touch the recipient to achieve the desired effects during a healing session. Techniques may be performed inches and sometimes feet from the recipient's body, or may involve gentle, light, or near-body touch to clear, balance, energize, and support another's energy system. These therapies are modern interpretations of several ancient healing practices, traditionally known as the "laying on of hands." TT, HT, and Reiki, however, must not be confused with faith healing, because the context in which they are practiced is not religious but scientific.

The goals of these hand-mediated therapies are to facilitate self-healing at all levels of body, mind, emotions, and spirit. This may result in relaxation, stress reduction, and promotion of self-healing. All three are forms of treatment and are not designed to diagnose physical conditions but are to be used in conjunction with other therapies. This means that they are not meant to replace conventional surgery, medicine, or drugs in treating organic disease (Quinn, 2006).

BACKGROUND

Healing Touch is an international, multi-level educational program that is taught in either the Healing Touch Program or Healing Touch International, Inc. Healing Touch is also taught in many countries throughout the world. Healing Touch (HT) was developed by Janet Mentgen, BSN, RN, HNC, CHTP/I, a Colorado nurse, who practiced and taught medically based energy therapy since 1980. In 1989, her five-course sequence in HT became the first certified program offered by the Amereican Holistic Nurses Association (AHNA). "Healing touch utilizes light or near-body touch to clear, balance and energize the human energy system in an effort to promote healing for the mind, body and/or spirit. The goal of Healing Touch is to restore harmony and balance in the human energy system by creating an optimal environment for the body's innate tendency for healing to occur" (HT Program, 2008, p. 1).

Therapeutic Touch was developed by Dolores Krieger, PhD, RN, Professor Emeritus, New York University, who launched the TT movement in 1970 after studying with Dora Kunz, a past president of the Theosophical Society of America and a natural healer. TT refers to the Krieger–Kunz method of Therapeutic Touch (Krieger, 1979; Kunz, 1991) and was originally developed as an energy field interaction between nurse and client.

Reiki (pronounced "ray-kee") originated in Japan/Tibet. Reiki is composed of two Japanese words: *Rei*, or universal spirit/God's Wisdom or the Higher Power, and *ki*, meaning life force energy. Reiki means universal life energy (NCCAM, 2008) and spiritually guided life force energy. The origin of Reiki can be traced to an ancient Buddhist practice rediscovered by Dr. Mikao Usui, a Japanese physician and monk and perhaps earlier from the Tibetan sutras (texts of Buddhism) (NCCAM, 2008). He first used Reiki on himself and his family and then began to share his knowledge with the larger public. Chujiro Hayashi, who was a student of Usui, futher developed this healing practice, and Hawayo Takata, an Japanese-American student of Hayashi's, introduced Reiki to Western cultures in the late 1930s (NCCAM, 2008).

All hand-mediated biofield therapies reflect the unitary-transformative perspective, which encourages each person to relate with others and their world as unitary"pan-dimensional" beings in a pan-dimensional universe (Newman, 1997; Rogers, 1992; Watson, 1999). Within this worldview, a unitary human being (human field) "is an irreducible, indivisible, pan-dimensional energy field identified by pattern and manifesting characteristics that are specific to the whole and which cannot be predicted from knowledge of the parts" (Rogers, 1992, p. 29). The kaleidoscopic role of nursing within this perspective is to view the client as expert. Caring–healing relationships are based on an ethic of caring consciousness, mutuality, relatedness, and connectedness. Creative unfolding of our caring–healing relationships occurs through our loving, caring–healing consciousness, intentionality, presence, and authenticity (Watson, 2005, p. 225). Both HT and TT programs of study have formally incorporated this philosophical stance, while Reiki is derived from Usui's philosophy, which is also "based on the idea that there is a universal (or source) energy that supports the body's innate healing abilities" (NCCAM, 2008, para. 9).

PREPARATION

Nurses who prepare to practice hand-mediated biofield therapies take time to assess and further develop their caring–healing way of being–belonging–doing with others. As a reflective nursing practice, learning may involve study/reflective practice, such as mindfulness meditation, centering and grounding work, listening and communicating with the intent to understand others at a deeper level, considering ways to create sacred space, and connect with nature as healer. Nurses who seek certification as HT practitioners from either the Healing Touch Program or Healing Touch International practice a variety of biofield techniques to assist the patient/client to self-heal. They also reflect on their own development through reflective practice and activities, such as journaling, reading books about techniques, healing traditions, self-healing, and possible theoretical explanations. The preparation may take two or more years of study as practitioners meet requirements for each of the five levels prior to certification. Most programs strongly emphasize development of the nurse as healer by considering the relationship they have with clients and with themselves, with a focus on "being mindful of the intention to deliver the best nursing care for the body, mind, spirit and emotional well-being of the patient and using verbal and nonverbal communication that reflects a nurse who is caring, calm, and receptive" (Mentgen, 2001, p. 148).

Therapeutic Touch does not require extensive formal training. It can be learned by almost anyone who is motivated by compassion and committed to helping others. Family members can be taught how to use it effectively with their loved ones. In fact, one of the leading researchers and teachers of this method, Janet Quinn, PhD, RN, has created a videotape home-study course for family caregivers as well as a series of three videotapes for nurses who wish to incorporate TT in their practice (see the Resource section at the end of this chapter). Both HT and TT were developed by nurses, and all nurses, regardless of clinical specialty, can use HT and TT in any setting. It is an independent nursing intervention and as such does not need a physician's order. But as with any independent nursing intervention, it does require client consent.

Reiki is usually learned from a Reiki Master. There are two degrees in Reiki healing, as well as a Master degree that prepares one to teach others. Most people can complete the first degree in a weekend course. The content includes historical information, the concept of energy healing, how to transfer energy from oneself to another person, and the hand positions used in healing. The second degree, also done over a weekend, includes learning how to do distant healing and further enhancement of one's physical, mental, emotional, and spiritual healing abilities. The Master degree takes years of additional study and a training mentorship with a Master Reiki practitioner. AHNA often approves Reiki programs for continuing education units.

CONCEPTS

By any name—qi, ki, prana, subtle energy—a life force energy is universally recognized in biofield therapies as the core of life and the driving force in healing. The belief is that all living beings are complex networks of interwoven vibratory energy systems composed of an energy field (aura), energy centers (chakras), and energy tracts (meridians) and that energy centers control the energy flow into and out of the body. It is at this level of the subtle energy system that both health and illness originate. Energy field theory is based on quantum physics law, which assumes that matter is energy and that all living things generate vibratory fields interconnected by mathematical laws.

At this time few Western scientific studies prove the existence of this human energy field, but that it exists is the working hypothesis of biofield therapies. Many of the most sophisticated instruments widely used in conventional medicine for diagnosis and treatment are energy medicine devices. The electrocardiogram, electroencephalogram, electromyogram, and ultrasound and magnetic resonance imaging devices—all measure the electromagnetic frequencies emitted by various parts of the body. People can detect a far greater spectrum of energies than can scientific measuring devices. Elmer Green of the Menninger Foundation believes that people's ability to sense and work with subtle energies is based on a communication system in the body that links the endocrine glands, nervous system, and the biofield (Green & Green, 1989). William Collinge, author of *Subtle Energy* (1998), believes that many phenomena that are dismissed as coincidences are examples of extrasensory perception, déjà vu, and precognition that are part of a subtle perceptual system outside usual perception. He believes that everyone has the ability to sense energies that are not detectable technologically, but that many Western individuals reject their intuitive experiences because of a belief that anything that cannot be measured does not exist. It is this energy field that skilled biofield practitioners can literally feel and modulate.

The energy principles shared by practitioners of biofield energy-based healing approaches include the following (Mentgen, 2001):

- Energy permeates all animate and inanimate matter.
- All healing is self-healing, but it can be assisted by others.
- Human beings are composed of interpenetrating layers or fields of energy and each layer vibrates to a different frequency.
- The world and everything in it is interdependent.
- A person can influence the energy system without being able to feel or see it.
- All life experiences are recorded and stored within the energy system.
- Potential illness appears in the energy system before signs of illness appear.
- A person's health and quality of life are affected by the health and quality of the energy system and vice versa.
- The energy system is influenced by the environment, thoughts, emotions, actions, and intentionality.
- Energy can be experienced as movement, temperature, or density. (p. 146)

Researchers and proponents of biofield therapies believe that conscious caring–healing intent is necessary as well as a conscious use of self as a link between the universal life energy and the other individual. Prior to the actual intervention, practitioners focus completely on the well-being of the recipient in an act of unconditional love and compassion. Compassion, basic to all nursing intervention, involves two things: intention and action. Practitioners of biofield therapies always set their intention in mind first before entering and intervening in others' energy fields (Quinn, 2006).

In the early days, most biofield therapists thought they acted solely as a conduit or a channel for environmental energy. Because people are open systems, the transfer of energy is a natural, continuous event. Therefore, it is conceivable that one person could transfer energy to another through conscious intent. That view has since been modified to include repatterning the recipients' energy systems by providing a template of sorts upon which the repatterning occurs. When two people are close to one another, their energy fields overlap. As they intermingle, each energy field influences the other. Through proximity or actual touch, two people create a larger, joint energy field by connecting their individual energy fields. In intentional healing situations, practitioners regulate their own internal energy frequencies, allowing recipients to draw upon the healers' resources and energy patterns. It has been found that in an intentional healing situation, with or without physical contact, a state of coherence and synchrony between the brain waves of the healer and the recipient develops, and they literally become unified in one energetic field (Oschman, 2000).

VIEW OF HEALTH AND ILLNESS

Within individuals, energy flows like a river. If it encounters no obstructions, it is smooth, gliding, and barely perceptible. People whose energy flows smoothly usually report good health and a feeling of peace with themselves and with others. Health, then, is defined as an abundance of qi and a balance or harmony of body, mind, and spirit. In addition, healthy people experience an equilibrium between their own energy systems and those of the environment. If obstructions or imbalance in energy occur, such as trauma, pain, rage, sadness, or any physical, mental, emotional, or spiritual problem, the balanced stream of energy is disrupted, and illness or disease may result.

The locus of healing is within each person and cannot be "given" to a client by a biofield therapist. People must, and do, heal themselves. Healing environments are created when nurses enter into caring moments with clients. This moment provides a spirit-to-spirit connection in which the nurse becomes a resource that clients use to heal themselves. As recipients become engaged in the healing process, they often find new ways of coping with their illness.

TREATMENT

Each of the biofield therapies discussed in this chapter utilizes the following treatment practices:

1. Creating a caring–healing environment (e.g., promoting/supporting a quiet, safe, private, dignified environment with consideration of heating, ventilation, lighting, tidiness, and cleanliness of the environment; promoting the person's comfort with appropriate positioning and attention to their specific needs for order, beauty, and peace).

BOX 14.1

How to Center

- Sit or stand comfortably and close your eyes or focus on one spot on the floor.
- Breathe in and out, slowly and deeply, concentrating on how the breath feels as it goes in and out.
- Breathe in relaxation and peace while breathing out stress and tension.
- Imagine a fairly large tree; really sense the tree as it sounds, as it smells, and according to the season.
- Get close to the tree and put your hands on the tree; lean up against the tree and put your full weight on the tree.
- Look up through the branches and feel the sun shining down; feel the sun traveling down through the tree and coming in through your head, down through your body, and out your legs.
- Focus once again on your breathing and know that you can come back to this place at any time.
- With practice and experience, you will be able to center yourself within one or two deep breaths.

Source: Therapeutic Touch video courses by Janet Quinn, PhD, RN.

2. Centering before beginning the biofield practice. *Centering* is a general term for any method that people use to quiet themselves physically, mentally, and emotionally. Centering can be achieved by many methods, such as deep breathing, visualization, and focusing, which allow the practitioner to relax and focus on the intent of the healing session. Being centered allows healers to operate intuitively, with awareness, and to channel energy throughout their bodies. Box 14.1 describes one centering method.

3. Interview with client prior to caring–healing practice of Healing Touch, Reiki, or Therapeutic Touch.

4. Client may choose to sit or lie down, always fully clothed.

5. Assessment: Steps in the biofield caring–healing process include initial and ongoing assessment of the energy field. Once centered, nurses use their hands to *assess* the recipient's energy field. Some nurses are able to feel the energy field when they first learn their biofield therapy, while for others it takes months of practice to experience the sensations. Different people describe different sensations commonly characterized as heat, cold, tingling, buzzing, emptiness, or pressure. The energy field is assessed for bilateral similarities or differences in the flow of energy. A healthy energy field is symmetrical with a smooth, flowing texture.

Practitioners often combine both physical and nonphysical contact during the course of treatment. Clients do not have to believe in the efficacy of the biofield therapy to receive benefit. The one absolutely essential ingredient in each of these biofield therapies is the goodwill and compassion of the practitioner (see Figure 14.1).

6. The practitioner chooses specific healing interventions based on the interview findings, assessment of the energy field, and specific needs of each client. These specific techniques are carried out with a caring–healing presence and active listening process.

7. Completion and grounding: The practitioner reassesses the biofield of the client prior to "grounding" or helping the client become aware. Often this is accomplished by the nurse gently holding the tops of both feet and shoulders for a minute or two. Another way is to brush down the arms and legs toward the ground until clients start moving their hands and feet and they reconnect completely with their body. Verbal cues such as "Feel your fingers and toes and gently move them" may also be helpful.

8. Feedback, documentation, and planning: Discharge planning begins with the first visit. The practitioner listens to what the client wishes to share about his or her experience and answers any questions the client may have. Counseling and/or education is provided in a mutual process that is based on client goals and the knowledge and skills of the nurse. Examples of areas for dialogue can include but are not limited to stress management, lifestyle, nutrition, quality of life, and self-care processes such as journaling, meditation, exercise/yoga along with other resources that the client finds helpful (i.e., need for referral to other practitioners such as psychotherapist, massage therapist, physician, and so on). Planning may include setting time for future visits with the nurse or teaching the client and/or family a specific biofield technique. The total number of visits with the nurse is based on the client's responses to the biofield therapy. Documentation begins with the initial client interview and continues through the visit.

TT, HT, and Reiki are used only as forms of treatment, not to diagnose physical conditions. They work in conjunction with other medical or therapeutic techniques to promote healing and relieve side effects of conventional therapies. Indications include irritability and anxiety; lethargy, fatigue, and depression; premenstrual syndrome; nausea and vomiting; chemotherapy and radiation sickness; wound and bone healing; and acute musculoskeletal problems such as sprains and muscle spasms. These healing practices are often effective in many types of pain. Side effects of biofield therapies are temporary lightheadedness and/or a temporary sensation of heat. Very gentle treatments are used for infants, the elderly, and those experiencing a critical illness. The primary contraindication to TT, HT, and Reiki is someone who does not want it, which falls under the doctrine of informed consent (Quinn, 2006).

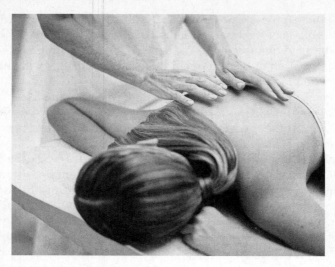

FIGURE 14.1   No Touch Energy Transfer

Source: Getty Images, Inc.-Stone Allstock/Julie Toy

Practitioners believe that when they work with energy fields, they are dealing with that person as a whole, and healing may occur at many levels. Recipients may experience emotional and spiritual growth as well as physical improvement, while in some cases the therapy may not seem to work at all. Even when these methods do not help people resolve a particular problem, the session is soothing and relaxing.

RESEARCH

Research on biofield therapies is in the early stages of development. "Studies of Therapeutic Touch, Healing Touch, and Reiki are quite promising. However, at this point, they can only suggest that these modalities have efficacy in reducing anxiety; improving muscle relaxation; aiding in stress reduction, relaxation, and sense of well-being; promoting wound healing and reducing pain" (Engebretson & Wardell, 2007, p. 243). The National Center for Complementary and Alternative Medicine at the National Institutes of Health is currently funding a number of projects for each of these biofield therapies. The following is a small sample of current studies:

- An experimental, randomized, controlled trial was conducted to determine the efficacy of Healing Touch in 237 patients undergoing coronary artery bypass graft surgery. Participants were randomly assigned to one of three groups: HT group, visitor group, and control group. HT was done three times: the day before surgery, right before surgery, and the day after surgery. Significant differences were noted in anxiety scores when compared to the visitor and control groups. There were no significant differences in the use of pain medication, anti-emetic medication, or the incidence of atrial fibrillation (MacIntyre et al., 2008).

- A recent analysis of randomized, experimental, and controlled studies found 12 articles that met the criteria using HT, TT, or Reiki treatments for people with cancer. Although there were varying levels of evidence, it was agreed that these biofield therapies reduced pain and anxiety in the treatment groups (Jackson et al., 2008).
- Bossi, Ott, and DeCristofara (2008) reviewed the literature regarding Reiki as an intervention for people with various problems. Findings included a significant drop in heart rate, the facilitation of the relaxation response, and a reduction in pain, depression, and anxiety.
- Fibroblasts, tendon cells, and bone cells in culture were treated with TT, sham TT, or untreated for a 2-week period of time. TT significantly increased proliferation of all three types of cells compared to the sham TT and the untreated groups (Gronowicz, Jhaveri, Clarke, Aronow, & Smith, 2008).
- 148 people in alcohol recovery were randomized to HT or the Big Book control group. Those receiving HT had a greater reduction in both physiological and psychological levels of stress compared to the Big Book group (Dubrey, 2006).

USING RESEARCH TO HEAL

Wardell, D. W., Rintala, D., & Tan, G. (2008, May/June). Study descriptions of Healing Touch with veterans experiencing chronic neuropathic pain from spinal cord injury. *Explore*, 4(3): 187–195.

What Is This Study About?

Many patients with spinal cord injury experience chronic pain syndromes that conventional pain treatment is unable to relieve. Therefore, the purpose of this study was to gain information about the influence of HT on the energy field for these patients and practitioners, using a qualitative case study approach (total seven cases). The researchers obtained data from 42 HT sessions from seven veterans with spinal cord injury who were experiencing chronic neuropathic pain and its sequelae.

What Were the Results of the Study?

The two cases demonstrated "changes in the energy field and the chakra patterns over time." Within the series of sessions, there were different patterns or even repetitions of previous 'cleared' patterns. This might help explain the variable nature of healing, as often times other unresolved issues would surface. Even when subjects did not report a positive response to the HT sessions, they did report changes, which may account for some of the responses that did not directly deal with the pain experience. The changes might have also been due to the desire and intent of the Clinical Healing Touch Practitioner (CHTP) to effect change. However, it was evident that the CHTPs were able to discern changes pre-session

(continued)

and post-session that did not always indicate a complete clearing or balancing of the field. HT did have an effect on the perception of pain for the beneficial and equivocal cases. This might be clinically significant when dealing with intractable and chronic pain. However, further study would be needed to determine long-term benefits and efficacy. Patient satisfaction questionnaires, to date, have indicated a high degree of satisfaction in improving relaxation and decreasing pain" (Wardell, Rintala, & Tan, 2008, p. 194).

What Additional Questions Might I Have?

Knowing that this study utilized local and full body techniques, which varied from session to session based on the patient's needs, seems to suggest that the use of standard protocols within study designs may be problematic. Are there other examples when the use of standard protocols within a study design would be appropriate?

How Can I Use This Study?

Nurses can consider the appropriateness of Healing Touch in collaboration with patients experiencing pain, as a complementary caring–healing modality, in conjunction with other pain treatments. This is also a study that would be useful for students who are learning about various biofield techniques as it presents a number of different techniques, along with hand-drawn pictures of various patients' energy fields before and after HT sessions.

INTEGRATED NURSING PRACTICE

Hand-mediated biofield therapies of TT and HT have been pioneered by nurses and are easily learned by nurses. Although many nursing curricula currently include some components of biofield therapies, most of us did not receive information about the use of hand-mediated biofield therapies in nursing school. If you have not been taught any of these therapies, you may want to participate in courses that are shown on the websites for Healing Touch, Therapeutic Touch, and/or Reiki (see Resource list).

You can use TT, HT, and Reiki in almost any clinical setting, including hospitals, nursing homes, home health care, hospice, and private practice. TT, HT, and Reiki are used in Lamaze classes, labor rooms, newborn nurseries, neonatal intensive care units, pediatric units, medical surgical units, recovery rooms, palliative care, and in behavioral medicine. These therapies are helpful for people with a variety of health needs. In the current health care environment, people with acute and chronic disorders are rapidly discharged back to the community. Family and friends are often overwhelmed by caregiver responsibilities. Often they feel helpless in the face of their loved one's obvious suffering or pain. Teaching caregivers one or more biofield modalities can be a powerful nursing intervention that counteracts the sense of helplessness many of them experience. As caregivers discover that biofield therapies can minimize the experience of pain and increase the sense of relaxation, they often feel they have something "worthwhile" to offer. In addition, the use of biofield therapies can be helpful to the caregiver, who is most likely exhausted from trying to carry on the normal daily routine, as well as care for the sick or injured person. Because one of the steps of biofield therapies is centering, the process demands that caregivers take a few minutes for themselves as they concentrate on their well-being and sense of peace. As caregivers increase their self-awareness, they are quicker to recognize tension and stress in their bodies, which should encourage them to develop stress management skills. TT, HT, and Reiki produce a sense of well-being and relaxation for both the nurse and the recipient. For some nurses, it is the first time they have been given permission to be quiet, take a breath, and center during working hours. When you walk into a client's room or home in a peaceful state of mind, that gentleness, that kindness permeates the environment. Recipients react positively to the treatments, but also to the individual attention from nurses as they build relationships with clients, offer noninvasive nurturing touch, and reduce clients' stress and anxiety (Brill & Kashurba, 2001). As Dr. Janet Quinn (1992) has said, "We can participate in creating environments that will support healing. We can become midwives to this process of healing, creating and being safe, a sacred space into which the healing might emerge. We can, literally, become the healing environment" (p. 28). Practicing one or more of the biofield therapies is one of the ways we, as nurses, create healing environments.

TRY THIS

Experience Your Energy Field

- Vigorously rub your hands together for 20–30 seconds.
- Hold your palms together, parallel but not touching.
- Slowly separate them a couple of inches.
- Slowly bring them close together again.
- Repeat this process several more times, each time separating your palms by an additional two inches until they are eight inches apart.
- You should be able to detect your energy field as you bring your palms together; you may feel a sense of bounciness, sponginess, or elasticity; some people describe it as the feeling of two magnets repelling each other.

References

Bossi, L. M., Ott, M. J., & DeCristofaro, S. (2008). Reiki as a clinical intervention in oncology nursing practice. *Clinical Journal of Oncology Nursing*, 12(3): 489–494.

Brill, C., & Kashurba, M. (2001). Each moment of touch. *Nursing Administration Quarterly*, 25(23): 8–14.

Collinge, W. (1998). *Subtle Energy*. New York: Warner Books.

Dubrey, R. J., Sr. (2006, December). The role of Healing Touch in the treatment of persons in recovery from alcoholism. *Counselor*, 58–64.

Engebretson, J., & Wardell, D. D. (2007). Energy-based modalities. *Nursing Clinics of North America*, 42(2): 243–259.

Green, E., & Green, A. (1989). *Beyond Biofeedback*. New York: Knoll Publishers.

Gronowicz, G. A., Jhaveri, A., Clarke, L. W., Aronow, M. S., & Smith, R. H. (2008). Therapeutic Touch stimulates the proliferation of human cells in culture. *The Journal of Alternative and Complementary Medicine*. 14(3): 233–239.

Healing Touch Program (2008). *Healing Touch Program: Creating healing relationships*. Arvada, CO: Healing Touch Program.

Jackson, E., Kelley, M., McNeil, P., Meyer, E., Schlegel, L., & Eaton, M. (2008). Does therapeutic touch help reduce pain and anxiety in patients with cancer? *Clinical Journal of Oncology Nursing*, 12(1): 113–120.

Kreiger, D. (1979). *The Therapeutic Touch. How to Use Your Hands to Help or to Heal*. New York: Prentice Hall.

Kunz, D. (1991). *The Personal Aura*. Wheaton, IL: Quest.

MacIntyre, B., Hamilton, J., Fricke, T., Ma, W., Mehle, S., & Michel, M. (2008). The efficacy of Healing Touch in coronary artery bypass surgery recovery: A randomized clinical trial. *Alternative Therapies*, 14(4): 24–32.

Mentgen, J. (2001). Healing touch. *Nursing Clinics of North America*, 36(1): 143–157.

National Center for Complementary and Alternative Medicine (2007). Energy medicine: An overview. NCCAM Publication No. D235. http://nccam.nih.gov/health/backgrounds/energymed.htm. Accessed September 5, 2008.

National Center for Complementary and Alternative Medicine (2008). *An Introduction to Reiki*. NCCAM Publication No. D315. http://nccam.nih.gov/health/reiki.htm. Accessed September 5, 2008.

Newman, M. A. (1997). Evolution of theory of health as expanding consciousness. *Nursing Science Quarterly*, 7: 153–157.

Oschman, J. L. (2000). *Energy Medicine: The Scientific Basis of Bioenergy Therapies*. New York: Churchill Livingstone.

Quinn, J. F. (1992). Holding sacred space. The nurse as healing environment. *Holistic Nursing Practice*, 6(4): 26–36.

Quinn, J. F. (2006). Therapeutic Touch. In M. Snyder & R. Linquist (Eds.), *Complementary/Alternative Therapies in Nursing* (5th ed., pp. 225–241). New York: Springer Publishing Company.

Rogers, M. E. (1992). Nursing science and the space age. *Nursing Science Quarterly*, 5(1): 27–34.

Watson, J. (1999). *Postmodern Nursing and Beyond*. Edinburgh: Churchill Livingstone.

Watson, J. (2005). *Caring Science As Sacred Science*. Philadelphia, PA: F. A. Davis.

Resources

American Holistic Nurses Association
323 N. San Francisco St., Suite 201
Flagstaff, AZ 86001
800.278.2462
www.ahna.org

Canadian Holistic Nurses Association
c/o Marie Knapp
RR7
Owen Sound, OT, Canada
519.371.1255
www.chna.ca

Canadian Reiki Association
  P.O. Box 54570
  7155 Kingsway
  Burnaby BC V5E 4J6
  www.reiki.ca

Healing Touch Canada
  RR2
  Warsaw, ON K0L 3A0, Canada
  705.652.0506
  www.healingtouchcanada.net

Healing Touch International
  445 Union Blvd.
  Lakewood, CO 80228
  303.989.7982
  www.healingtouch.net

Nurse Healers Professional Associates
  International
  Box 419
  Craryville, NY 12521
  877.326.4724
  www.therapeutic-touch.org

International Center for Reiki Training
  21421 Hilltop St., Suite 28
  Southfield, MI 48034
  800.332.8112
  www.reiki.org

15

Combined Physical and Biofield Therapies

In every culture and in every medical tradition before ours, healing was accomplished by moving energy.

ALBERT SZENT-GYORGYI

The two methods described in this chapter, Applied Kinesiology and Polarity Therapy, are a combination of physical and biofield interventions. *Applied Kinesiology* is both a diagnostic method and treatment modality using energy, lymphatic, neurovascular, and muscle systems. *Polarity Therapy*, a nondiagnostic healing system, is based on the theories of Traditional Chinese Medicine and Ayurvedic medicine and combines bodywork, diet, exercise, and counseling in the treatment of clients.

BACKGROUND

George Goodheart and Alan G. Beardell, American chiropractic physicians, developed **Applied Kinesiology** in the 1960s. In the 1970s, John Thie, also a chiropractor, took their work, simplified it for the general public, and called this modified approach "Touch for Health." **Polarity Therapy** is a system of health care developed in the 1920s by an Austrian-American holistic physician, Randolph Stone, who was a chiropractor, osteopath, and naturopath. He studied and tested health theories from around the world, combining ancient and modern techniques. His first work was published in 1947, and by 1954 he had completed the seven books that contain his findings.

PREPARATION

Health care professionals may go on to study Applied Kinesiology only after completion of their basic professional education. Chiropractors, nurses, osteopaths, naturopaths, dentists, and physicians practice Applied Kinesiology. Interested professionals take the training in a postgraduate setting, usually in weekend classes. The basic course takes more than 100 hours of classroom study and numerous hours of practice in the clinical setting after which students can test for basic proficiency. Another 200 hours of classes and the writing of at least two research papers are undertaken to reach the next step in which a diplomate written and oral exam is taken. Organized courses in Applied Kinesiology are taught in Europe, Canada, the United States, and Australia. There is no licensure per se; providers of Applied Kinesiology practice on their professional license.

Polarity Therapy is practiced by a variety of health care professionals who have completed their basic education. To achieve the level of associate polarity practitioner, the applicant must take 155 classroom and clinical hours of study in a program approved by the American Polarity Therapy Association (APTA). Those wishing to become registered polarity practitioners must take an additional 520 hours of study for cumulative hours totaling 675. No licensure was available as of 2004. Some states, however, are considering licensing polarity therapists under massage therapists, even though they are distinct therapeutic practices (American Polarity Therapy Association, 2003).

CONCEPTS

As in many alternative practices, the concept of energy is at the heart of Applied Kinesiology and Polarity Therapy. The belief is in a life force of subtle energy that surrounds and permeates all living things, often referred to as a *biofield*. It is unclear at this time whether the biofield is electromagnetic or a field in physics other than an already known field. The present hypotheses are that the biofield is a form of bioelectricity, biomagnetism, or bioelectromagnetism. The exact nature is not yet established (Smith, 2008).

Meridians

Applied Kinesiology works closely with the meridian system and pressure points. *Meridians* are a network of energy circuits that run vertically through the body. Each meridian passes close to the skin's surface at places called *pressure points*. Since each meridian is associated with an internal organ, the points offer surface access to the internal organ system. Each of the 14 meridians has related specific neurovascular points and neurolymphatic points (Smith, 2008).

Neurovascular Points

Neurovascular points are located mainly on the head. A few seconds after placing one's fingers on these points, a slight pulse can be felt at a steady rate of 70 to 74 beats per minute. This pulse is not related to the heartbeat, but is believed to be the primitive pulsation of the microscopic capillary bed in the skin.

Neurolymphatic Points

The lymphatic system in the body flows only in one direction and acts as a drainage system for the body. It produces antibodies, makes white blood cells, and transports fats, proteins, and other substances to the blood system. Neurolymphatic reflexes, located mainly on the chest and back, regulate the energy to the lymphatic system. These reflex points act like switches that get turned off when the system is overloaded. They are usually tender spots and those which are the most sore are in greatest need of massage.

Polarity

The term **polarity** refers to the universal pulsation of expansion/contraction or attraction/repulsion known as yin and yang energy in Traditional Chinese Medicine. These polarized forces together make up the whole of anything. For example, all tissues in one's body can be understood in terms of charged energy categorized as positive, negative, or neutral. These three are in constant dynamic tension with each other, creating the basis for health or illness. Polarity between different body parts appears to be equivalent to polar differences in electromagnetic fields. The head and the right side of the body represent the positive pole and the feet and left side represent the negative pole. The center of the body, along with the spinal cord, is neutral and contains five energy centers that correspond to the chakras of Ayurvedic medicine. Polarity therapists think of the right hand as the giving energy hand and the left as the receiving energy hand. It is believed that energy is affected and possibly distorted by life experiences, diet, movement, sound, attitudes, relationships, trauma, and environmental factors, and that these distortions may be corrected by a variety of healing methods.

VIEW OF HEALTH AND ILLNESS

Well-being and health are determined by the nature of the flow of energy within and without the body. When energy flows smoothly without significant blockage or fixation, the person experiences health in an ongoing and dynamic way. Disease and pain occur when energy is blocked, fixed, or unbalanced. When someone's physical body, thoughts, and emotions are out of alignment with the energy necessary to meet a life challenge, an energy imbalance results. Within the Applied Kinesiology framework, one of the signs of an imbalance is a weakening of the muscles and a change in the posture. If these minor problems are not corrected, the imbalances may develop into physical, mental, and emotional discomfort or pain. Pain and discomfort are seen as signals to people to learn, change, and realign their lives.

Diagnostic Methods

An Applied Kinesiology exam depends on knowledge of functional neurology, anatomy, physiology, biomechanics, and biochemistry. It is combined with standard procedures, laboratory findings, X-rays, and history taking. Generally, problems can be related to a chemical imbalance, a structural imbalance, mental stress, or any combination of these states. General examination procedures are used to assess the health of the client and are followed by specific examination procedures such as testing reflexes or assessing balance.

Every muscle in the body is related to a specific organ or gland through the sharing of lymphatic vessels or meridians. Because organs and glands have few pain and sensory fibers, people are largely unaware of energetic imbalances in these parts. Unbalanced organs or glands, however, refer pain externally to the corresponding surface meridians and muscles, indicating the cause of the problem. For example, the deltoid muscle in the shoulder shares a relationship with the lungs. If a person has abnormal lung function, such as bronchitis, pneumonia, congestion, or the flu, the problem may exhibit as a weakness in one or both deltoid muscles. When the lung problem is cleared up, the deltoid muscle returns to a normal state (Hislop & Montgomery, 2007).

Manual muscle testing is done to augment the other examination procedures. Goodheart and Beardall designed specific methods for testing the function of the 576 muscles of the body. Muscle weaknesses are often so subtle that physical therapists would consider the muscle strength to be within normal limits. No more than 15 percent difference should be discernible between the right and left sides. The testing positions are intended to isolate the muscle from the group with which it normally works, making it less strong than if it were used in the usual way. Small children, the elderly, and the frail will not be as strong as a healthy adult. It is more difficult to test a person who has great strength, such as an athlete, because the weakness cannot be distinguished by the tester (Hislop & Montgomery, 2007).

A number of causes result in weak muscles, including immobility, lack of exercise, poor posture, gland/organ dysfunction, dysfunction of the nerve supply, impairment of lymphatic drainage, decreased blood supply, blockage of meridians, and chemical imbalance. Testing of individual muscles is combined with knowledge of the basic mechanics and physiological functioning of the body to provide practitioners with information necessary to formulate a diagnosis.

TREATMENT

Applied Kinesiology and Polarity Therapy practitioners believe that the body, mind, emotions, and spirit are interdependent. It is believed that people are responsible for their own health and that they can take simple steps to improve and maintain their level of wellness. The practitioner's role is to facilitate and support clients' self-healing capabilities.

Applied Kinesiology uses various methods to strengthen those muscles and related organs that were found to be weak during the diagnostic phase. Improvement in the flow of energy can be measured by increased muscle strength, which is assumed to lead to an increase in energy to the corresponding organs.

Neurovascular holding points are located mainly on the head. The practitioner makes simple contact with the pads of the fingers for anywhere from 20 seconds to 10 minutes, depending on the severity of the problem. This method appears to improve the blood circulation to both the muscle and the related organ, and the weak muscle will have increased strength when retested.

Neurolymphatic points are located mainly on the chest and back. Practitioners work on the points that are related to a specific weakened muscle by a deep massage of the points for 20 to 30 seconds. This massage is believed to turn on the blocked reflexes, allowing the lymph flow to return to normal. The weak muscle will have improved strength when retested. Figure 15.1 illustrates the neurolymphatic points for the lungs.

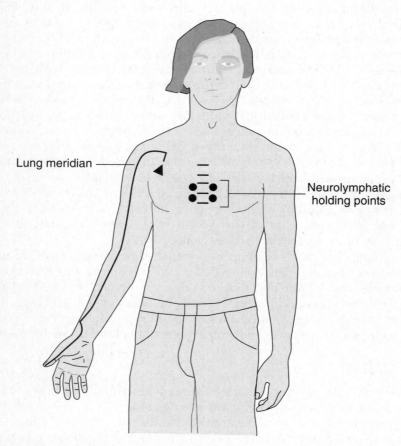

FIGURE 15.1 Lung Meridian and Neurolymphatic Holding Points

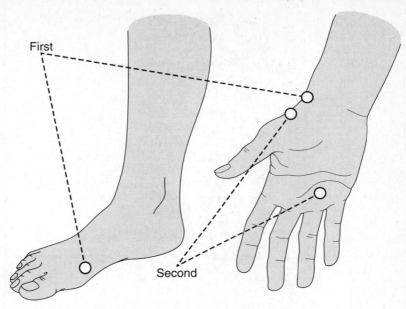

FIGURE 15.2 Pressure Points for the Lungs

Meridians are traced in the designated direction using both sides of the body. Practitioners use the flat of their hands to give better coverage. It can be done over clothing without actually touching the client. Tracing the meridian adds the practitioner's flow of energy to the recipient's energy in a blocked meridian and may restore the normal flow of energy. Figure 15.1 also illustrates the lung meridian.

Acupressure points are held on the same side of the body as the muscle that is weak. The first arm and leg points are held at the same time, one with each hand. Light pressure is maintained for about 30 seconds or until a pulse is felt in the leg. The hands are then moved to the second acupressure points and held, again waiting for the pulse in the leg (Hislop & Montgomery, 2007). Figure 15.2 illustrates the pressure points for the lungs.

In a typical Polarity Therapy session, the practitioner assesses energy flow using palpation, observation, and interview with the recipient clothed for the entire session. Sessions usually take 60 to 90 minutes and involve both touch and verbal interaction (see Figure 15.3). Touch contact may be light, medium, or firm and is used to stimulate and balance the body's biofield. During the session, the practitioner supports the client in increasing self-awareness of subtle energy sensations, which may be experienced as tingling, warmth, or wavelike movement. Clients are also helped to process feelings and develop specific strategies for reducing stress and increasing wellness. Clients are encouraged to take responsibility for their lives and create positive thinking, which is the cornerstone of good health (Oschman, 2000).

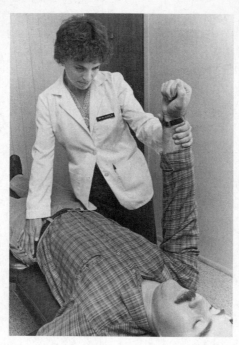

FIGURE 15.3 A Polarity Therapy Practitioner Stretches the Arm of a Male Client

Source: Pearson Education/PH Collage/Laimute Druskis

Adherents of both Applied Kinesiology and Polarity Therapy believe that nutrition plays a major role in health and well-being. Kinesiology assesses people's nutritional status, including food intolerances, vitamin and mineral deficiencies, and other chemical sensitivities. Polarity nutrition views food as energy and develops an ongoing, changing nutritional awareness rather than a rigid set of rules. Many practitioners support the value of a vegetarian diet with no meat, fish, fowl, or eggs. They also advocate periodic use of a "cleansing diet," consisting of fresh and cooked vegetables, as well as herbal cleansing practices and formulas (American Polarity Therapy Association, 2003).

Exercise is an important part of these therapies. Applied Kinesiology practitioners encourage clients to walk for exercise. Walking is one of the few exercises that benefit all parts of the body. All of the muscles are flowing when people walk with their arms swinging. Polarity yoga is a series of simple self-help energy techniques that create relaxation and balance. This bodywork includes gentle rocking and stretching postures combining breathing and self-massage, both of which affect the flow of energy.

Applied Kinesiology can relieve pain, stress, and muscular disorders. It is used to detect allergies, nutritional deficiencies, back or neck pain, fatigue, headache, tension, and the common cold and is believed to have some benefit for those with learning disorders. Polarity Therapy induces profound relaxation, new insight into energy flow patterns, and positive changes on the physical, mental, and emotional levels.

RESEARCH

The National Institutes of Health are currently funding seven studies on Polarity Therapy and one study on Kinesiology (http://clinicaltrials.gov, 2008). Cuthbert and Goodheart (2007) conducted a literature review of studies related to manual muscle testing and Applied Kinesiology. Twelve randomized controlled trials met the criteria for the review. The analysis demonstrated good reliability and validity in the use of Applied Kinesiology for people with neuromusculoskeletal problems.

INTEGRATED NURSING PRACTICE

As a nurse, you need advanced study to apply the specific techniques of Applied Kinesiology and Polarity Therapy. As a practitioner in Applied Kinesiology, you may actively intervene or make suggested changes to address food allergies, chemical imbalances, or nutritional deficiencies as determined by your clinical assessment. If appropriate, clients are encouraged to take care of their physical body with moderate exercise such as walking or swimming.

As a Polarity Therapist, you may suggest dietary changes that help balance the body. You may also suggest specific cleansing diets, herbs, and procedures to rid the body of toxic accumulations of waste products. Clients who have restricted breathing patterns may be given breathing exercises. Bodywork in Polarity Therapy involves many techniques, most of which are gentle, such as cranial holds, rocking movements, or reflexology movements. As a Polarity Therapist, you also pay close attention to people's thoughts and feelings. Negative thoughts and feelings can be detrimental to a state of well-being.

TRY THIS
Emotional First Aid

The next time you are upset, try this procedure to decrease your stress.

- Hold the frontal eminences on your forehead either with the first two fingers of your hands—the right and left at the same time—or place the palm of your hand flat on your forehead.
- While applying light pressure, in your mind go over exactly what you are thinking and how you are feeling about the problem. Continue holding these points and going over what is bothering you for a few minutes or until you feel the emotions becoming less strong.
- Let go with your hands and look around you. Mentally review the issue again. If stressful feelings are still there or have changed to other stressful feelings (fear changed to anger, for example), go back and begin the process again. After a further few minutes, release the pressure and check your feelings about the situation again.
- Hopefully your mind feels clearer and the same emotions no longer have the same stressful impact.

TRY THIS

Redirecting the Flow of Energy

Sit facing a partner and, placing both hands in the air, move your hands close to your partner's hands without touching. Experiment with distance and where you can feel the energy pulsating between your hands. Imagine that your partner's energy is coming in your left hand from your partner's right hand and your energy is flowing from your right hand into your partner's left hand. Imagine the circular circuit between the two of you as the energy flows up the left arm, across the heart, and down the right arm. Imagine how connected you feel at this given moment.

References

American Polarity Therapy Association. (2003). *Foundation of Professionalism in Polarity Therapy Practice*. Boulder, CO: Author.

Cuthbert, S. C., & Goodheart, G. J., Jr. (2007). On the reliability and validity of manual muscle testing: A literature review. *Chiropractic & Osteopathy*, 15(4): 1–22. www.chiroandosteo.com/content/15/1/4. Accessed December 02, 2008.

Hislop, H., & Montgomery, J. (2007). *Daniels and Worthingham's Muscle Testing: Techniques of Manual Examination*, 8th ed. Philadelphia, PA: Saunders.

Oschman, J. L. (2000). *Energy Medicine: The Scientific Basis of Energy Therapies*. New York: Churchill Livingston.

Smith, K. (2008). *Awakening the Energy Body*. Rochester, VT: Bear & Company. http://clincialtrials.gov. Accessed August 22, 2008.

Resources

American Polarity Therapy Association
  122 N. Elm St., Suite 512
  Greensboro, NC 27401
  336.574.1121
  www.polaritytherapy.org

Ontario Polarity Therapy Association
  416.621.6857
  www.polaritytherapy.ca

The Kinesiology Federation
  P.O. Box 28908
  Dalkeith EH22 2YQ UK
  084.5260.1094
  www.kinesiologyfederation.org

Touch for Health Kinesiology
  Association
  3225 West St. Joseph
  Lansing, MI 48917
  800.466.8342
  www.tfhka.org

Mind–Body Techniques

I still need more healthy rest in order to work at my best. My health is the main capital I have and I want to administer it intelligently.

ERNEST HEMINGWAY

Peace is present right here and now, in ourselves and in everything we do and see. The question is whether or not we are in touch with it.

THICH NHAT HANH

16

Yoga

*You have to trust your inner knowing. If
you have a clear mind . . . you won't have
to search for direction. Direction will
come to you.*

PHIL JACKSON

Yoga, part of Ayurvedic medicine, has been practiced for thousands of years in India, where it is a way of life that includes ethical models for behavior and mental and physical exercises aimed at producing spiritual enlightenment. Although yoga developed from Hinduism, it is not a religion, but rather a journey of the body, mind, and spirit on a path toward unity. It is a method for life that can complement and enhance any system of religion, or it can be practiced completely apart from religion.

The Western approach to yoga tends to be more fitness oriented, whereas the Eastern approach to yoga is to prepare people for the experience of self-realization. Most Westerners begin yoga with the goal of managing their stress, learning to relax, and increasing their vitality and well-being. After learning yoga, many become more interested in the underlying principles of physical fitness and keeping the mind focused, calm, and clear. Yoga is meant to prepare the body and mind for a useful, dedicated life.

BACKGROUND

The word *yoga* means to direct and concentrate one's attention and comes from the Sanskrit word *yuj*, meaning "to yoke" or "to join." Yoga was first described by Patanjali, an Indian sage who, thousands of years ago, wrote the *Yoga Sutra*, which recorded information that had been passed down orally for many years. This text has helped to define and shape the modern practice of yoga. Yoga first came to the United States in the 1890s, when Swami Vivekananda became a popular teacher and guide. In the 1960s, the Maharishi Mahesh Yogi, the creator of Transcendental Meditation, became a popular figure for America's "hippie generation," and the vogue has continued to grow since then.

The various methods of yoga all have the same goal: to attain a state of pure bliss and oneness with the universe. *Raja yoga* emphasizes control of the intellect to attain enlightenment, accomplished through meditation, concentration, and breath control. *Kriya yoga* is the practice of quieting the mind through scriptural study, breath control, mantras, and meditation. *Karma yoga* focuses on service to all beings as the path to enlightenment. *Bhakti yoga* emphasizes devotion to the divine. *Inana yoga*'s goal is wisdom and the direct knowledge of the divine. *Tantra yoga* involves the study of sacred writings and rituals. *Mantra yoga* is the study of sacred sounds. *Kundalini yoga* is the study of energy movement along the spine. *Iyengar yoga*, a form of *hatha yoga*, strives for perfection in the postures using props such as belts or ropes. *Silver yoga* is designed to accommodate those with reduced body flexibility such as senior people or those with physical challenges (Platania, 2009; Stone & Iyengar, 2009).

Although these many branches of yoga exist, this chapter focuses on **hatha yoga** as the form of yoga most frequently practiced by Westerners. In this particular type of yoga, the path to enlightenment is through control over the physical body as the key to control of the mind and freedom of the spirit. Physical exercises, breath control, and meditation tone and strengthen the whole person—body, mind, and spirit.

PREPARATION

No national licensure or standard certification is required for yoga instructors. Becoming a yoga instructor or yoga therapist requires much more personal dedication than many other alternative therapy practitioners. To be admitted to most training programs, prospective yoga instructors must have been practicing yoga daily for 6 months to a year, abstain from drugs, alcohol, and tobacco, and follow a vegetarian diet.

CONCEPTS

Classical yoga incorporates *eight limbs* or *paths* that provide structure for one's daily life. These physical and psychological practices are believed to contribute to a higher level of personal development. The outer aspect of yoga consists of right living (abstinence and personal discipline), right care of the body (body control), and enhancement of vital energy (breath control). Yoga also has an inner dimension that emphasizes its key purpose. Detachment, concentration, and meditation together form a single process toward the development of pure consciousness (Carapellese & Slonina, 2009). Box 16.1 lists the eight limbs of yoga.

BOX 16.1

The Eight Limbs of Yoga: Guidelines for Living

1. Abstinences (yamas)
      Nonviolence (ahimsa)
      Truthfulness (satya)
      Nonstealing (asteya)
      Chastity or nonlust (brahmacharya)
      Nongreed (aparigraha)
2. Personal Disciplines (niyamas)
      Purity (shauca)
      Contentment (santosha)
      Self-discipline (tapas)
      Self-study (svadhyaya)
      Centering on the divine (ishvara-pranidhana)
3. Body Control (asanas)
4. Breath Control (pranayama)
5. Detachment (pratyahara)
6. Concentration (dharana)
7. Meditation (dhyana)
8. Pure Consciousness (samadhi)

Abstinences

Abstinences are about what not to do in life. The first abstinence pertains to nonviolence. Nonviolence not only means not physically hurting others but also having nonviolent words and nonviolent thoughts. Truthfulness, the second abstinence, results in personal integrity and strength of character. Nonstealing, the third abstinence, includes not stealing others' material belongings as well as not taking credit for things one has not done, not stealing the center of attention, and so forth. The fourth abstinence, chastity or nonlust, means holding people in high esteem and loving and respecting others. The fifth abstinence is nongreed, which means living simply and viewing possessions as tools to use in life. Nongreed leads to the avoidance of jealousy and envy (Jayanti, 2009).

Personal Disciplines

Personal disciplines are about what to do in life. Purity, the first discipline, is achieved through the practice of the five abstinences. The abstinences clear away negative ways of being, leading one straight to purity. Purity also relates to cleanliness and respect for all life. Contentment, the second discipline, means finding happiness with who one is and with what one has. The third discipline, self-discipline, means being able to make a commitment and adhere to it. The fourth discipline, self-study, means studying oneself through introspection. Centering on the divine, the fifth discipline involves devotion. These disciplines work with any religion because individuals are encouraged to focus on how the divine is in them, part of them, and all around them (Jayanti, 2009).

Body Control

Body control, an important part of hatha yoga, is attained through a number of poses or **asanas.** These body positions are what most Western people think of when they hear the word *yoga* (see Figure 16.1). These poses help people learn to control their bodies, making them stronger, more flexible, better functioning, and more resistant to disease and other problems. Poses are also meant to facilitate meditation. The poses are frequently classified into the following groups: standing poses, inverted poses, twists, backward bending poses, forward bends, and poses for restoration. Another way of classifying poses is balance, strength, flexibility, and relaxation. The belief in nonviolence also applies to the poses, which means that physical exercise is never done to the point of pain, because pain is indicative of doing violence to the body (Stone & Iyengar, 2009).

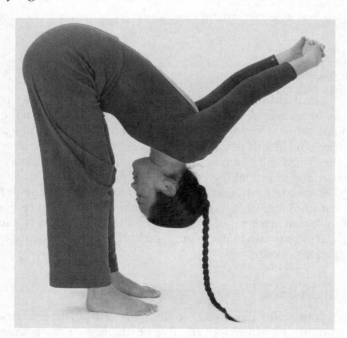

FIGURE 16.1 Woman Bent Over with Her Arms Stretched Over Her Head

Source: Dorling Kindersley Media Library/Dorling Kindersley

Breath Control

Breath control teaches people to direct energy or prana for optimal physical and mental benefit. When air is inhaled, so is vital energy that flows into the body to nourish and enliven. The purpose of balancing the breath is to make respiratory rhythm more regular, which in turn has a soothing effect on the entire nervous system. It is the best antecedent to meditation, because it focuses attention inward and reduces scattered thinking (Platania, 2009).

Detachment

The practice of detachment is related to the senses. It is the withdrawal of the senses from everything that stimulates them. The goal of detachment is to gain mastery over external influences. This detachment can happen during breathing exercises, during meditation, and while doing the poses. The process of detachment can also be an effective technique for pain control (Jayanti, 2009).

Concentration

Teaching the mind to focus on one thing instead of many is the goal of concentration. Concentration is sustaining attention while at the same time quieting the mind and relaxing the breathing. Frequently people focus on one object such as a candle flame, the figure of a circle, or a single sound. The purpose is to learn to push away many thoughts that usually float around in one's mind. Concentration works directly on the body, allowing each yoga pose to accomplish the maximum possible benefit (Jayanti, 2009).

Meditation

Breath control, detachment, and concentration lead to the state of meditation. Meditation occurs when people become absorbed into the object upon which they are concentrating. At this point, nothing else exists. It is through the process of meditation that people are able to clear their minds of clutter and thus think more quickly and see things more clearly in daily life (Kabat-Zinn, 2007). Meditation is covered as a separate topic in Chapter 17.

Pure Consciousness

The other seven limbs of yoga lead to pure consciousness. It means a total merging with the object of meditation and, in such a way, becoming one with the universe. Generally speaking, it is "mind without thought." Many religions throughout history have pure consciousness as part of their tradition. Christianity refers to it as "pure love" and Judaism as the "divine nothingness" or "the naught." It is more than a mental or emotional experience. Physically, breathing slows drastically, the heart rate drops, and EEGs demonstrate unique patterns unlike any of the other three common states of consciousness— waking, sleeping, or dreaming. It is an ideal state, a state of pure bliss that is elusive for most people. A few rare and diligent yogis have been able to maintain this state for extended periods of time. Most others get occasional glimpses of it while meditating (Kabat-Zinn, 2003).

VIEW OF HEALTH AND ILLNESS

In yoga, health is related to the **five sheaths of existence.** The first sheath is the physical body; the second is the vital body, life force, or prana; the third sheath is the mind, including thoughts and emotions; the fourth sheath is the higher intellect; and the fifth sheath is bliss, filled with positive energy and inner peace. It is believed that imbalances in any of these sheaths can result in illness. For example, intense anger, a disturbance in the third sheath, disrupts one's breathing pattern, which leads to an imbalance in prana or life force. The disrupted breathing allows the invasion of a virus leading to a disruption in the first sheath, manifesting as a cold. Living one's life in moderation is thought to keep all five sheaths in balance, which contributes to health and well-being.

Yogic thought places *food* or *ahara* on three levels. The first is the physical food that nourishes the body. The second is impressions or the sensations of sound, touch, sight, taste, and smell that nourish the mind. The third level is associations or the people who nourish the soul. Health and well-being are withdrawal from wrong food, wrong impressions, and wrong associations, while simultaneously opening up to the right food, right impressions, and right associations. Just as a healthy body resists toxins and pathogens, a healthy mind resists the negative influences around it (Stone & Iyengar, 2009).

The yogic perspective of health and illness is related to internal and external balance. Although it is recognized that viruses, bacteria, genetics, and accidents can cause illness, disorders can also be brought on by:

- Insufficient prana, or life force
- Blocked prana
- Inappropriate diet
- Lack of cleanliness
- Unhappiness
- Pessimism and negativity

Healthy habits, maintenance of the body, peacefulness of mind, and calmness of spirit protect people from ill health. Yoga is a great preventive medicine. It helps the body cleanse itself of toxins by removing obstacles to the proper flow of the lymphatic system. Lymph is pumped through the body by movement—musculoskeletal movement, respiratory movement, circulatory movement, gastrointestinal movement, and so forth, all of which are part of yoga. Yoga also increases the flow of vital energy throughout the body by opening up and increasing the flexibility of body joints, considered to be minor chakras. Yoga poses and breathing techniques allow energy and lymph to flow freely throughout the entire body, resulting in a body that works better, feels better, and fights disease more effectively. Health, from a yogic perspective, can be described as the body easeful, the mind peaceful, and the life useful (Carapellese & Slonina, 2009; Platania, 2009).

TREATMENT

People can do as much or as little yoga as they wish. Some start with all three practices—poses, breath control, and meditation. Others start with the poses and may or may not develop interest in breathing and meditation.

As practiced in the United States, a typical yoga session lasts 20 minutes to an hour. Some spend 30 minutes doing poses and another 30 minutes doing breathing practices and meditation. Others spend the majority of the time doing poses and end with a short meditation or relaxation procedure. Some people practice one to three times a week in a class, while others practice daily at home. Yoga should not be done within one to two hours after a heavy meal for sake of abdominal comfort when doing the poses. Caffeine and other stimulants should be avoided because they may interfere with the goal of relaxation. Yoga should never be done under the influence of alcohol or recreational drugs because they may decrease concentration, coordination, and strength, thus increasing the risk of physical injury. Yoga is best done in comfortable, loose clothing using a nonslippery surface such as a rug, mat, or blanket. Because it is important that the process has one's full attention, the room should be void of all extraneous noise, even soft background music.

Yoga is tailored to the individual and can be done with great benefit at the beginner level as well as at the most advanced level. Participants must remember that yoga is not a competitive sport and thus a person's level does not matter. If people are stiff and out of shape, sick, or weak, sets of easy exercises help loosen the joints and stimulate circulation. If practiced regularly, these simple exercises alone make a great difference in people's health and well-being.

Poses can be slow and careful or more vigorous. Beginning poses are used to relax tension in the muscles and joints and center the mind. Attention is paid to how the body feels and what it is doing. Every movement is made gently and slowly. Strain or force is to be avoided because yoga is a nonviolent approach that is done comfortably. Strength training is isometric because the muscles are tensed in opposition to each other. After one assumes the pose, it is held for as long as it can be done comfortably, usually about six breaths. Each pose, in a well-structured workout, includes a pose and its opposite, such as a forward bend and a backward bend, so the body stays physically balanced. Breathing should be easy, fluid, and continuous and used to facilitate the poses (Carapellese & Slonina, 2009).

Every yoga session should end with a few minutes of complete and total relaxation. This period is an important part of bringing the mind and body together to maximize the benefits. Some people end the session with chanting to reach a deeper state of relaxation. The instructor ends the session with the word *namaste:* "The divine in me bows to the divine in you."

Yoga offers a number of health benefits. The physical and psychological benefits include the following (Chen & Tseng, 2008; Mayo Clinic, 2008):

- Increases flexibility of muscles and joints.
- Improves range of motion.
- Tones and strengthens muscles.
- Improves endurance.
- Increases circulation.
- Lowers blood pressure.
- Increases lymph circulation.
- Improves digestion and elimination.
- Promotes deeper breathing.
- Increases brain endorphins, enkephalins, and serotonin.
- Increases mental acuity.
- Augments alpha and theta brain wave activity.
- Promotes relaxation.
- Manages stress.

Yoga is not a cure-all for disease. It can help, however, to relieve symptoms, decrease pain, and improve the quality of life. It helps prevent disease by reinforcing lifestyle changes such as positive health habits and attitudes. Overall, yoga is safe. If people have a weak link—whether it is the lower back, knees, or shoulders, they are at higher risk of injury and need to be more careful when doing yoga. There has been one case of retinal vein occlusion and one case of optic neuropathy in persons who routinely practiced the headstand posture (de Barros, Bazzaz, Gheith, Siam, & Moster, 2008; Shah & Shah, 2009). The two main causes of yoga-related injuries are unqualified teachers and overzealous students. Poorly trained instructors teach improper form. Overzealous students see yoga as a competition and push themselves beyond their physical limits.

RESEARCH

A tremendous amount of scientific research documents the benefits of yoga. The following is a small selection of current studies:

- A systematic review of randomized controlled clinical trials on the practice of yoga in the management of type II diabetes found improvement in short-term outcomes, but the results were inconclusive and not significant for long-term outcomes (Aljasir, Bryson, & Al-Shehri, 2008).
- A systematic review of the impact of yoga on psychological adjustment of cancer patients found some positive results, but drawbacks in methodologies limited the extent to which yoga can be effective in this group of patients (Smith & Pukall, 2008).
- Older adults where randomized into either a silver yoga exercise group or a control group. The yoga group participated in a 70-minute, 3 times per

week, 6-month long program. The yoga group demonstrated significantly improved sleep quality, depression, and self-perception of health status compared to the control group (Chen et al., 2009).

- A convenience sample of older women involved in a silver yoga exercise program found that percentage of body fat, systolic blood pressure, balance, and shoulder flexion and abduction significantly improved with three 70-minute sessions per week for 4 weeks (Chen & Tseng, 2008).
- People with Class I–III heart failure were randomized to yoga treatment or standard medical therapy. Yoga significantly improved exercise tolerance and reduced inflammatory markers. There was also a trend toward improvement in quality of life (Pullen et al., 2008).
- 131 people with mild to moderate stress levels were randomized in a comparative trial of yoga or progressive muscle relaxation. Yoga was more effective than relaxation in improving mental health. Yoga and progressive relaxation showed equal improvement in physical function, role function, general health perceptions, emotional role function, social function, body pain, and vitality (Smith, Hancock, Blake-Mortimer, & Eckert, 2007).

INTEGRATED NURSING PRACTICE

The regular practice of yoga builds and tones muscles, increases flexibility, improves endurance, and promotes a state of relaxation. The physiologic responses are the opposite of the fight-or-flight stress response. Stretching and deep breathing bring on a profound sense of relaxation. Gentle stretching and range-of-motion joint exercises decrease muscle tension and joint stiffness. The mindful focus on awareness of self, breath, and energy minimizes anxiety associated with stress. Just getting your body down on the floor tends to clear the mind. Perhaps it is because being on the floor is so unusual to us that it changes our attitude toward and our awareness of our body (Kabat-Zinn, 2003).

Hatha yoga is designed by and for healthy, flexible people. Even when experiencing a serious illness, however, most people can work on breath control even if they do not feel up to doing the poses. The breathing exercises and relaxation response nourish the body, quiet the mind, and contribute to a more balanced state. Encourage individuals to check with their primary care practitioner if they have recently had surgery, have a debilitating physical handicap, or have cancer, diabetes, epilepsy, heart disease, high blood pressure, HIV, multiple sclerosis, or any other serious condition. Yoga, combined with a low-fat diet and moderate aerobic exercise, can significantly reduce blockages in coronary arteries (Ornish, 2008). Other studies have shown yoga to be effective in treating arthritis, diabetes, mood disorders, asthma, hypertension, menstrual cramps, back pain, and chronic fatigue.

Yoga can benefit people of any age, from children to older adults. Children take naturally to yoga and usually find it to be much fun. Getting the whole family involved is one way to maintain the routine. Some adults find yoga complements their aerobic routine, while others engage in yoga as a great nonaerobic conditioner. It is possible to learn yoga from books or compact disks (see Resources section at the end of this chapter), but it is easier to learn from a teacher. Yoga classes are available in many places, such as health clubs, community centers, universities, and hospitals.

As a nurse, you can encourage people to utilize yoga as a way to start on the path of taking responsibility for their well-being. Consistent practice of yoga changes people's attitudes about their bodies and their beliefs about what they can do to take care of themselves, both of which are crucial to well-being. For some, the physical exercise may be a way to attain a specific goal such as improving flexibility, improving muscle tone, or losing weight. Others have no specific goal other than the exercise itself and becoming aware of their self, breath, and energy. The relaxation that accompanies yoga can stimulate self-healing and contribute to a sense of inner peace.

Almost anyone can be taught the Mountain Pose, which is a standing position of postural awareness. When this pose is practiced well, the body is prepared for almost all daily movement: standing, sitting, walking, and running. Like the mountain poised between heaven and earth, this pose establishes a grounding through the legs and feet and encourages the lift of the spine. Instruct people to stand sideways near a full-length mirror so they can check their alignment, which may feel strange at first (see Figure 16.2). Once people are in alignment, they should notice their physical sensations. Is weight balanced evenly between the feet? Are the legs firm but not tight? Are shoulders relaxed? Does the spinal cord feel light and the head feel balanced on the torso? Is breathing comfortable and easy? Encourage people to practice the Mountain Pose several times a day. Standing well reduces strain on the joints, ligaments, and muscles, especially on those of the spinal column and lower extremities. It also aids respiration, digestion, and elimination. The Mountain Pose conveys a sense of poise and self-esteem.

Benefits from any fitness program, including yoga, can occur only with continued practice. Try some of these suggestions to help people develop a regular pattern:

- Encourage clients to make time for yoga practice every day, to give themselves permission to take care of themselves and take time to relax. They may find that doing a few poses before bedtime or early in the morning works best. Even if they practice for only 5 minutes, a daily practice is the foundation on which to build.
- To maintain their practice, many people find it helpful to go to a yoga class at least once a week. The support of practicing with others and the information they get from teachers help strengthen their commitment to yoga.

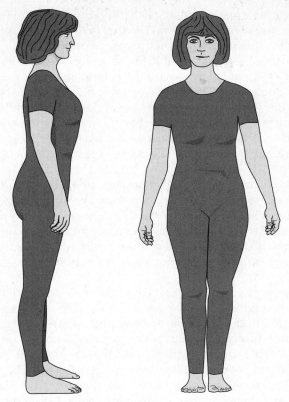

FIGURE 16.2   Mountain Pose (Tadasana)

- Suggest that they create a dedicated yoga space. They may have to temporarily push things aside to have enough space for their practice. Or they may simply choose a place to spread their yoga mat on the floor. Having a regular space for practice helps people focus on the poses without being distracted by their surroundings.
- Have people start with the poses they like. If they like a pose, they will do it even if it is difficult. You may suggest that they take one pose they like from each class and practice it at least once a day, which takes only a few moments. They can then gradually begin to combine the poses to form their own yoga session.

One of the many applications of yoga is in pregnancy and childbirth. In fact, many of the techniques taught in childbirth classes, such as focus, relaxation, and systematic breathing, have their roots in yoga. The gentle stretching of the poses helps ease the muscle aches of pregnancy and strengthens the muscles that will be used during delivery. The breathing techniques may lessen the shortness of breath that often accompanies advanced pregnancy.

Yoga practiced while pregnant is slightly different from regular yoga in that some poses are contraindicated. These poses are the extreme stretching positions and any position that puts pressure on the uterus. Full forward bends will probably be uncomfortable for both woman and baby. Remind the woman that her center of balance has shifted completely, and thus, she must be careful with balance poses. Pregnant women should never lie on the stomach for any pose. After the 20th week, they should lie on their left side rather than their back. If any pose feels uncomfortable, the woman should stop at once. If a pregnant woman experiences dizziness, sudden swelling, extreme shortness of breath, or vaginal bleeding, she should see her midwife or doctor immediately (Becker, 2000).

With midwife or doctor approval, most women can usually start gentle yoga poses two weeks after delivery, a few weeks longer if they have had a cesarean section. They should start with a few poses and gradually work back to their regular routine. If their postpartum bleeding gets heavier or brighter red, they need to stop and call their midwife or doctor. Filling their body with energy through breathing exercises may promote self-healing after childbirth.

As people learn yoga, they will find that each sequence of poses helps them focus on something specific; for example, one sequence can improve balance, while another may release anger and negative feelings; some sequences will tone internal organs, increase lung capacity, or build upper-body strength. People choose the sequences that are right for them. It is most important to remind people that it is not a matter of being a beginning, intermediate, or advanced student but rather that they keep practicing, doing as much as they can whenever they can. Yoga moves at their pace, in the time they have.

TRY THIS

Heart Breathing

- Sit comfortably and close your eyes.
- Simply notice your breathing without trying to change it. Pay attention to your in-breath and your out-breath.
- Now imagine that the breath is pouring into your heart with each inhalation and flowing out of your heart with each exhalation. Just feel the breath flowing in and out of your heart. Imagine the breath is pure love.
- Do this breath awareness for 5 to 10 minutes.
- Now let your attention return to your environment, slowly open your eyes, get up, and move on.
- Think about the feeling throughout the day.

USING RESEARCH TO HEAL

Chen, K. M., Tseng, W. S., Ting, L. F., & Huang, G. F. (2007). Development and evaluation of a yoga exercise program for older adults. *Journal of Advanced Nursing*, 57(4): 432–441.

What Is This Study About?

Evidence-based research studies have established the beneficial effects of yoga in reducing cardiovascular risk, blood pressure, respirations, and enhancing pain management in the older population. Therefore, the purpose of this study was to report the development and evaluation of a new yoga exercise program specifically designed for this population.

How Was the Study Done?

This was a two-phase study aimed at establishing a yoga program for older adults in Taiwan. Phase I of the research requested 10 yoga experts (n = 2 certified yoga instructors; n = 2 gerontological nurse practitioners; n = 2 physical therapists; n = 2 osteopathic physicians; n = 2 physical educators/trainers) to assist in the development of the Silver Yoga Program (based on hatha yoga and raja yoga). All experts were provided with a hard copy and video containing detailed descriptions and demonstrations of the proposed program for their input regarding safety, clarity, and feasibility of the yoga protocol. Phase II of the study consisted of using a descriptive design and convenience sample to receive inputs from 14 older women regarding the program implementation. Inclusion criteria for study participants was: (1) all participants lived in the community aged 60 and over, (2) no previous yoga experience, (3) cognitively intact, (4) independent in activities of daily living, and (5) mobility did not require any form of assistance. Participants in the study were interviewed after 1 month of instructor-led Silver Yoga group practice. This group practice was conducted three times a week for 70 minutes. Data collection included 4 months of participation in the program. Institutional Review Board approval was granted for this study.

What Were the Results of the Study?

Phase I: Eight poses (4 sitting positions and 4 standing positions) were designed aimed at loosing up the body for a safe transition into hatha yoga (combination of stretching postures and diaphragmatic breathing techniques). In addition, relaxation activities and guided imagery mediation (raja yoga) were recommended to be incorporated into the program. *Phase II*: Participants in the Silver Program reported that relaxation and guided-imagery meditation were fairly easy to follow but the hatha yoga postures were challenging. After 1 month of being in the study, 50% of the participants reported sleeping improvements. In addition, improvements were noted in flexibility, physical health, body weight, and experiences of shoulder pain by select participants. Most participants preferred the yoga practice three times a week for 70 minutes. Ten participants expressed a preference for the yoga practice group to be between 15 and 20 persons.

(continued)

What Additional Questions Might I Have?

Would a larger sample size in Phase II have revealed different results? Would a male sample have experienced similar results when participating in these two types of yoga? Would other forms of yoga be useful with older adults? Could the incorporation of yoga in persons with mobility challenges be beneficial to this population?

How Can I Use This Study?

Nurses can use the findings of this study in assisting older adults to maintain flexibility and perhaps overcome health problems such as insomnia. Increased use of yoga may be helpful in reducing frequent orthopedic injuries experienced in the older adult population.

Source: Contributed by Dolores M. Huffman, PhD, RN, Associate Professor of Nursing, Purdue University Calumet.

References

Aljasir, B., Bryson, M., & Al-shehri, B. (2008). Yoga practice for the management of type II Diabetes Mellitus in adults: A systematic review. *Evidence-based Complementary and Alternative Medicine*. Published online eCAM, doi:10.1093/ecam/nen027. Accessed May 7, 2008.

Becker, I. (2000). Uses of yoga in psychiatry and medicine. In P. R. Muskin (Ed.), *Complementary and Alternative Medicine and Psychiatry* (pp. 107–146). Washington, DC: American Psychiatric Press.

Carapellese, L., & Slonina, E. (2009). *Anywhere, Anytime, Any Body Yoga*. Alameda, CA: Hunter House.

Chen, K. M., Chen, M. H., Chao, H. C., Hung, H. M., Lin, H. S., & Li, C. H. (2009). Sleep quality, depression state, and health status of older adults after silver yoga exercises: Cluster randomized trial. *International Journal of Nursing Studies*, 46: 154–163.

Chen, K. M., & Tseng, W. S. (2008). Pilot-testing the effects of a newly-developed silver yoga exercise program for female seniors. *Journal of Nursing Research*, 16(1): 37–45.

de Barros, D. S., Bazzaz, S., Gheith, M. E., Siam, G. A., & Moster, M. R. (2008). Progressive optic neuropathy in congenital glaucoma associated with the Sirsasana yoga posture. *Ophthalmic Surgery, Lasers, & Imaging*, 39(4): 339–340.

Jayanti, B. K. (2009). *Practical Meditation: Spiritual Yoga for the Mind*. New York: Sterling Ethos.

Kabat-Zinn, J. (2003). Mindful yoga movement & meditation. *Yoga International*, 70: 86–93.

Kabat-Zinn, J. (2007). *Arriving at Your Own Door: 108 Lessons in Mindfulness*. New York: Hyperion.

Mayo Clinic. (January 18, 2008). Yoga: Improve your stress management and relaxation skills. www.mayoclinic.com/health/yoga/CM00004. Accessed April 15, 2008.

Ornish, D. (2008). *The Spectrum: A Scientifically Proven Program to Feel Better, Live Longer, Lose Weight, and Gain Health*. New York: Ballantine Books.

Platania, J. V. (2009). *Yoga for Beginners: 5000 Years of History and Philosophy*. New York: For Beginners.

Pullen, P. R., Nagamia, S. H., Mehta, P. K., Thompson, W. R., Benardot, D.,

Hammoud, R., et al. (2008). *Journal of Cardiac Failure*, 14(5): 407–413.

Shah, N. J., & Shah, U. N. (2009). Central retinal vein occlusion following Sirsasana (headstand posture). *Indian Journal of Ophthalmology*, 57(1): 69–70.

Smith, C., Hancock, H., Blake-Mortimer, J., & Eckert, K. (2007). A randomized comparative trial of yoga and relaxation to reduce stress and anxiety. *Complementary Therapies in Medicine*, 15: 77–83.

Smith, K. B., & Pukall, C. F. (2008). An evidence-based review of yoga as a complementary intervention for patients with cancer. *Psycho-oncology*, 18(5): 465–475.

Stone, M., & Iyengar, B. K. S. (2009). *Yoga for a World Out of Balance*. Boston, MA: Shambhala.

Resources

American Yoga Association
    P.O. Box 19986
    Sarasota, FL 34276
    941.927.4977
    www.americanyogaassociation.org

Center for Mindfulness in Medicine,
    Health Care, and Society
    University of Massachusetts
    Medical School
    55 Lake Ave. North
    Worcester, MA 01605
    508.856.2000
    www.umassmed.edu/cfm

Tapes and compact disks available.
    International Centre for Yogic Arts
    and Sciences
    164 Eglinton Ave. East, Suite 100
    Toronto, ON, Canada, M4P 1G4
    416.544.9642
    www.icyas.com

The British Wheel of Yoga
    25 Jermyn St.
    Sleaford, Lincolnshire, NG34 7RU, UK
    01529.306.851
    www.bwy.org.uk

Yoga Research and Education Center
    10336 Loch Lomond Rd, Suite 221
    Middletwon, CA 95461
    www.yrec.org

17

Meditation

To train the mind, you must exercise the patience and determination it takes to shape that steel.

THE DALAI LAMA

You must learn to be still in the midst of activity and to be vibrantly alive in repose.

INDIRA GANDHI

Meditation is a general term for a wide range of practices that involve relaxing the body and stilling the mind. The root word, *meditari*, means "to consider," or one could say, "to pay attention to something." As the founder and director of the Stress Reduction Clinic at the University of Massachusetts Medical Center, Jon Kabat-Zinn (1994) states, "Meditation is simply about being yourself and knowing something about who that is. It is about coming to realize that you are on a path whether you like it or not, namely, the path that is your life. . . . Meditation is the process by which we go about deepening our attention and awareness, refining them, and putting them to greater practical use in our lives" (pp. xvi–xvii).

In 1975, Dr. Herbert Benson wrote the book *The Relaxation Response*, which drew the attention of Western health care practitioners to the physical and psychological benefits of relaxation. As Benson pointed out, the components of relaxation are quite simple: a quiet space, a comfortable position, a receptive attitude, and a focus of attention. The relaxation response involves physiological and psychological effects that appear common to many forms of focused attention in addition to meditation: prayer, yoga, biofeedback, and the presuggestion phase of hypnosis. These practices are covered in other chapters in this text. Benson (1975) described meditation as a process that anyone can use to calm down, cope with stress, and, for those with spiritual inclinations, feel as one with God or the universe. Meditation can be practiced individually or in groups and is easy to learn. It requires no change in belief system and is compatible with most religious practices.

BACKGROUND

Most meditative practices have come to the West from Eastern practices, particularly those of India, China, Japan, and Tibet. Meditative techniques, however, can be found in most cultures of the world where prayer, meditation, ritual, or contemplation are all initiated by shifting into a relaxed state. Nearly all major religions include some form of meditative practice. Christianity, Judaism, Buddhism, and Islam all use repetitive prayers, chants, or movements as part of their worship rituals. Although religious practices in the West are not typically labeled "meditative," they in fact are. The Catholic practice of using rosary beads while saying the "Hail Mary" is a familiar example. The repetition of the words combined with the movement of the beads induces a state of relaxation and a quieting of the mind.

Until recently, the primary purpose of meditation has been spiritual or religious. Since the 1970s, it has been explored as a way of reducing stress on both body and mind. Many conventional health care practitioners recommend it for widely diverse situations, from natural childbirth to managing hypertension to pain control. For many years, nurses have taught clients progressive relaxation in a wide variety of clinical settings.

PREPARATION

Practicing meditation does not require a teacher, and many people learn the process through instructions from books, recordings, or compact disks. Some people, however, find that the structure of a meditation class is helpful. Many varieties of teachers and classes are available. Currently no certification process is available for a meditation teacher. The general standard is some years of daily meditation practice before one teaches others. Both Christian and Buddhist traditions offer regular classes and retreats designed to teach meditative practices and the process of being a spiritual being in a material world. In the Hindu tradition, people learn meditation from a guru who is a spiritual teacher or guide. Whatever the tradition, teachers encourage self-responsibility and the practice of mindfulness in everyday life (Levy, 2008).

CONCEPTS

Meditative State

Meditation is about being aware of who one is in the here-and-now rather than about feeling a particular way. It means letting go of any expectations of the process and simply observing what happens as it unfolds. People are sometimes concerned that they do not have the skills to meditate. As Dr. Jon Kabat-Zinn (1994) states, "Thinking you are unable to meditate is a little like thinking you are unable to breathe, or to concentrate or relax. Pretty much everybody can breathe easily. And under the right circumstances, pretty much anybody can concentrate, anybody can relax" (p. 33). All forms of meditation require regular, daily practice over a period of time to experience the many benefits.

Attention and Concentration

Basic to all meditative techniques is the intentional focus of attention on one thought, word, sound, image, or physical sensation for a sustained period of time. The mind is fully alert but not focused on the external world or events. The normal rapid series of thoughts and feelings is replaced with inner awareness and attention. Rather than the mind jumping around between the past and the future, attention is in the present reality. It is impossible to make the mind empty, but it is possible to focus on one thing, which helps the mind let go of the tendency to worry, plan, think, analyze, remember, or solve problems. A passive, nonjudgmental attitude is necessary during meditation. When thoughts intrude, they are noticed, and then let go as the attention returns to the original focus.

In some types of meditation, the focus is on the breath, the primary purpose being to calm the mind and body. It is a process of keeping the attention on the breath while breathing deeply, slowly, and regularly. The awareness is on the breath moving in and the breath moving out and allowing all other thoughts, feelings, or sensations to pass by as this focus is maintained. Through regular meditation practice, it becomes a habit to breathe more consciously and deeply throughout the day, so that in the long run, the breath becomes a calming force in daily life (Gardner-Nix, 2009).

Some people use a mantra as their focus of attention. A **mantra** is a sound or sounds that resonate in the body and evoke certain energies. Mantras, such as OM, soothe the mind and awaken the senses. Another beginning mantra is OM SHANTI SHANTI SHANTI. *Shanti* means peace, and when repeated three times, it balances the body, mind, and spirit.

A mandala meditation uses an object to focus the mind through sight. A **mandala** is a circular geometric design that draws the eye to the center and is meant to suggest the universe's circular patterns from atoms to solar systems. Mandalas appear as labyrinths in the floors of some cathedrals in Europe. The faithful follow the course of the labyrinth into the center as penitence or in spiritual contemplation. Mandalas have recently become popular in the United States among some Christian religious groups who are renewing the contemplative aspects of their faith. Using mantras and mandalas together is an effective focus for meditation (Artress, 2006; Sands, 2005).

Figure 17.1 is the mandala that appears in the floor of Chartres Cathedral in France. Using a pencil, trace the walking path to the center and then back to the outer world again.

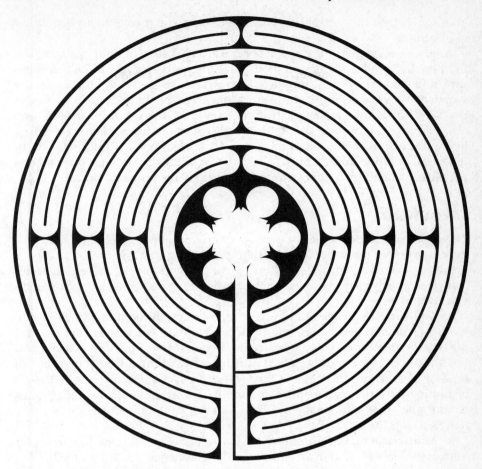

FIGURE 17.1   Mandala in the Floor of Chartres Cathedral

Meditation is both simple and difficult—simple because it is nothing more than maintaining focused attention; difficult because of the habitual, lifelong pattern of letting the mind wander wherever it wants. With extended practice, the mind tends to become better and better at staying focused. The stability and calmness that come with focused attention are the foundation of meditation.

VIEW OF HEALTH AND ILLNESS

Many disorders or diseases are aggravated or caused by stress. They are labeled as disorders of arousal, in which the limbic system of the brain has become overstimulated. In addition, overactivity of the sympathetic nervous system and exhaustion of the adrenal glands are related to stress. It is thought that excessive limbic activity may inhibit immune function, which may account for the association of chronic stress and increased susceptibility to infection.

A relaxed state is the opposite of the aroused state of fight or flight. The fight-or-flight reflex increases blood pressure, heart rate, breathing, metabolism, and blood flow to the muscles. The response triggered by all the relaxing practices does the opposite and results in a lower blood pressure and slower heart rate, breathing, metabolism, and blood flow. Relaxation and meditation also decrease the production of adrenergic catecholamines, thereby decreasing limbic activity. Since the state of mind, the emotional, attitudinal, and intellectual components of oneself, initiates activities in the nervous system, people can consciously choose to trigger the benefits of meditation.

TREATMENT

The relaxation response can be evoked by any number of techniques, including progressive relaxation, meditation, prayer, jogging, swimming, Lamaze breathing exercises, yoga, t'ai chi, and qigong. The beauty of these techniques is their simplicity. They allow the mind to have a focus while enhancing one's vitality and well-being.

The varieties of meditation have many different names. Some are religious practices and some are not. Some are complicated while some are simple. Each type of meditative practice involves a form of mental focusing and the adoption of a nonjudgmental attitude toward intruding thoughts. All types appear to produce similar physical and psychological changes. People beginning the practice of meditation should look around for a form that seems comfortable, that suits them, and that does not conflict with their belief system (Kelsang, 2009).

Transcendental Meditation® (TM) was developed by the Indian leader Maharishi Mahesh Yogi in an effort to make the ancient practice of meditation more attainable to Westerners. TM is a sound-focused form of meditation and is simple and easy to learn. To prevent distracting thoughts, a person is given a mantra (a word or sound) to repeat silently over and over again while sitting in a comfortable position. When thoughts other than the mantra come to mind, the person is to notice them and then gently return the focus to the mantra. It is expected that people will practice TM for 20 minutes, once or twice a day. The trademarked Transcendental Meditation is a commercial enterprise that is a fairly expensive undertaking. Classes are typically found in Ayurvedic schools and health care centers. Local centers may be found on the Internet at www.tm.org.

The essence of **Buddhist meditation** is training the mind in compassion and in wisdom. The goal is to develop compassion for all living things. Meditation begins with a time of contemplation, which typically includes points such as these (Thondup, 2009):

• Just as I wish to be free from suffering and experience only happiness, so do all other beings.

- I am no different from any other being; we are all equal.
- My happiness and suffering are insignificant when compared with the happiness and suffering of all other living beings.

The next step is a process of meditating on any determinations that might have been made during contemplation. The practice is concluded by dedicating one's life and purpose to the welfare of all living beings. It is believed that many of the daily problems people experience will disappear, because most of them arise from regarding oneself as more important than others.

Mindfulness, an ancient Buddhist practice, is both a philosophy and a meditation practice. Its primary principle is "being in the moment." Most often people go through daily routines with little awareness or attention. People read while they eat, exercise while watching TV, or cook while talking to their children, and the nuances of these experiences are lost. This situation might be called living mindlessly by ignoring present moments. **Mindfulness** is the opposite of living on "automatic pilot." It is the art of conscious living through focusing full attention on the activity at hand. While it may be simple to practice mindfulness, it is not necessarily easy. Habitual unawareness is persistent, and mindfulness requires effort and discipline. Thus, to eat a peach mindfully would involve being actively aware of every sensation, every smell, every taste, noticing its texture, its color, its weight, and how it feels on the tongue. This technique can be practiced with any activity (Kabat-Zinn, 1994).

Mindfulness meditation is a daily practice that encourages living in the moment. It begins by sitting quietly with eyes closed and focusing on breathing. The flow of thought during the meditation is observed as thoughts come and go. The key to mindfulness meditation is the ability to accept rather than judge the wandering thoughts, bringing attention back to the breathing as needed.

Mindfulness-based stress reduction (MBSR) is a structured 8-week therapy program utilizing mindfulness medication, yoga, and group discussion. Mindfulness-based relapse prevention (MBRP) is a program focused on breathing and physical sensations as a way to cope with triggers to substance abuse relapse (Marlatt & Chawla, 2007; Praissman, 2008).

Tibetan meditation is a breath-focused form of meditation. The person simply focuses attention on each in-breath and out-breath. When thoughts about anything other than the breath intrude, they are noted by silently saying "thinking," and then attention is returned to the breath. It is recognized that thought cannot be completely halted and that thoughts are a natural process and are simply to be noted in a nonjudgmental way.

Forms of **moving meditation** include the Chinese martial art t'ai chi, the Japanese martial art Aikido, the Indian practice of yoga, and the walking meditation in Zen Buddhism. Instead of focusing on a word or on breathing, movement meditations use physical sensations as the focus of concentration. In walking meditation, for example, attention is given to the feeling of each step as it is taken. Intruding thoughts are simply noticed, and attention is returned to the step. Research has found that focused walking, in contrast to unfocused walking, is associated with reduced anxiety and fewer negative thoughts. In **rhythmic meditation** participants pay attention to their hand and body movements while their eyes are open (Rungreangkulkij & Wongtakee, 2008).

If practiced regularly, even 15 minutes twice a day, meditation produces widespread positive effects on physical and psychological functioning. The autonomic nervous system responds with a decrease in heart rate, lower blood pressure, decreased respiratory rate and oxygen consumption, and a lower arousal threshold. People who meditate say that they have clearer minds and sharper thoughts. The brain seems to clear itself so that new ideas and beliefs become available. This clearer mind may be accompanied by a cognitive restructuring in which people interpret life events in a more positive, more realistic fashion. Meditation's residual effects—improved stress-coping abilities—are a protection against daily stress and anxiety. All other self-healing methods are improved with the practice of meditation (Miller, 2006).

Some adverse effects of meditation are possible. Relaxation exercises should not be practiced while driving or operating potentially dangerous machinery. Some people have been stressed so long that they are unfamiliar with deep relaxation and therefore, feel threatened by it. In meditation, people are taught to accept nonjudgmentally whatever thoughts occur. Sometimes, however, extremely upsetting thoughts arise and it is impossible to remain nonjudgmental, which could lead to disparaging thoughts about one's abilities. The adverse effects for more experienced meditators are temporary fear, anxiety, confusion, depression, and self-doubt. For an unknown reason, these kinds of thoughts are more likely to arise during the first 10 minutes of meditation.

RESEARCH

Since the 1960s, a large body of research has been documented regarding meditation and the relaxation response. It is almost impossible, however, to double-blind and placebo-control meditation studies, which makes it difficult to fit into evidence-based practice. A small sampling of the research demonstrates the following:

- In a literature review, Praissman (2008) found that people with mood disorders experienced an improvement in depressive and anxiety symptoms in response to a mindfulness-based stress (MBSR) reduction program. This same program demonstrated less anxiety for persons with cardiovascular disease, improved quality of life for people with early-stage breast cancer and prostate cancer, and reduced stress and improved sleep in people with cancer.
- A pilot study comparing MBSR to cognitive-behavioral stress reduction (CBSR) found that those assigned to MBSR had greater improvement in all variables when compared to CBSR (Smith et al., 2008).

- A convenience sample of 22 people with unrelieved anxiety symptoms found that mindfulness-based cognitive therapy (MBCT) experienced significant relief from anxiety symptoms and insomnia (Yook et al., 2008).
- College students were randomly assigned to one of three groups: MBSR, Eight-Point Program (EPP), or a wait-list control group. The MBSR and the EPP have a similar practice of sitting meditation, focused attention, and motivational support. When compared to the control group, those in MBSR and EPP experienced significant decreases in perceived stress and significant increases in forgiveness. There were marginally larger reductions in rumination. These results remained the same at the 8-week follow up (Oman, Shapiro, Thoresen, Plante, & Flinders, 2008).

INTEGRATED NURSING PRACTICE

Progressive relaxation and meditation are used in a wide variety of clinical settings such as rehabilitation facilities, cardiac care units, postoperative units, stress management centers, behavioral counseling settings, and centers dedicated to health and wellness promotion. Thousands of hospitals, clinics, private practitioners, and universities offer training in meditation. In addition, recordings, compact disks, and books are available that make meditation more accessible to people with busy schedules. Many people practice meditation to reduce stress, anxiety, anger, and other negative emotions. But increasingly, nurses are prescribing meditation as part of the treatment for a large and growing number of medical conditions.

Mindfulness-based stress reduction (MBSR) programs have been developed by Jon Kabat-Zinn at the University of Massachusetts Medical Center and are taught by nurses and other health care professionals worldwide. People participate for many reasons, including job, family, or financial stress; chronic pain and illness; anxiety and panic; sleep disturbances; fatigue; hypertension; and headaches. A number of midwifery practices include MBSR as a complement to childbirth education and parenting classes. The course schedule consists of eight weekly classes and one daylong class.

Progressive relaxation is a way of decreasing muscular tension. The relaxation response can be elicited by teaching clients two common techniques: progressive relaxation and body scan. Both focus on reducing muscle tone in the major muscle groups and take about 7 to 10 minutes. If possible, help client find a quiet place with a comfortable temperature to do the exercise. It can be done in any comfortable position, although typically it is done with people lying on their backs and begins with a focus on the breath, breathing gently, slowly, and deeply. The awareness is then shifted to different parts of the body in turn, by instructing the client to tense a muscle group as tight as possible, hold the tension for several seconds, and then consciously relax it. This sequence is repeated for each of the major muscle groups in the body, usually beginning at the toes and slowly working up the body. Progressive

USING RESEARCH TO HEAL

Lazar, S. W., Kerr, C. E., Wasserman, R. H., Gray, J. R., Greve, D. N., Treadway, M. T., et al. (2005). Meditation experience is associated with increased cortical thickness. *NeuroReport*, 16(17): 1893–1897.

What Is This Study About?

The use of meditation as a form of mental exercise is gaining popularity in the Western culture. Long-term meditation has shown to change resting electroencephalogram patterns. However, the question persisted if long-term use of meditation is correlated with structural changes in the brain. Therefore, the purpose of this study was to visualize the differences in the thickness of the cerebral cortex of Insight meditation practitioners as opposed to persons with no experience in meditation or yoga.

How Was the Study Done?

This was a correlational study using 20 practitioners with extensive experience in Insight meditation (this type of mediation does not use mantra or chanting but places an emphasis on attention and "mindfulness"). The participants were recruited from local mediation communities and Insight meditation was incorporated into their daily life. Two participants were full-time meditation instructors, 3 were part-time yoga or meditation teachers, and 16 meditated approximately 40 minutes daily as they pursued careers in health care and law. A control group (n = 15) was matched for sex, age, race, and education. The majority of participants was male, in their late 30s, White, and had completed over 17 years of education. Institutional Review Board approval was granted for this study. Magnetic resonance imaging (MRI) was used to assess cortical thickness in the participants.

What Were the Results of the Study?

Significant differences in the distribution of cortical thickness in the brain existed between the two groups. The participants using Insight meditation showed increased cortical thickness in brain regions associated with attention, interoception, and sensory processing moreso than in the control group. It was noted that prefrontal cortical thickness was most obvious in older participants. In addition, the thickness of two regions correlated with meditation experience. Therefore, the data suggest structural evidence for experience-dependent cortical plasticity related to meditation. In addition, those participants engaged in regular meditation practice showed a significant drop in respiration rate during formal practice.

What Additional Questions Might I Have?

What would be the results for those using other types of meditation? Would a larger sample size significantly alter the results of the study?

How Can I Use This Study?

Professional nurses can implement the findings from this study in health promotion across the lifespan in an effort to impact age-related declines in cortical structure.

Source: Contributed by Dolores Huffman, PhD, RN, Associate Professor of Nursing, Purdue University Calumet.

BOX 17.1

Body Scan Meditation

- Lie on your back with your legs uncrossed, your arms at your sides, palms up, and your eyes closed.
- Focus on your breathing; breathe in peace and breathe out tension.
- As you begin to feel relaxed, direct your attention to your feet, paying attention to any sensations. Let your feet relax, and feel the warmth spread throughout your feet.
- Then move your focus to your ankles. Follow the same procedure as you move up your lower legs, knees, thighs, hips, and so on all around the body.
- Pay particular attention to any areas that are painful or are the focus of any medical condition, such as the lungs or heart.
- Finish the body scan by paying particular attention to the neck and head. Experience the warmth of the relaxation.

relaxation is designed to help people with chronic tension experience the difference between a muscle that is tense and one that is relaxed. In the body scan exercise, clients are instructed to focus their attention on body parts, one at a time, often beginning at the feet and moving toward the head, and to consciously relax each part. Box 17.1 provides directions for the body scan technique.

You can also teach clients to anchor the relaxation response with a sensory stimulus, such as an aroma of lavender or rose, or a touch, such as pressing two fingers together. The sensory anchor should be done within 30 seconds of the relaxation exercise. After doing the sensory anchor for 2 weeks, the individual should be able to instantaneously relax by reexperiencing the particular sensory trigger, be it an aroma or a physical sensation.

Meditation is the next step following the mastery of progressive relaxation and body scan. Explain the two basic steps to clients: the repetition of a word, sound, prayer, phrase, or muscular activity and the disregard of everyday thoughts that interfere with the process. Box 17.2 lists focus words or prayers that you may suggest to clients. The word or phrase is silently repeated with each in-breath and out-breath. Some people choose to use one word for the in-breath and another for the out-breath. Some meditators choose an object of personal significance on which to focus. Every detail of the object is studied, including gradations of shape, color, texture, and so on. Flowers, candle flames, or religious statues are common choices.

Before sitting down to meditate, it is helpful to make sure that the area is clean and uncluttered, which helps keep the mind clear and fresh. No props are required for meditation, although some people may choose to include incense, candles, or religious symbols in their meditative practice. Beginners often start

BOX 17.2

Focus Words or Prayers

Secular Focus Words
>One
>Ocean
>Love
>Peace
>Well-being
>Let it be
>Relax

Religious Focus Words or Prayers
>Christian
>>"Our Father who art in heaven"
>>"The Lord is my shepherd"
>>"Hail, Mary, full of grace"
>>"Lord Jesus Christ, have mercy on me"
>Jewish
>>"Sh'ma" (Hear, O Israel: the Eternal One is our God, the Eternal One alone)
>>"Shalom" (Peace)
>>"The Lord is my shepherd"
>Islamic
>>"Insha'allah" (There is no God but God)
>>"Allah-u-akbr" (God is the Greatest)
>Hindu
>>"Namaste" (The Divine in me bows to the Divine in you)
>Tibetan Buddhist
>>"Om Mane Padme Om" (Blessed is the jewel in the lotus)

Source: Benson, H. (1997). *Timeless Healing*. New York: Fireside Books.

with 5 to 10 minutes of meditation and increase the time gradually. It is most important that time is scheduled each day, and many people find that meditating first thing in the morning, before the busy day begins, works well. Other people prefer to meditate in the evening. The key is to find a time when one is unlikely to be disturbed. It is best to wait about 2 hours after a big meal, during which time the blood flow is diverted from the brain to the gut, which makes falling asleep during meditation more likely.

All sitting meditative practices begin with finding a comfortable but erect position. The posture itself is a meditation. Slumping reflects low energy and passivity, while a ramrod-straight posture reflects tension and effort. It is easiest to meditate if the spine is straight and the body posture is symmetrical. Some people sit on the floor cross-legged using a firm cushion under their backside to support the spine. Others sit in a chair with a straight back, with both feet on the ground. The face relaxes, shoulders drop, and head, neck, and back move into easy alignment. The eyes may be either open or closed. Hands may be resting in the lap or held with palms together. It is believed that having the palms together with the fingertips touching completes a circuit of energy extending from the heart down the arms and through the chakras in the center of the palm of each hand as well as the chakras in the fingertips. People often experiment with various ways of positioning their hands during meditation until they determine which position is best for them (Gardner-Nix, 2009; Harrington, 2008).

Benson (1997, p. 136) describes the process he teaches his patients and the one he uses himself:

Step 1. Pick a focus word that is compatible with your belief system.

Step 2. Find a comfortable position in which to sit.

Step 3. Close your eyes.

Step 4. Let your muscles relax.

Step 5. Breathe slowly and naturally, and as you do, repeat your focus word silently to yourself.

Step 6. If you get distracted, simply bring your mind back to your focus word and your breathing.

Step 7. Continue for 10 to 20 minutes.

Step 8. Do not stand immediately. Continue sitting quietly for a minute or so, allowing other thoughts to return. Then open your eyes and sit for another minute before rising.

Step 9. Practice this technique once or twice daily.

Once people are adept at meditation, they can be taught to use *minis*. Minis are small versions of meditation. Instruct clients to breathe deeply, releasing tension, while saying the chosen focus word, sound, phrase, or prayer. Minis are very helpful in the midst of busy, stressful times (Benson, 1997).

One type of meditation is an awareness of breathing meditation. In this form, the person concentrates on the sensation of the breath as it enters the nose and fills the chest and abdomen, and again as it passes out of the body. Alternatively, one can imagine the breath coming in from the toes, up the legs, through the belly, and into the chest and out the same pathway. It is helpful to imagine healing and relaxation flowing into the body with each in-breath, and stress or pain leaving the body with each out-breath. When thoughts arise, they are noticed, and then let go as attention is brought back to the breathing.

Another awareness of breathing practice you can teach clients is a simple technique used in Zen meditation. Instruct clients to sit in a comfortable position with the spine straight. Ask them to gently close their eyes while breathing naturally and easily. To begin the exercise, have them count "one" to themselves as they exhale. On the next exhale, count "two," and so on up to "five." Then a new cycle is begun, counting "one" on the next exhale. Tell clients never to count higher than "five" and count only on the exhale. They will know their attention has wandered when they find themselves up to "eight" or "ten." When this occurs, have them gently refocus and restart on the count of "one." This form of meditation should be done for about 10 minutes (Weil, 1995).

Any repetitive behavior can be used as a meditative focus. One of the most universally used practices is walking meditation. In walking meditation, one is not walking to get any place. Having no place to go makes it easier to be where one is. It is often done some place in nature, on a track, on a walking mandala, or even pushing a shopping cart through a supermarket. It can be practiced at any pace, from very slow to very brisk. The practice is to take each step as it comes and to be fully present with it. One notices the movements of each foot, how it lifts, moves forward in space, and then descends again. Just as in other forms of meditation, when one begins to think, the thoughts are let go and awareness is returned to the physical sensations of walking.

An excellent book for nurses is Sherry Kahn's text, *The Nurse's Meditative Journal* (1996). This book provides you, the nurse, with step-by-step instruction in meditation and journal writing as an aid in self-exploration and growth. Your ability to focus in the midst of chaos and understand in the midst of confusion can bring comfort to your clients and inspire your professional peers to find these same qualities within themselves.

There are as many ways to meditate as there are people. When people say they have tried meditation and cannot do it, they just have not found the right practice for them. One person may want to sit, one do repetitive prayers, one swim or run, one walk, and one do yoga or t'ai chi. Encourage clients to explore a variety of techniques and develop the habit of meditation on a daily basis.

TRY THIS

Loving–Kindness Meditation

Begin by focusing on your breathing and take a few slow, easy breaths. Feel yourself relaxed. Imagine a white light above you and slightly in front of you, pouring a waterfall of love and light over you. Let the light enter the top of your head and wash through you. See yourself totally enclosed in a cocoon of white light and repeat these loving–kindness blessings for yourself, with all the respect and love that you would have for your only child:

> May I be at peace
> May my heart remain open
> May I awaken to the light of my own true nature
> May I be healed
> May I be a source of healing for all beings.

Next, bring one or more loved ones to mind. See them in as much detail as possible. Imagine the white light shining down on them and surrounding them. Then bless them:

May you be at peace
May your heart remain open
May you awaken to the light of your own true nature
May you be healed
May you be a source of healing for all beings.

Next, think of a person or persons whom you hold in judgment or with whom you are angry and to whom you are ready to begin extending forgiveness. Place them in the white light and see the light washing away all their negativity, just as it did for you and your loved ones. Bless them:

May you be at peace
May your heart remain open
May you awaken to the light of your own true nature
May you be healed
May you be a source of healing for all beings.

See our beautiful planet as it appears from outer space, a delicate jewel spinning in space. Imagine the green earth, the blue seas, the birds, the animals, the fish. Earth is a realm of opposites—of day and night, good and evil, sickness and health, riches and poverty, female and male. Hold the earth as you offer these blessings:

May there be peace on earth
May the hearts of all people be open to themselves and to each other
May all people awaken to the light of their own true nature
May all creation be blessed and be a blessing to all that is.

Sources: Borysenko, J., & Borysenko, M. (1994). *The Power of the Mind to Heal.* Carlsbad, CA: Hay House; Collinge, W. (1998). *Subtle Energy.* New York: Warner Books; and Kabat-Zinn, J. (1994). *Wherever You Go, There You Are.* New York: Hyperion.

References

Artress, A. (2006). *The Sacred Path Companion: A Guide to Walking the Labyrinth to Heal and Transform.* New York: Riverhead Trade.

Benson, H. (1975). *The Relaxation Response.* New York: Morrow.

Benson, H. (1997). *Timeless Healing.* New York: Fireside Books.

Borysenko, J., & Borysenko, M. (1994). *The Power of the Mind to Heal.* Carlsbad, CA: Hay House.

Collinge, W. (1998). *Subtle Energy.* New York: Warner Books.

Gardner-Nix, J. (2009). *The Mindfulness Solution to Pain.* Oakland, CA: New Harbinger.

Harrington, A. (2009). *The Cure Within.* New York: W.W. Norton & Co.

Kabat-Zinn, J. (1994). *Wherever You Go, There You Are: Mindfulness Meditation in Everyday Life.* New York: Hyperion.

Kahn, S. (1996). *The Nurse's Meditative Journal.* Albany, NY: Delmar.

Kelsang, G. (2009). *The New Meditation Handbook.* Glen Spey, NY: Tharpa Publications.

Levy, R. (2008). *Miraculous Health*. New York: Atria Books.

Marlatt, G. A., & Chawla, N. (2007). Meditation and alcohol use. *Southern Medical Journal*, 100(4): 451–453.

Miller, R. L. (2006). *Calm Healing*. Berkeley, CA: North Atlantic Books.

Oman, D., Shapiro, S. L., Thoresen, C. E., Plante, T. G., & Flinders, T. (2008). Meditation lowers stress and supports forgiveness among college students: A randomized controlled trial. *Journal of American College Health*, 56(5): 569–578.

Praissman, S. (2008). Mindfulness-based stress reduction: A literature review and clinician's guide. *Journal of the American Academy of Nurse Practitioners*, 20: 212–216.

Rungreangkulkij, S., & Wongtakee, W. (2008). The psychological impact of Buddhist counseling for patients suffering from symptoms of anxiety.

Archives of Psychiatric Nursing, 22(3): 127–134.

Sands, H. R. (2005). *Walking the Healing Labyrinth*. London: Gaia Books.

Smith, B. W., Shelley, B. M., Dalen, J., Wiggins, K., Tooley, E., & Bernard, J. (2008). A pilot study comparing the effects of mindfulness-based and cognitive-behavioral stress reduction. *The Journal of Alternative and Complementary Medicine*, 14(3): 251–258.

Thondup, T. (2009). *The Healing Power of Loving-Kindness*. Boston, MA: Shambhala.

Weil, A. (1995). *Natural Health, Natural Medicine*. Boston: Houghton Mifflin.

Yook, K., Lee, S. H., Ryu, M., Kim, K. H., Choi, T. K., Suh, S. Y., Kim, Y. W., et al. (2008). Usefulness of mindfulness-based cognitive therapy for treating insomnia in patients with anxiety disorders. *Journal of Nervous and Mental Disease*, 196: 501–503.

Resources

American Chronic Pain Association
P.O. Box 850
Rocklin, CA 95677
800.533.3231
www.theacpa.org

American Meditation Institute
60 Garner Rd.
Averill Park, NY 12018
518.674.8714
www.americanmeditation.org

Canadian Meditation Institute
2039-26 Ave. 5W
Calgary, Alberta, T2T IE5
Canada
403.802.0852
www.canadianmeditation.org

Maharishi Medical Centers in the United
States
www.maharishi-medical.com

Mind–Body Medical Institute
151 Merrimac St.
Boston, MA 02414
617.643.6090
www.massgeneral.org

Upaya Zen Center
1404 Cerro Cordo
Santa Fe, NM 87501
505.986.8518
www.upaya.org

18

Hypnotherapy and Guided Imagery

Tension is who you think you should be.
Relaxation is who you are.

ANCIENT CHINESE PROVERB

We are more often frightened than hurt.
Our troubles spring more often from
fancy than reality.

SENECA

Hypnotherapy is the application of hypnosis in a wide variety of medical and psychological disorders. Hypnosis is a state of attentive and focused concentration during which people are highly responsive to suggestion. **Guided imagery,** a state of focused concentration, is a similar process that encourages changes in attitudes, behavior, and physiological reactions. Many people consider guided imagery to be a form of hypnosis.

Hypnotherapists and guided imagery therapists help people learn methods to take advantage of the mind/body/spirit connection through the medium of relaxation and imagination. The basic difference between meditation and hypnosis or guided imagery is that in meditation, one empties one's mind of images, whereas in hypnosis or guided imagery, one creates vivid mental images.

BACKGROUND

Around the world, shamans and traditional healers have used the power of suggested mental images for thousands of years. Hypnotic trances have been used in a variety of healing practices and religious rituals such as holding sweat lodge ceremonies, drumming, and chanting. Inducing trance states and using therapeutic suggestion were central practices of the early Greek healing temples. People in the fourteenth century thought illness was related to evil spirits, and evil spirits were often treated with imagery and hypnotic techniques. During the Renaissance (fourteenth to sixteenth centuries), it was believed that dysfunctional imagination was the root of all pathology. It was even believed that the mother's imaginings during pregnancy could alter the growth and development of her fetus (Nash & Barnier, 2008).

Hypnotherapy began in the late eighteenth century in Europe with an Austrian physician, Franz Anton Mesmer, who is considered the father of hypnosis. He is remembered for the term *mesmerize*, which described a process of inducing a trance through a series of passes he made with his hands and/or magnets over people. He worked with psychic and electromagnetic energies that he called *animal magnetism*. The medical community eventually discredited him despite his considerable success in treating a variety of ailments. In the mid-nineteenth century, James Braid, an English physician, successfully used hypnosis in pain control and as an anesthetic in surgery. Even after witnessing live demonstrations of a patient undergoing painless surgery, his colleagues dismissed him as a fake. Not long afterward, the discovery of chloroform led to the near abandonment of hypnotic anesthesia.

In the late nineteenth and early twentieth centuries, Emile Coue, a French physician, formulated the *laws of suggestion*, discussed later in this chapter and used to this day by hypnotherapists. He also discovered that giving positive suggestions when prescribing medication proved to be a more effective cure than prescribing medication alone. Sigmund Freud at first found hypnosis extremely effective in treating hysteria, and then, troubled by the sudden emergence of powerful emotions in his patients, he abandoned it in favor of psychoanalysis. Carl Jung did not actively use hypnosis, but he encouraged his patients to use active imagination to change old memories. He often used the concept of the inner guide in his healing work. Milton Erickson, an American psychologist and psychiatrist, is considered the father of modern hypnotherapy. He demonstrated how traumatic amnesia and psychosomatic symptoms can be resolved with hypnotherapy and was influential in the official acceptance of hypnotherapy by the American Medical Association in 1958 (Nash & Barnier, 2008).

Guided imagery is a process of using all of the senses to relax, maintain health, and heal the body and mind. Since the 1970s, many books have been written on the use of guided imagery to improve health, expand thinking, and achieve life goals. Some are directed toward children and adolescents, some toward adults, and some toward people in old age.

PREPARATION

At present, no laws limit the use of hypnosis to clinical practitioners. Although anyone can hypnotize other people, hypnotherapy is best practiced by a health care professional. Nurses, physicians, dentists, psychologists, occupational

BOX 18.1

Program Content for Nurses' Certificate Program in Imagery

- Core concepts in integrative medicine, psychoneuroimmunology, and holistic healing
- Principles and theory of the guided imagery process
- Stress management strategies and self-care as an integral aspect of professional practice
- A variety of breathing and relaxation techniques
- Eight distinct integrative imagery techniques in the practicum

This program is approved for 108 continuing education hours by the American Holistic Nurses Association.

therapists, social workers, and counselors are eligible to take approved professional training in hypnotherapy. The American Society of Clinical Hypnosis and The American Council of Hypnotist Examiners share in the education and accrediting of people who meet professional requirements. In addition to successful completion of an examination, certified hypnotherapists complete 200 hours of instruction and certified clinical hypnotherapists complete 300 hours of instruction. Most practitioners do not identify themselves as hypnotists but as nurses, doctors, dentists, and others who use hypnosis as one of several modes of intervention.

The American Holistic Nurses Association and Beyond Ordinary Nursing offer a Nurses' Certificate Program in Imagery. The program consists of 108 hours of in-depth, hands-on training to provide nurses with experience in relaxation and therapeutic imagery skills. These skills are used to promote healing, decrease pain and symptoms, minimize side effects, manage chronic illness, prepare for procedures, surgery, or childbirth, and access inner wisdom and resources. An overview of the program content is found in Box 18.1.

CONCEPTS

Trance

To understand hypnotic trance, one must understand the functional difference between the conscious and subconscious mind. The *conscious mind* contains the short-term memory and the intellect. It functions like a computer, always analyzing, criticizing, and discriminating one's thoughts and perceptions. The language of the intellect is logic and reason. The *subconscious mind* contains emotions, creativity, imagination, intuition, long-term memory, and control of body functions. It also contains the habit center where persistent habits such as nail biting or test anxiety are located. The subconscious does not respond to reason and facts as does the intellect. The language of the sub-conscious is imagery and metaphor. During times of emotional turmoil or sudden trauma, people often become aware of the subconscious mind's power over body functions and intellect when they are unable to eat, sleep, or talk, and cannot think clearly. After years of ignoring feelings or "stuffing" them into the subconscious, in a hypnotic trance, people can access the sub-conscious mind, which allows them to tap into their creativity, access buried memories, change habits, unmask erroneous beliefs, repair self-esteem, and restore health.

A **trance state** is a form of heightened concentration. People in trance are aware of what is going on around them but choose not to focus on it and can return to normal awareness whenever they choose. The majority of peo-ple will tend to remember most of what happens in a controlled hypnother-apy or guided imagery session. Trance is not a form of sleep or stupor as is easily determined by observing the range of activities possible by people in a hypnotic trance.

There are three levels or stages of trance. The first is a *superficial trance* in which people are very aware of their surroundings and may accept sugges-tions such as eating less or quitting smoking, but do not necessarily carry them out. The second level, known as *alpha trance*, is significantly deeper. Heart rate, blood pressure, and respiration become slow. Hypnotic sugges-tions at this level are more effective. The third level, called *somnambulism*, is the level most beneficial to health and well-being. It is at this level that posthypnotic suggestions are most effective and people can remember past events with extreme clarity (Bailey, 2009).

People naturally flow in and out of hypnotic trances. When driving a fa-miliar route, people may slip into a trance. They can arrive at a destination and not be exactly sure about how they got there. During the trance they drive appropriately, stop at stop signs, obey traffic laws, and so on, but have no con-scious awareness of doing these things. Another example of hypnotic trance occurs during movies. People enter the theater having set aside a specific pe-riod of time wherein they can enjoy themselves. The process of settling into theater seats relaxes moviegoers and puts them in a receptive frame of mind. The lights go down to reduce the distractions from the outside world and the big screen becomes the most noticeable aspect of one's perceptual world. Within moments, the audience is transported to another place and time. If the movie is frightening, many people experience a racing heart, rapid breathing, and muscle tension—yet they are well-aware that no physical danger exists. They are responding to images and sounds alone. Movies work by similar mental mechanisms as hypnosis. First participants decide to let go of normal concerns and open the mind to a new experience. Then certain procedures re-lax the beta level of brain activity. Then, through the thoughtful use of metaphor and imagery, deeper levels of consciousness are reached. Finally, new images and perceptions can be introjected (Hamilton, 2001).

A trance is characterized by muscle relaxation, predominating alpha brain waves, feelings of well-being, diminished ability to vocalize, and an ability to accept new ideas if not in conflict with personal values. The perception of time is often distorted; 30 minutes may seem like 5 minutes. Feelings are more accessible while entranced, as well as memories from long ago. As one's awareness phases in and out, parts of the session may not be consciously remembered but are retained in the subconscious. People in trance describe their arms and legs as feeling heavy like lead or light and tingly, almost numb. Some experience slight twitches as the nervous system relaxes, and respiration shifts to abdominal breathing. Coming out of the trance, people awaken with very pleasant, almost euphoric feelings of well-being.

Laws and Principles of Suggestion

The first **law of suggestion,** as formulated by Coue, is that of *concentrated attention*. When people focus their attention repeatedly on a goal or idea, that event tends to be realized. Based on this belief, practitioners repeat hypnotic suggestions three or four times during a session. The law of *dominant affect* states that stronger emotions tend to take precedence over weaker ones. An effective hypnotherapist, after assessing the client's emotional state, connects the hypnotic suggestion to the dominant emotions. The *carrot principle* is applied when the practitioner interjects comments about the person's goals with the hypnotic suggestions, thus linking motivation to the suggestions. The principle of *positive suggestion* is applied to help people override existing attitudes. Dr. Coue was known for encouraging his patients to say to themselves 20 to 30 times each night before going to sleep, "Everyday in every way, I am getting better and better." If someone is seeking hypnosis in an effort to lose weight, the suggestion is not "You will not be hungry," which is unlikely and a negative rather than a positive statement. Rather the positive suggestion might be, "You will be surprised to find how comfortable you will be. You treat your body with kindness and respect."

Memories

It is true that under hypnosis people often recall past forgotten events. It is also true that people under hypnosis often "remember" things quite vividly that never actually happened, but which have great personal significance nonetheless. These might be called fantasized life events. In a deep trance state, memories and fantasies may be intense, and the two may be indistinguishable. People are able to remember great detail of actual events and are also uniquely capable of making up details and experiencing them as if they were remembered. Recognizing the potential difficulties arising from what some call "false memory syndrome," several states in the United States now limit legal testimony to that obtained prior to any systematic hypnotic treatment. In 1985, the American Medical Association cautioned against the systematic use of hypnosis for memory recall for both its unreliability and its potential to create vivid false memories.

BOX 18.2

Sensory Imagery

- Relax and take some easy, deep breaths.
- Focus on letting the tension go out of your body.
- Imagine holding a juicy, yellow lemon. Feel its coolness, its texture, and its weight in your hand.
- Imagine cutting the lemon in half. Notice the cut surfaces—the bright yellow outer layer, the whiteness of the inner peel, and the pale yellow of the pulp.
- Cut one of the halves in two and pick up the freshly cut lemon quarter and imagine smelling the lemony scent.
- Now imagine biting into the lemon and sucking its sour juice into your mouth.
- What happened when you imagined biting into the lemon? Did you salivate or grimace? Did you have any other physical reaction?

Imagery

Imagery is a two-way communication between the conscious and unconscious mind and involves the whole body and all of its senses. Most of us image frequently throughout the day, and worry is the most common form of imagery that affects our health. In our imagination, we react to current stressors and anticipated dangers. Our bodies become aroused and tense, and we activate the fight-or-flight mechanism. Guided imagery can help us learn how to stop troublesome thoughts and focus on images that help us relax and decrease the negative impact of stressors. Those of you who think you may not be able to image should do the exercise in Box 18.2 to demonstrate the power of imagery.

In guided imagery, the images may be created by the therapist based on the needs and desires of the client. Clients can also create the images as a way to understand the meaning of symptoms or to access inner resources. Imagery stimulates changes in many body functions such as heart rate, blood pressure, respiratory patterns, brain wave rhythms and patterns, electrical characteristics of the skin, local blood flow and temperature, gastrointestinal motility and secretions, sexual arousal, and levels of various hormones and neurotransmitters. Box 18.2 provides an example of sensory imaging and allows you to experience your physical response to imaging.

TREATMENT

Hypnotherapists do not "put" people into trances. They arrange circumstances to increase the likelihood that people will shift themselves into a trance state. About 20 percent of the population has a high capacity for trance; these people may go under hypnosis deeply. Another 20 percent had a slight capacity for trance, is easily distracted, and may not respond to hypnotherapy at all. People who cannot be hypnotized include those with organic brain disease, those with low IQs, and those who do not want to be hypnotized. The remaining 60 percent of the population falls somewhere between these extremes (Barrett, 2009).

For people seeking hypnotherapy or guided imagery, the question arises as to whether the use of audio recordings would offer equal benefit. The answer to that question depends on several factors, including the nature and depth of the problem one wants to resolve. General self-hypnosis recordings will give one only general results. Personalized audio recordings, created by a therapist using the person's own images, are more effective. Working with an experienced practitioner is most effective because the procedure is individualized according to the client's expectations and preferences.

The first and most important step in hypnotherapy is establishing a relationship with the client. It is a cooperative venture, and if the suggestions are to be effective, the therapist and client must work together. The relationship is one in which clients permit themselves to be as receptive as possible, and the therapist commits to working for the clients' well-being. People who benefit most from hypnotherapy are those who understand that hypnosis is not a surrender of control; it is only an advanced form of relaxation. The therapist gets to know clients, develops treatment plans, explains the hypnotic process, dispels myths and fears, answers questions, encourages positive attitudes about hypnosis, and with people's permission, trains them in self-inductive procedures. This process is as applicable for a short-term case of test anxiety as it is for a lengthy terminal illness. A measure of trust is needed to start the process and develop the relationship.

The **induction phase** is generally a period of relaxation or focus on the breathing that disengages people from other concerns and helps them focus their attention. In other words, the induction phase is similar to meditation and elicits the same physiological response. The induction starts with "easy" suggestions, such as focusing on breathing and closing the eyes. Directions are given to relax physically and mentally and to focus on the therapist's voice and words.

Training in induction may take one or two sessions. When the client is comfortable with entering the trance experience, the **hypnotic suggestion** begins. Based on the assessment process, the practitioner suggests an image known to be pleasurable to the client and related to the desired outcome. Hypnotic communications contain cues and explicit instructions for focusing attention and imagining in line with the aims of suggestions. The imagery is intensified by incorporating the five senses: The person is asked not only to visualize the scene but to smell the scents, touch things in the environment, hear the surrounding sounds, and even taste anything appropriate. The client is asked to focus attention on as many details about the situation as possible and is walked through the session focusing on the desired events. The suggestions of the hypnotherapist are translated by the client into ideas. These ideas then lead to corresponding behaviors in the nontrance state (Bandler, 2008).

Trance removal is that time when clients are given suggestions that will return them to a nontrance state. The hypnotherapist, for example, may count to ten, asking clients to open their eyes at the count of five, and to be fully alert at ten. Clients most commonly report that they feel relaxed during the session but may not be certain that they were hypnotized, since they could hear every word the therapist said. Many hypnotherapists provide guided audio recordings for their clients so they can practice the therapy at home.

Hypnosis cannot make people do anything against their will. If they really do not want to change, hypnosis will be a waste of time and money. If, for example, a person seeks hypnotherapy to stop smoking at a spouse's insistence but is poorly motivated, hypnotherapy will not be effective. Occasionally clients may demand that the hypnotherapist perform some magical incantation and remove 30 pounds or make the person never smoke again. This demand is the equivalent of insisting that their primary care provider cure them of hypertension while refusing to change their diet or follow a recommended medication schedule.

In some medical facilities, hypnosis and imagery are now routinely used with a variety of conditions, usually in conjunction with other forms of medical, surgical, psychiatric, or psychological treatment. They can be used with nonmedical clients as well, working through problems of living, situations of performance anxiety, and in changing bad habits. Depending on the complexity and seriousness of the complaint, treatment typically runs from two to ten sessions.

Jeanne Achterberg (2008), well known for her use of imagery in the treatment of cancer, believes that imagery is as essential as radiation and chemotherapy and must not be thought of as a "last alternative." She believes that imagery plays an important role in the biochemical healing process. She hypothesizes that images produced in the mind are converted to biochemical messages that somehow initiate a path of cancer-cell destruction or organ-cell reconstruction. Possibly, this healing process inhibits the nervous and endocrine systems from secreting stress hormones. Of course, it is difficult to prove definitively that imagery is a direct cause of healing when it occurs, because imagery is never the sole treatment used.

Hypnotherapy and guided imagery can be used to help people gain self-control, improve self-esteem, and become more autonomous. People who are imprisoned by negative beliefs see themselves as hopeless, helpless victims. With guided imagery, they can learn how to substitute positive, empowering messages. Hypnosis and imagery can also be used as a mental rehearsal for procedures, treatments, or surgery. Clients are shown how to use their own images about the healing process or, alternatively, they are guided through a series of images intended to distract them from painful procedures or anxiety-producing situations. The practitioner may have them imagine themselves in a state of good health, well-being, or successfully achieved goals.

Virtual reality environments are a recent modification of guided imagery. With the use of head-mounted displays, people experience high immersion into the virtual world. This is effective in reducing pain and anxiety from treatments or disease. Increasingly, interactive tools are providing successful distraction that allow people to cope more effectively with their treatment protocol (Wiederhold & Wiederhold, 2007).

People, especially children, are often able to rid themselves of warts by visualizing their disappearance in one way or another. Hypnosis and imagery are often used as a clinical treatment for Reynaud's disease, a condition in which the capillaries of the extremities constrict, with the result that hands and feet are cold and painful. When they learn to "think warm," people may find that the circulation to their hands and feet improves, resulting in less pain. Similarly, hand-warming frequently cuts down on both the incidence and severity of migraine headaches. The use of hypnosis in promoting feelings of comfort, distraction, and dissociation through imagery in those with chronic pain has been well established. Clients are often able to change their perceptual experience of pain by substituting numbness, a sense of pressure, or other sensation for an unwanted pain. In 1995, a National Institutes of Health (NIH) panel endorsed hypnosis as a useful adjunct to conventional treatments. Current clinical studies at NIH include hypnosis for overactive bladder, ulcerative colitis, hot flashes, Posttraumatic Stress Disorder (PTSD), and sleep disturbance.

Contraindications for hypnosis and imagery include poor motivation, such as "My husband sent me so I would lose weight," or an unwillingness even to try the treatment because of extreme fear or compelling religious objections. The procedure is unsuitable for people with active psychosis or somatic delusions. It is generally considered that these individuals are often bombarded with too many images already, and are unable to differentiate between voluntary and involuntary images.

RESEARCH

One of the difficulties in conducting research on hypnotherapy is that it is not simply one form of treatment. Hypnosis does not represent one standard set of suggestions, which may account for the large number of studies that favor anecdotal, rather than controlled, evidence. For hypnosis to be most effective in a clinical setting, hypnotic suggestions are best formulated on the basis of the individual person's interests, style, motivation, and receptivity to hypnosis. It is not like administering a drug, where doses are standardized. In hypnosis, the personal and subjective matter a great deal.

Numerous studies indicate that mental imagery can bring about significant physiological and biochemical changes. Some of these findings are from well-controlled studies, while others are reports of single cases or small studies that have not been replicated. Nevertheless, the overriding conclusion points to a relationship between imagery of body change and actual body change.

The following is a small sample of current studies in imagery and hypnotherapy.

- A pilot study involving nursing students and imagery training for the mastery of procedures found that those who engaged in imagery for blood pressure measurement performed significantly better than those students who did not participate in imagery training. In terms of aseptic techniques, there was no significant difference (Wright, Hogard, Ellis, Smith, & Kelly, 2008).

- Ten research groups are studying or have studied the impact of immersive virtual reality (VR) for pain associated with wound care of burn injuries and post-burn physical therapy. Reports suggest that the treatment is safe and effective (Sharar et al., 2008).
- Hypnotherapy has strong supportive evidence for improving the management of symptoms in people with irritable bowel syndrome (Kearney & Brown-Chang, 2008).
- In a randomized, controlled study of breast cancer survivors with hot flashes, those who received hypnosis had a significant improvement in frequency and severity of hot flashes compared to the no treatment control group (Elkins et al., 2008).
- In a randomized, controlled study of people with fibromyalgia, those who received audiotaped guided imagery demonstrated significant improvement in functional abilities compared to the Usual Care control group (Menzies, Taylor, & Bourguignon, 2006).

USING RESEARCH TO HEAL

Baird, C. L., & Sands, L. P. (2006). Effect of guided imagery with relaxation on health-related quality of life in older women with osteoarthritis. *Research in Nursing & Health*, 29: 442–451.

What Is This Study About?

Pain associated with osteoarthritis (OA) is a very common chronic health problem in older adults and significantly impacts their reported quality of life. The incidence of this disease is increasing, and it is identified as a national health priority in the United States. Therefore, the main purpose of this research study was to test the effectiveness of guided imagery with relaxation (GIR) to enhance health-related quality of life (HRQOL).

How Was the Study Done?

This was a randomized longitudinal pilot study focused on testing the effectiveness of GIR to improve HRQOL in women living with osteoarthritis. A convenience sample of 28 women was randomized to either the GIR intervention or the control group for 12 weeks. Institutional Review Board approval was granted. All participants were over 65 years of age with a diagnosis of OA and experiencing joint pain. The women ranged in age from 65 to 93 years and were considered highly educated and living in the central Midwest. The two groups were not significantly different in age, education, marital status, presence of other rheumatologic conditions, or presence of other diseases. Groups were similar in baseline pain, mobility, and HRQOL. All participants were to complete a daily journal concerning symptoms related to OA. The GIR intervention group listened to a 12-minute audiotape twice a day and made a notation of GIR in their journal. All intervention participants were instructed on GIR followed by a practice session. The GIR audiotape focused on vivid imagery about beautiful scenes, sounds and comfortable feelings individualized to each participant's preference. The script included deep breathing and an emphasis on using all senses when focusing on a relaxing scene. All scenarios were specific in describing movement of the participant's painful joint as part of the GIR. HRQOL score was derived from the following scales of the AIMS2: mobility, walking and bending, hand and finger function, arm function, self-care tasks, household tasks, social activity, support from family and friends, pain, tension, and mood.

What Were the Results of the Study?

Participants assigned to the intervention group significantly improved their HRQOL scores from baseline to 12 weeks. Women in the control group experienced no change in HRQOL scores from baseline to 12 weeks. GIR implementation revealed promise for improving the HRQOL of women with OA, including decreased daily social and emotional functioning.

What Additional Questions Might I Have?

Would one GIR session daily reveal similar results? Would additional daily session's demonstrated greater effectiveness? What is the long-term effect of GIR for women living with OA? Would a greater sample size result in similar or different findings? Can GIR be effective for persons living with other painful degenerative diseases?

How Can I Use This Study?

Professional nurses may use the findings of this study to support the use of GIR in improving the quality of life for those living with OA. GIR may be considered a cost-effective intervention that can be taught to women with OA.

Source: Contributed by Dolores M. Huffman, PhD, RN, Associate Professor of Nursing, Purdue University Calumet.

INTEGRATED NURSING PRACTICE

As a nurse, you can employ guided imagery for personal and professional development. On a regular basis, take time to envision what kind of nurse you would like to be. Envision yourself as healthy, alert, balanced, compassionate, and competent in the clinical arena. You can also use imagery to learn new procedures or techniques. After learning the goals, steps, and processes of a new activity, you can envision yourself doing the procedure safely and skillfully several times as you integrate knowledge with psychomotor skills. This "rehearsal" is a powerful tool to improve your technical nursing practice.

Some people fear that hypnosis and guided imagery may cause them to lose control of their minds to an outside force. This fear, most likely, results from stage hypnosis demonstrations. Volunteers may seem to be under the

BOX 18.3

Hypnotherapy: Myths and Realities

Myth	Reality
People are asleep during hypnosis.	People are awake and aware throughout the entire process and are highly selective about where they focus their attention.
Hypnotized people have lost control and are under someone's power.	All hypnosis is self-hypnosis since people cannot be hypnotized against their will. Hypnotized people are fully able to stop the process at any time.
People can be influenced to tell secrets.	Because the subconscious only offers information it deems appropriate and ready to contribute, people cannot be forced to reveal any secrets they would not disclose in a fully alert state.
People might get "stuck" in a hypnotic trance.	Because individuals control the situation, they can end the hypnotic trance at any time.

control of the stage hypnotist. In volunteering, they know they will be expected to do silly things in front of an audience, and it is a chance for those with extrovert tendencies to perform, have fun, and be a star. The volunteers are often truly hypnotized and doing exactly what they want to do—giving themselves permission to be outrageous. They would not, however, do something against their moral beliefs (Levy, 2008). Box 18.3 lists the myths and realities of hypnotherapy.

The reality of therapy is quite the opposite of this fear, because the individual is always under self-control. When clients learn a technique like imagery, it is entirely within their control for use when, how, and where they want. It is a tool that can be used whenever a person feels particularly anxious, upset, or uncomfortable. That type of empowering, in itself, is healing, because people feel better and do better when they have a sense of mastery over what is happening to them.

Hypnosis is used in many different clinical settings. Hypnosis is effective in surgery and in childbirth and in the management of cancer, stress, weight loss, smoking withdrawal, and posttraumatic stress disorder. Some people use hypnosis to improve self-confidence and in spiritual growth.

Many kinds of imagery work well with clients. *Feeling-state imagery* is designed to simply help clients change their mood in a general way. You can suggest to people that they let their imaginations take them to a favorite place, real or imagined. For example, some may imagine themselves at a beach and floating gently on the water, while feeling peaceful and relaxed. Others may imagine themselves as a young child sitting on the lap of a beloved grandparent. Clients can use this kind of imagery to move from a feeling state of tension and fear to one of peace and calm.

End-state imagery occurs when clients imagine themselves already in the situation or circumstances that they wish for. It may be seeing themselves as healthy, strong, and free from disease. Others may imagine themselves as successful, happy, and well-loved.

Symptoms of disease are often thought to result from blocked energy. *Energetic imagery* involves imagining the life force energy, or qi, flowing smoothly and easily throughout the body. Clients can be taught to imagine that they are pulling up energy from the earth through the soles of their feet to replenish the body's energy.

Cellular imagery relates to imagining events at the cellular level. For example, you may teach clients to imagine their natural killer cells surrounding and attacking cancer cells. Cellular imagery is usually specific and focused on exactly what needs to be fixed. Remind clients that imagery does not have to be visual. Some people "hear" their imagery, others "feel" it, and some "taste" or "smell" it. Some people might choose to put a hand over the affected area and send healing images to the cells in that area.

Similar to cellular imagery, *physiologic imagery* involves the entire body. Thus, clients might be directed to imagine that their blood vessels are relaxed and wider in an effort to lower their blood pressure. People with back pain may imagine that all the muscles in their back are relaxing and softening. People with diabetes may put their hands over the abdomen and imagine insulin moving out of the pancreas to connect with hungry cells throughout the body.

Psychological imagery involves people's perception of themselves. For example, people who feel overly responsible may feel as though they have the weight of the world on their shoulders. Those who feel abandoned may feel the pain as a heartache. In guiding the imagery, you may direct them to focus on their sensation, put their hands on the hurting places, and breathe into the pain. Psychological imagery can also be interactive. When conflict is the issue, people can imagine a dialogue with the adversary that may bring a fresh perspective and new solutions to problems.

The goal of *spiritual imagery* is to make contact with God or the Divine or gain entrance into a larger world. Clients may use spiritual imagery to find guidance or inspiration. Some clients find it comforting to imagine that they are being held in the hands of God where they are perfectly safe.

Eight characteristics help to make imagery effective as a healing tool, especially with regard to cancer (Achterberg, 2008; Naparstek, 1994; Norris, 1992):

- Images must be personal. Images created by others appear to be less effective in the healing process.

- Images must feel right to the person and be congruent with who they are and their values. For example, for those people who see themselves as gentle and conciliatory, combative or warlike images are not appropriate.
- Imagery works best in a permissive, unforced atmosphere. What seems to be most effective is an attitude of allowing the imagery to happen.
- Images must be energetic and physical. People do best when they allow themselves to feel the sensations of their images.
- Images must be anatomically correct and accurate. The type of imagery is chosen on the basis of knowing the nature of the disease and understanding exactly what body part and/or system is affected.
- Skill at using imagery increases with practice. As people use imagery more, their response to it intensifies. Suggest to clients that they use imagery in 5- to 20-minute blocks of time, one or two times a day.
- Imagery should have an end-stage component. Encourage clients to see the imagery as a mission accomplished.
- If people are receiving medical treatment concurrently, they should include it in the imagery. Clients who incorporate their chemotherapy or radiation treatment do better than those who ignore these medical procedures in their imagery.

Prior to beginning guided imagery, you should assess a client's belief system, desired outcome, and basic understanding of the pathophysiology involved, as well as an understanding of the effects of medications, treatments, or surgery. This information is necessary to formulate appropriate script content. Establish a quiet, safe environment free of unwanted distractions. Prior to the induction phase, take a few moments to center yourself. Let your mind and body release tension and tightness. Focus on letting your vocal cords relax to enhance a calming pitch, volume, and tone to your voice. Ask clients to assume a comfortable position, reclining if possible, and to close their eyes. Guide them through a progressive relaxation or body scan as described in Chapter 17. Instruct them to go to a safe, comfortable place—an actual location or one conjured up in the imagination. Ask them to use all of their senses to explore this place—what they see, hear, smell, taste, or feel. For example, you might ask them to identify the time of day or year, what flowers or trees they smell, the taste of any food that is around, and birds, train whistles, or any other sounds they hear.

Next, have clients focus on the problem at hand (e.g., the diagnosis of cancer, being HIV positive, wound or bone healing, or improved organ function). At this point you begin your script, directing them toward their previously discussed goals. You might say something like: "Imagine the broken edges of your bone. Now, bring lots of red blood cells to the area for extra nutrition and oxygen. Imagine new cells being formed and the bone edges growing together." After this type of individualized script, you should include an end-stage script, which might be something like: "Imagine that your broken leg is totally healed now. You have returned to your favorite ski hill. See yourself skiing down the slope. Your leg is strong and healthy and pain free."

Following this phase of guided imagery, talk with clients about the meaning of what occurred during the session, and reinforce the positive aspects of the experience. Some nurses make recordings of the individualized session to which clients may choose to listen as they practice on their own every day.

Gawain (2002) has developed an exercise from which most people can benefit. The pink bubble technique can be done as a one-time experience or regularly over a period of time. It is best to do the technique in the morning when you first wake up and/or in the evening right before sleep. This technique works as follows:

- Assume a comfortable position, breathe slowly, and go through a progressive relaxation or body scan procedure.
- Imagine something you would like to have or would like to have happened.
- Imagine that it has already happened. Picture the object or the situation as clearly as possible, with yourself in the picture.
- Surround this image with a pink bubble.
- Let go of the bubble and watch the bubble float off into the universe. See it becoming one with the higher power of the universe.

You can use guided imagery in many different clinical settings. In general, imagery can be used to move toward the following outcomes:

- Induce a state of physiologic relaxation.
- Reduce stress.
- Control habits: smoking, overeating, nail biting.
- Reduce pain.
- Reduce anxiety (and test anxiety).
- Understand symptoms.
- Stimulate healing responses.
- Increase tolerance of nursing and medical procedures.
- Enhance motivation and self-care.
- Find meaning in illness.
- Resolve conflicts.
- Enhance self-esteem and self-confidence.
- Increase problem-solving ability.
- Access positive inner resources.

Shames (1996) describes numerous ways for nurses to incorporate the use of imagery with nursing procedures. She suggests that people receiving intravenous fluids envision the fluid flushing out cellular toxins while simultaneously nourishing the cells. You can teach people taking antibiotics to imagine the medication attacking and destroying bacteria. Individuals

TRY THIS

Renovating Your Day

This exercise is designed to empower yourself with your thoughts by transforming negative thoughts and events through visualization. Do this every day for a week, prior to bedtime. Mentally go through your day and decide what you could have changed that would have brought better results. Then imagine that change occurring. For example, if someone said something to you that you did not like, imagine that something more positive was said. If you did not like your test score, visualize the grade as a better one.

experiencing illness or distress can be instructed to take a deep breath and send healing oxygen and a sense of peace to the lungs. On the out-breath, they can image all the toxins or tension leaving the body and disappearing into the air. When a specific organ or part of the body is disrupted, people can bring their awareness to that part and imagine healing resources migrating there to nourish and support the function. People experiencing pain can envision the pain flowing out of the body through the feet and fingertips. Some imagine the capillaries and veins expanding to become large pipes, carrying the pain out. Similarly, people can imagine the soothing effects of pain medication on the affected area and feel the softening and relaxing of the body as the pain lessens. Shames's book, *Creative Imagery in Nursing*, is a wonderful resource and provides many suggestions for clinical application of guided imagery. This technique allows you to use your creativity, intuition, and imagination as you support others on their healing journeys.

TRY THIS

Shrinking Antagonistic Forces

If you are angry with or intimidated by another person, shrink that person and put him or her in the palm of your open hand. Dialogue with that person but have that person talk in a different voice, such as a high, squeaky, or cartoon voice. See that person getting smaller and smaller until the person disappears or you blow him or her off into space.

Source: Harding, M. (2003). *Hypnosis and Imagery*. Personal communication.

References

Achterberg, J. (2008). *Intentional Healing: Consciousness and Connection for Health and Well-Being*. (Audio CD). Louisville, CO: Sounds True.

Bailey, G. (2009). *Creating Trances and Hypnosis Scripts*. Ropley, Hampshire, UK: O Books.

Bandler, R. (2008). *Richard Bandler's Guide to Trance-formation: How to Harness the Power of Hypnosis to Ignite Effortless and Lasting Change*. New York: HCI Publications.

Barrett, D. (2009). *Hypnosis and Hypnotherapy*. Westport, CT: Praeger Publishing.

Elkins, G., Marcus, J., Stearns, V., Perfect, M., Rajab, M. H., Ruud, C., et al. (2008). Randomized trial of a hypnosis intervention for treatment of hot flashes among breast cancer survivors. *Journal of Clinical Oncology*, 26(31): 5022–5026.

Gawain, S. (2002). *Creative Visualization*, 2nd ed. Novato, CA: New World Library.

Hamilton, N. (March 1, 2001). *Understanding Hypnosis*. Personal communication.

Harding, M. (October 14, 2003). *Hypnosis and Imagery*. Personal communication.

Kearney, D. J., & Brown-Chang, J. (2008). Complementary and alternative medicine for IBS in adults: Mind–body interventions. *Natural Clinical Practice. Gastroenterology & Hepatology*, 5(11): 624–636.

Levy, R. (2008). *Miraculous Health*. New York: Atria Books.

Menzies, V., Taylor, A. G., & Bourguignon, C. (2006). Effects of guided imagery on outcomes of pain, functional status, and self-efficacy in persons diagnosed with fibromyalgia. *The Journal of Alternative and Complementary Medicine*, 12(1): 23–30.

Naparstek, B. (1994). *Staying Well with Guided Imagery*. New York: Warner Books.

Nash, M., & Barnier, A. (2008). *The Oxford Handbook of Hypnosis*. Oxford, UK: Oxford University Press.

Norris, P. (1992). *Psychoneuroimmunology: Visualization and Imagery*. Paper presented to the Association for Applied Psychophysiology and Biofeedback, Colorado Springs, CO, March 19, 1992.

Shames, K. H. (1996). *Creative Imagery in Nursing*. Albany, NY: Delmar Publishing.

Sharar, S. R., Miller, W., Teeley, A., Soltani, M., Hoffman, H. G., Jensen, M. P., et al. (2008). Applications of virtual reality for pain management in burn-injured patients. *Expert Review of Neurotherapeutics*, 8(11): 1667–1674.

Wiederhold, M. D., & Wiederhold, B. K. (2007). Virtual reality and interactive simulation for pain distraction. *Pain Medicine*, 8(53): 182–188.

Wright, C., Hogard, E., Ellis, R., Smith, D., & Kelly, C. (2008). Effect of PETTLEP imagery training on performance of nursing skills: Pilot study. *Journal of Advanced Nursing*, 63(3): 259–265.

Resources

Academy for Guided Imagery
10780 Santa Monica Blvd., Suite 290
Los Angeles, CA 90025
800.726.2070
www.academyforguidedimagery.com

American Council of Hypnotist Examiners
700 S. Central Ave.
Glendale, CA 91204
818.242.1159
www.hypnotistexaminers.org/

American Society of Clinical Hypnosis
140 N. Bloomingdale
Bloomingdale, IL 60108-1017
630.980.4740
www.asch.net

Beyond Ordinary Nursing
205 De Anza Blvd., #201
San Mateo, CA 94402
650.570.6157
www.integrativeimagery.com

Canada Society of Clinical Hypnosis
2036 West 15th Ave.
Vancouver, BC V6J 2L5, Canada
604.688.1714
www.hypnosis.bc.ca

Simonton Cancer Center
P.O. Box 6607
Malibu, CA 90264
800.459.3424
www.simontoncenter.com

19

Dreamwork

*Go confidently in the direction of your
dreams. Live the life you have imagined.*

HENRY DAVID THOREAU

*One of the most adventurous things left
us is to go to bed. For no one can lay a
hand on our dreams.*

E. V. LUCAS

*Throw your dreams into space like a kite,
and you do not know what it will bring
back, a new life, a new friend, a new love,
a new country.*

ANAIS NIN

In some ways, a great deal is known about **dreaming**, because
it has been important to people for all time and across all cultures. In the twentieth and twenty-first centuries, the biology
of the brain has been explored and increasingly understood.
While this basic knowledge provides some facts underlying
dreaming, it does not tell us what dreaming is. Thus, in a sense,
little is known about dreaming, and scientists cannot yet agree on
the basic nature of dreaming. Some believe dreams are nothing
more than random firing of neurons during sleep. Others believe
dreams are symbolic stories or metaphors people tell themselves
that represent personal and social mythology. The contemporary
psychobiologic view of the dream process blends both the neuro-
scientific findings with psychoanalytic thought and believes that
dreaming is one of the ways that people reflect on and make
sense out of their waking life events. In other words, when the

brain is experiencing the physiologic state of dreaming, the mind exploits this to work on current life problems (Reiser, 2001).

BACKGROUND

Virtually every culture has believed dreams carry important messages. To the ancient Greeks, dreams were great healers. People who were sick slept in special healing temples in hopes of receiving therapeutic dreams from the gods. The Talmud, the Hebrew sacred book of practical wisdom, states clearly that the Jews gave great importance both to the dream and to the dream interpreter. Mohammed began writing the Koran after an angel visited him in a dream. Tibetan Buddhists saw no distinction between dreaming and waking and considered all of life a dream.

Plato saw dreams as a release for fervent inner forces. Hippocrates thought dreams were windows on illness, and that normal dream content indicated a state of wellness and bizarre content a state of illness. Aristotle believed that the beginning of illness could be felt in dreams before actual symptoms appeared. Likewise, Artemidorus, a physician in the Middle Ages, believed that dreams were like magnifying glasses that detected the small beginnings of physical illness.

The most famous dream book was written by Artemidorus of Daldi in the second century, and the dreams recorded are remarkably similar to contemporary ones. Chengis Khan is reported to have received his battle plans from his dreams, while Hannibal attributed the battle plan to attack Rome over the Alps with elephants as something that came to him in a dream.

During the late Middle Ages, dreams began to fall into disfavor with Christians in spite of the fact that throughout the Bible, God spoke directly to people through dreams and visions. St. Frances of Assisi founded the Franciscan Order as a dream directive from Jesus Christ.

In the United States, the traditional Iroquois were (and are) a people of dreams. Children were taught that dreams were the most important source of practical and spiritual guidance. The people of an Iroquois village began each day with dream-sharing. The entire village became involved in dreamwork, especially if a dream seemed to contain a warning of death or disease. "Big" dreams were thought to come about in one of two ways. During sleep, the dreamer would have an out-of-body experience and travel to many places, past, present, and future. Alternatively, the dreamer could receive a visit from a spiritual being. Dreams were considered to be central to healing by providing insight into the causes of illness, often before physical symptoms appeared. Dreams continue to be important tools for many traditional healers in the Native American population (Buhner, 2006).

In 1900, Sigmund Freud wrote *The Interpretation of Dreams* and proposed that dreaming might represent a unique avenue by which unconscious motivation could be explored. Freud's theory was that dreams were disguised wish fulfillments of infantile sexual needs, which were repressed by censors in the waking mind. Freud's protégé, Carl Jung, believed that humans were spiritual rather than instinctual and saw dreams as a compensatory mechanism whose function was to restore psychological balance. Jung said that the conscious and unconscious minds speak entirely different languages. The conscious mind is analytical, critical, and rational, whereas the unconscious mind thinks in metaphor, simile, symbols, and intuition (Marszalek & Myers, 2006).

Dr. Nathaniel Kleitman is considered to be the father of modern scientific dream research. In 1957, he and Eugene Aserinsky identified rapid eye movement (REM), demonstrating the activity of the brain during sleep. This active sleep stage has consequently been called **REM sleep.** Today hundreds of sleep clinics operate in the United States, and sleep disorders constitute the second most common health complaint after the common cold (Goll & Goll, 2006).

PREPARATION

In a society that discounted dreams, Sigmund Freud introduced the concept of therapeutic **dreamwork.** He and his followers, however, began to associate dreams with illness rather than wellness and reserved dream interpretation for professionals who were deemed the only people competent to understand the latent content of dreams. This approach said, in effect, that individuals were not experts about their own dreams. In contrast, Carl Jung (1965) stated that he "avoided all theoretical points of view and simply helped the patients to understand the dream-images by themselves, without application of rules and theories. . . . That is how dreams are intended" (Jung, 1965, pp. 170–171). Many contemporary therapists believe that dreams belong to individuals, and they are the final authority on the meaning of their own dreams. This viewpoint is not intended to minimize the fact that the meaning of many dreams is obscure and that other people may be able to help unlock hidden meaning.

Among indigenous peoples, shamans are recognized as dream counselors but not as "experts" in the Western sense. They are often called to their vocation by dreams. Shamans have a special relationship with the dream-world, and through dreams are able to look into the future, communicate with spirits, and clarify the meaning of other's dreams (Buhner, 2006).

CONCEPTS

Biology of Dreaming

Sleep can be divided into two distinct kinds: a quiet phase and an active phase. Changes in brain waves, eye movements, muscle tone, and the presence of dreams are used to define the two states. The quiet phase is divided into three substages. *Stage 1* is the transitional state between drowsy wakefulness and light sleep. It is characterized by slow drifting eye movements and vivid, brief dream images. Falling dreams typically occur during this stage and are often accompanied by muscle spasms of the arms, legs, or the whole body that seem to happen just as one hits the ground in the dream. These sudden contractions—myclonic jerks—are common in many mammals. *Stage 2* is genuine sleep and is characterized by unique patterns called *sleep spindles*, which are waxing and waning brain waves. After 20 to 30 minutes, people sink into *Stage 3*, delta sleep, named after the regular, slow brain waves that are characteristic of this stage of quiet sleep. Delta sleep lasts about 30 to 40 minutes, during which the muscles are relaxed, although most people make major postural adjustments every 5 to 20 minutes. The dreaming that occurs during delta sleep is more poorly recalled, less vivid and visual, less emotional, and more pleasant than REM sleep dreaming. The sleep pattern then retraces the same stages in reverse order.

About 90 minutes after the onset of sleep, several abrupt physiological changes occur as the sleeper enters REM sleep, or the active phase, for the first time of the night. It is the sleep phase of vivid, memorable dreaming. Brain waves become desynchronized in a fast activity pattern that is similar, but not identical, to that of the waking state. An accompanying profound loss of muscle tone throughout the body causes a general paralysis except for the muscles of the eyes, middle ear ossicles, and respiration. Sometimes, people awaken partially from REM sleep before the paralysis fades away, so that their body is still paralyzed, though they are otherwise awake. **Sleep paralysis,** as this state is called, can occur as people are falling asleep (rarely) or waking up (more frequently). Although the sensation may be terrifying, especially at the first occurrence, sleep paralysis is harmless.

During REM sleep, breathing may accelerate to a panting pace, and the rhythm of the heart may speed up or slow down. Typically, men have erections and women experience vaginal lubrication during every REM cycle, regardless of dream content. It is not unusual for men to ejaculate and women to experience orgasm during this time. During REM sleep, the cells of the brain, which have fired steadily throughout the wake state, fire in a wild and erratic pattern. Some neuroscientists believe dreaming is the attempt of the mind to impose meaning on these signals from random firings (Zillmer, Spiers, & Culbertson, 2007).

During a typical night's sleep, the average adult alternates between periods of REM sleep and quiet sleep at regular intervals four to six times each night. After the first REM period, the intervals between REM periods decrease throughout the night, while the length of each REM period increases. REM sleep is both the deepest and lightest stage of sleep. It is the stage when people are least likely to be aroused by environmental stimuli, and it is also the stage when people are most likely to awaken spontaneously. Interestingly, during REM sleep, each of us experiences "symptoms" of mental illness. Box 19.1 describes what happens when we sleep.

REM sleep is a primary means of brain development and maturation. Infants born 10 weeks prematurely spend 80 percent of their total sleep time in REM sleep and those born 2 to 4 weeks prematurely spend 60 to 65 percent in REM sleep. Full-term newborns spend about half of their sleeping time in REM sleep, which decreases to 30 to 35 percent by the age of 2. REM sleep stabilizes at about 25 percent by 10 years of age and shows little change until people are in

BOX 19.1

How the Brain Goes Out of Its Mind

Every 80 to 90 minutes, during REM sleep, we become completely psychotic.

Experience	Psychiatric Label
We see things that are not there.	Hallucinations
We believe things that could not possibly be true.	Delusions, magical thinking
We become confused about times, places, and persons.	Disorientation
Scenes simply appear and thoughts come and go.	Attention deficit
We think we are awake even though we are doing and seeing impossible things.	Lack of insight
We invent implausible narratives.	Confabulation, loose association
We forget almost everything on awakening.	Amnesia

This nocturnal madness is not only normal but probably essential to our health. Deprived of REM sleep, we become anxious and irritable and have trouble concentrating. Understanding this normal delirium may help you become more empathetic with the person experiencing those same symptoms while awake.

Sources: Hobson, J. A. (1996). How the brain goes out of its mind. *Harvard Mental Health Letter*, 12(8): 3–5; Barrick, M. C. (2001). *Dreams*. Corwin Springs, MT: Summit University Press.

their 70s or 80s, when it decreases to about 18 percent. The significance of the changing levels of REM sleep is unclear, but it may simply reflect that the parts of the brain controlling non-REM sleep have not yet matured (Zillner, Spiers, & Culbertson, 2007).

Dreaming and REM sleep are not the same. People also have dreams in non-REM sleep. In addition, some individuals do not dream during REM sleep, notably young children and people with certain kinds of brain injuries. Dreaming, as we know it, probably starts around age 3 with the development of language. Children under the age of 7 or 8 experience dreams in only 20 percent of their REM sleep compared to normal adults, who experience 80 to 90 percent dream time during REM sleep (Zillner, Spiers, & Culbertson, 2007).

REM sleep is important to memory. Brain activity in the hippocampus during REM sleep consolidates our experiences into long-term memory. This is evidenced by experiments interrupting either REM sleep or non-REM sleep

60 times a night. When REM sleep is interrupted, there is a complete block of learning, while interruption of non-REM sleep appears to have no effect on learning. Thus, it is believed that REM sleep is critical for organizing the pieces for long-term memory. The amygdala, where emotions are encoded and retrieved, is the source of emotional content of dreams (Nielsen & Stenstrom, 2005).

Deprivation of REM sleep does not lead to psychosis, bizarre behavior, or anxiety, as was once feared. The interference with REM sleep may come from alcohol, sedatives, caffeine, drugs, anxiety, or depression. People with major depression dream considerably less than average and have limited dream recall. A sign that the depression is lifting is an increase in REM sleep and the reporting of more dreams. The most important effect of REM deprivation is a dramatic shift in subsequent sleep patterns. Reduction of REM sleep for several nights is followed by earlier onset and longer and more frequent periods of REM sleep. The longer the deprivation of REM sleep, the larger and longer the REM rebound. This compensatory mechanism suggests that REM sleep is physiologically necessary (Zillner, Spiers, & Culbertson, 2007).

Functions of Dreaming

Dreaming is a process of making broad connections. Dreams connect with recent experiences, old memories, and imagination. Dreaming makes connections not made during the waking state. The waking state tends to be guided by a specific task or goal, whereas dreaming tends to wander and form unique combinations. For example, people who are awake and thinking of a house may recall a specific house in which they lived in the past. People who are dreaming and thinking of a house may see a generic house or a combination of several houses or even a hotel. During dreaming, consolidation of thoughts and memories occurs, and the bizarre twists and images of dreams often represent the processing and reclassifying of old information. Dream symbols bring together ordinary awareness and deeper levels of knowing. Images mean different things to different people. As Moss (1996) states, "A dream of teeth falling out might evoke fears of death or job loss in one person, the memory of a boyhood fistfight in another, and the need for a routine dental checkup to a third. A snake might warn of a sneak attack, arouse sexual fears or energies, or signal potential for healing or transformation" (Moss, 1996, p. 79). The dominant emotion of the dreamer guides the dreaming process to choose images in the memory related to that emotional concern. Dreams can be viewed as explanatory metaphors for the emotional state of the dreamer. "I leave my children in a house somewhere, and then I can't find them" may be a metaphorical description for the emotional state of guilt. If no single dominant emotion is present at the time, dreams may seem confused and almost random (Moss, 2007).

Jung believed that dreams are a remarkable way to reveal insights and solutions to deal with everyday problems encountered during the wake state. By and large, the language of dreams is anything but obvious, and for this reason it is easy to ignore the messages. What is bizarre to the conscious, rational mind is not so to the unconscious, which is rich in symbols. People who work on remembering and understanding their dreams often report that dreams provide insights to overcome and resolve problems and move ahead (Marszalek & Myers, 2006).

While some dreams seem to be sequences of disconnected images, ideas, feelings, and sensations, others are story-like sequences that are dramatic and intricately detailed. They may have plots as coherent, funny, and profound as the best stories and plays. Some dreams are not told in a single episode and the dream series is concluded the following night, and some may run for as long as a TV soap opera. It is known that dream content and process are similar to waking thought and behavior. That is, if we are outgoing and active in our waking moments, of if we are introspective and quiet in our waking moments, then we are usually the same in our dream lives (Goll & Goll, 2006).

Types of Dreams

Dreams offer nightly gauges on the dreamer's physical, emotional, and spiritual health. When disease begins to develop, dreams often provide warnings of specific problems before physical symptoms are apparent. The warning may be in the form of a broken heart, an exploding head, or limbs falling off. Such **early diagnosis dreams** are entirely natural and are reminders of how illness is related to one's entire being. It may be that when people are awake they tune out body messages, and when they are asleep their internal sensations get through more easily to the unconscious mind, which sends a message in a dream. Dreams may also give advice on preventive measures and ways to provide for one's well-being. Dreams frequently suggest specific courses of treatment for different problems. These suggestions may involve lifestyle changes, conventional medical treatments, alternative therapies, or counseling that addresses the hidden sources of disease. People may neglect the warnings but the unconscious is highly inventive in rescripting the message in ways that make it harder and harder to ignore (Moss, 2007).

Nightmares are terrifying dreams with complex imagery and story lines that are usually vividly recalled. The most common scripts of nightmares include being chased by a monster, being naked in public, falling through space, losing something precious, and being unprepared for an important exam. Nightmares are especially terrifying because in dreams, anything is possible. Most typically, the dreamer is alone with no chance for escape.

Because REM sleep becomes more physiologically intense as sleep continues, most nightmares occur in the early morning hours. Some factors that seem to contribute to nightmare frequency are fever, stress, and troubled relationships. Traumatic events can trigger a long-lasting series of recurrent nightmares. Alcohol, drugs, and some medications that suppress REM sleep can cause an increase in nightmares. The person sleeps soundly for the first 5 or 6 hours with little dreaming. When the effect of the substance has worn off, the brain makes up for the lost REM time. As a result, dreams are more intense than usual for the last few hours of sleep. Levodopa (L-dopa), used in the treatment of Parkinson's disease, and beta blockers, used in the treatment of cardiovascular disorders, seem to increase nightmares by increasing the activity during REM sleep (Rhudy, Davis, Williams, McCabe, & Byrd, 2008).

Night terrors awaken people with a scream as if they had just had a nightmare. Unlike a nightmare, however, the person frequently cannot remember anything except being afraid. Night terrors usually occur during non-REM sleep and are most common between the ages of 2 and 6 years. Although the cause is unknown, the incidence among adults increases with such factors as stress, lack of sleep, and alcohol and drug use.

Rapid eye movement sleep behavior disorder (RBD) has only recently been described in the literature. In this disorder people do not experience sleep paralysis, which allows them to act out the dream. Since these individuals often report action-filled and violent dreams, the acting out may cause self-injury or harm to others. People with Parkinson's disease are at higher risk for RBD (Chou, Moro-De-Casillas, Amick, Borek, & Friedman, 2007; Stores, 2008).

Traumatic dreams are a major symptom of posttraumatic stress disorder (PTSD). People exposed to extremely dangerous and life-threatening situations such as war, terrorist attacks, physical or sexual assault, hostage situations, or natural disasters may develop PTSD. Traumatic dreams occur in all stages of sleep and tend to return the victim to the traumatic event in all of its emotional horror. As the experience is gradually resolved, there is a decrease in frequency and an alteration in dream content. New stressors may reactivate the traumatic dream.

Recurrent dreams usually begin in childhood or adolescence, often at a time of significant stress. The emotional tone of recurrent dreams is negative 60 to 70 percent of the time, but the content of the dream does not directly reflect the original stress. Typical dreams include being attacked or chased by animals, monster, burglars, or natural forces. The dream often disappears when the original stressor or problem is resolved.

Conscious dreaming, sometimes referred to as **lucid dreaming,** is being aware that one is dreaming during the experience. People in this unusual state of consciousness are simultaneously aware of their bodies lying on a bed, aware of the content of their dreams, and aware of watching themselves dreaming. Conscious dreaming may be triggered by various things such as doing something impossible in the dream like flying or walking on water. Likewise, auditory signals such as a doorbell or a siren may startle people into becoming aware they are dreaming. Individuals who wish to explore and use dreams constructively in their lives can learn techniques to increase their conscious dreaming time.

Precognition is knowing about an event before it actually occurs. **Precognitive dreaming** involves seeing people and situations from the future and is an event where individuals are not bound by space-time. As people learn to recall their dreams and record them in a dream journal, they often begin to recognize and work with precognitive material in their dreams. Precognitive dreams may indicate what may happen if certain courses of action are pursued, or they may show a precise event that cannot be altered (Moss, 2007).

TREATMENT

Until recently, Western societies have discouraged dreamwork and dream-sharing. When dreams are recalled, the significance is often minimized. People tend to remember only bits and pieces from dreams and often jumble together parts from several dreams into a single confused story. By the time individuals are fully awake they have forgotten 90 percent, if not more, of their nighttime adventures. Thus, the remembered dream is often different from the fuller dream experience.

By paying closer attention to dreams, people often gain greater access to their inner lives. Some of the world's most successful business executives never make a decision until they have a chance to let it pass through their minds during sleep, allowing solutions to come during dreams. The first step in making sense of a dream is to own it. It belongs solely to the dreamer and is a personal story. Although many books have been written about dream symbols, they are best understood by the dreamer. Dreaming about a horse may be a symbol of comfort and security because the person always had a horse when she was growing up. A horse for another person may be a symbol of terror because he was kicked by a horse as a young child. Yet another person might see a horse as a symbol of a challenge since she has wanted to learn to ride for some time. Thus, dream dictionaries do not have the answers to people's dream symbols; they are personal images taken from one's life representing one's unique experiences.

Journaling helps to mobilize intuition as people begin to understand their personal symbols. Because the dream journal is intensely personal, it should be kept private unless the dreamer chooses to share it with others. The entries should be dated so they can be correlated to significant life events in the present or future and recurring themes, places, and situations should be noted. Giving dreams titles or headlines like a newspaper headline often reveals a dream message that may otherwise be overlooked. People are encouraged to go back over their journals at regular intervals to note connections between dreams and waking events.

In the midst of nightmares, people who realize they are dreaming frequently choose to wake up. Many therapists believe, however, that the essential issue is to discover what elements from the past, mixed with current events, are creating the nightmare. Insight into the source of the nightmare can help people face and overcome the terror while remaining in the dream. Nightmares can be transformed into more pleasant experiences. People are encouraged to remember that nothing in their dreams can hurt them.

Conscious dreaming, as a form of mental imagery, has the potential to aid in the promotion of health and in the healing process. Evidence supports the idea that the vividness of mental imagery determines how strongly it affects physiology. Dreams are the most vivid form of mental imagery most people experience and, therefore, they are also likely to be a source of highly effective healing imagery (Bulkeley, 2003).

Dreams can be immensely useful in gaining self-knowledge. Psychologist Ernest Rossi has proposed that an important function of dreaming is integration of split-off parts of one's personality. According to Rossi (1985):

> In dreams we witness something more than mere wishes; we experience dramas reflecting our psychological state and the process of change taking place in it. Dreams are a laboratory for experimenting with changes in our psychic life. . . . This constructive or synthetic approach to dreams can be clearly stated: Dreaming is an endogenous process of psychological growth, change, and transformation. (p. 142)

Individuals with posttraumatic stress disorder often relive the event through nightmares or flashbacks. Prazosin (Minipress), an alpha-blocker, shows promise in reducing nightmares in both combat and noncombat-related patients (Taylor, Freeman, & Cates, 2008).

RESEARCH

Dream research is often accused of working from biased or otherwise inadequate samples. Some question whether people who remember dreams are different from other people. Some fear people do not report their dreams honestly. Many studies of high and low dream recallers demonstrate only small differences between them on a variety of personality and cognitive tests. High recallers differ primarily in their interest in dreams and their motivation to recall them. In many studies, subjects provide dream reports anonymously, which reduces the tendency to misreport. For most people, dreams are something that happens to them, so they do not see the dreams as a reflection on their self-image and are thus quite willing to report whatever they experience (Dumhoff & Schneider, 2008).

There are four sources of dream reports: the sleep laboratory, the psychotherapy relationship, personal dream journals, and reports written on anonymous forms in group settings. Sleep laboratories awaken individuals during REM and non-REM periods, which allows for the maximum recall of dreams. The process, however, is time consuming and expensive. Psychotherapy is a longstanding source of dream reports. The patients, however, are a small and unrepresentative sample of the population. Dream journals are personal documents of dreams but may have gaps or omissions. Some individuals are not willing to provide their journals for scientific analysis. The easiest way to get large samples of dreams is in the classroom, meeting, conferences, waiting rooms, and so on. People are simply asked to provide their gender, age, and the last dream they remember having.

Four general methods are used to analyze dream content: free associations, finding metaphoric meaning, searching for repeated themes, and quantitative analysis. Free association, that is, saying whatever comes into their minds about each part of the dream, often reveals the day-to-day waking events incorporated into the dream. In psychotherapy, people may look for metaphors, often based on their own past life experiences. Researchers may also look for repeated themes in a dream series. Usually these themes are unique to each dreamer, which makes it impossible to generalize to other people. The major task in quantitative content analysis is the creation of carefully defined categories that lead to the same results when used by different researchers. Nominal scales simply record the presence or absence of a characteristic in a dream report. For example, there could be a general category of aggression and then each type of aggression can be assigned separate categories. Hall and Van de Castle developed the most comprehensive and widely used empirical system of content analysis in 1966. They cataloged more than 10,000 dreams from normal people and found that approximately 64 percent were associated with sadness, apprehension, or anger. Only 18 percent were happy or exciting. Only 1 percent of dreams involved sexual feelings or acts. DreamBank, a Web site at the University of California, Santa Cruz, has over 22,000 dream reports available for research regarding dream content (Domhoff & Schneider, 2008).

The following is a small sample of current research studies:

- It appears that body representation in the dream state is not sensitive to actual changes in body parts. People with amputations report that their bodies are intact during their dreams, even years after the actual amputation (Mulder, Hochstenbach, Dijkstra, & Geertzen, 2008).
- Children and adolescents who have experienced interpersonal violence have significantly more aggression in their dreams compared to peers who do not experience violence (Kamphuis, Tuin, Timmermans, & Punamaki, 2008).
- Forty-four people in the United States who had been recording all their dreams for years were asked to provide their 10 dream descriptions prior to 9/11 and the first 10 after 9/11. While they did not dream about the actual events of 9/11, their dreams were much more intense following 9/11 (Hartmann & Brezler, 2008).
- One third of people with Parkinson's disease (PD) experience rapid eye movement sleep disorder (RBD). This study compared dream content between people with and without RBD and men and women with PD. Those with RBD had more violent dreams compared to those without RBD. In addition, men with PD had more aggressive dreams than did women with PD (Borek, Kohn, & Friedman, 2007).
- 88 people with borderline personality disorder (BPD) were compared to 100 matched healthy control individuals to study the rate of nightmares and sleep quality. Those with BPD experienced significantly greater numbers of nightmares and disturbed sleep quality than did the control individuals (Semiz, Basoglu, Ebrinc, & Cetin, 2008).

INTEGRATED NURSING PRACTICE

Dreams are the doorway into the unconscious, which is also a domain of healing. Just as guided imagery can be used to direct people's attention to specific areas or organs of the body, so can dreams become a healing tool. For clients who are interested in **cultivating healing dreams,** they can follow a series of steps that you can teach them (Keegan, 1994):

- One half hour before bedtime, find a quiet place.
- Pay attention to the sounds and sensations of the outside environment as nature begins to settle down to rest.
- Spend a few minutes journaling the experiences and feelings you had during the day.
- Review your accomplishments of the day.
- Think for a moment of loving yourself and others with whom you interacted today.
- If you had conflict with others, put those thoughts and feelings away for now.
- Imagine yourself as part of the universe and feel a connection with all living things.
- Allow one issue of present concern to come to your conscious awareness.
- Ask for answers, solutions, or healing as you sleep and dream.
- On awakening, remember what you wanted to learn from your dreams and let the answers come to your awareness.

A similar process is called **dream incubation,** which is a somewhat more deliberate format. Examples of the types of requests to make of our dreams include these: How can I heal myself? Which path shall I choose? How can I solve (state problem)? How can I improve my relationship with (name)? How can I make (state project) a success? Should I do (state proposed action)? What shall I do now? Teach clients the following steps for dream incubation:

- Choose an important matter that you wish to explore.
- Write a short, simple question about which you want to know.
- Meditate on the question for a few minutes. Repeat the question several times, followed by "I give thanks for the answer, which will be in a dream that I remember."
- Envision yourself awakening, remembering, and receiving an answer.
- Write the question again.
- Place the paper with the question on it beneath your pillow.
- Upon awakening, follow the guideline in the "Try This" box on improving dream recall near the end of the chapter.
- Watch for extra information that may come later during the day.
- Do not give up if success is not immediate.

Help clients understand that they need not seek professional help for bad dreams unless they frequently disrupt one's sleep. Other distress signals include regular bouts of fatigue or depression when you wake up or consistently feeling worse than when you went to bed. Remind people that nothing in their dreams can hurt them. Suggestions for reframing nightmare themes are presented in Box 19.2. Alternatively, nightmares can be managed through a process called **dream reentry,** which is practiced in the waking state. People begin by selecting the nightmare to relive, then come up with alternative ways of acting in the nightmare to transform the events into a more enjoyable experience. They relive the nightmare in imagination, incorporating

BOX 19.2

Reframing Nightmares

Being Chased

Response: Stop running and face the chaser, which may cause it to disappear. If not, try to dialogue and reconcile with the person or animal. Alternatively, ask the adversary itself what you are running away from.

Being Attacked

Response: Demonstrate your readiness to defend yourself, rather than giving in or running away. Then try to dialogue with the attacker in a soothing manner. Alternatively, enlist friendly and cooperative dream characters to help overcome the threatening character.

Falling

Response: Rather than waking up, go with it, relax, and land gently. Think about landing in a pleasant and interesting place. Alternatively, transform falling into flying.

Trapped or Paralyzed

Response: Relax and tell yourself you are dreaming. Go along with images or things that happen to the body, because none of it can be harmful in reality. Adopt an attitude of interest and curiosity about what happens.

Being Unprepared for an Exam or Speech

Response: Leave the exam room or the lecture hall. Alternatively, answer the text questions creatively or give a spontaneous talk on any topic of interest. The key is in transforming the experience into one that is fun.

Being Naked in Public

Response: Remember, modesty is a public convention and dreams are private experiences. Have fun with the idea. Try having everyone else in the dream remove their clothing also.

Sources: Barrick, M. C. (2001). *Dreams.* Corwin Springs, MT: Summit University Press; Browne, S. (2002). *Book of Dreams.* New York: Dutton; and Bulkeley, K. (2003). *Dreams of Healing.* New York: Paulist Press.

the new action, and continue on with the dream until they see the result of their new behavior (Mellick, 2001).

Spiritual care, in many settings, includes listening to clients' dreams. During times of transition, growth, or suffering, spiritual issues or struggles often occur and may be found in dreams as people wrestle with what is most important in their lives. Nurses have a unique opportunity to listen attentively to clients and help them work through this process. Sharing dreams with another person or with a group can provide a variety of insights into the many levels of the dream. Dream-sharing also builds a sense of community as people discover they have a great deal in common. If you are a nurse who is sensitive and empathic and you have good listening, communication, and group skills, you can facilitate a dream-sharing group (Bulkeley & Bulkley, 2006).

If you want each member of the group to have time to work on a dream at every session, you will have to limit your numbers to six or eight. Members should be asked to make a commitment to attend regular sessions over a set time, usually for no less than 6 weeks. A typical group session is 2 to 3 hours. Dream-sharing requires mutual trust and respect. If people are going to share their innermost thoughts, they must have the assurance that they are in a place where they are protected and supported. The dream is always honored as a topic worthy of attention and thought. The protocol of dream-sharing is as follows (Kramer & Barasch, 2000):

- All members are given an opportunity to share dreams if they choose to, but are never pressured to do so.
- Dreams shared within the group should not be told to outsiders without the dreamer's permission.
- Sharing dreams does not mean giving up the right to privacy. Dreamers are free to share as much or as little about their dreams or personal lives as they wish.
- You are the final authority on the meaning of your dream.
- You cannot tell anyone else what her or his dream is about. You can only tell them what it would mean to you if it were your dream.

Even without a full understanding of what dreams signify, we can use their stories to know ourselves better. For many people—and you can be one of them—dreams really do come true.

TRY THIS

Improving Dream Recall

1. Clearly declare to yourself the intention to remember your dreams when you lie down to sleep.
2. Have your tools, notebook, and pen or tape recorder at your bedside.

3. If you awaken during the night while dreaming, record your dream immediately. Use a penlight to see if you do not wish to disturb your partner. If you tell yourself that you can go back to sleep and catch the dreams later, you will probably find you are wrong.

4. When you awaken in the morning, at first lie quietly before jumping out of bed. Then write whatever you remember, even if only one word or scene.

5. If you wake up with no dream memories, move your body back into the position you were in as you began to awaken, and you will be more likely to recall your most recent dream.

6. Don't censor your dreaming and don't try to interpret them right away. Bizarre, weird, or trivial dreams may become important later.

7. Pay attention to your feelings. They are often your best guide to the dream's meaning and urgency.

8. Keep a journal for a month of the dreams you do remember. Look for important ideas or themes running through the dreams.

9. The more you practice these skills, the more dreams you will remember.

References

Borek, L. L., Kohn, R., & Friedman, J. H. (2007). Phenomenology of dreams in Parkinson's disease. *Movement Disorders*, 22(2): 198–202.

Buhner, S. H. (2006). *Sacred Plant Medicine*. Rochester, VT: Bear & Company.

Bulkeley, K. (2003). *Dreams of Healing*. New York: Paulist Press.

Bulkeley, K., & Bulkley, P. (2006). *Dreaming Beyond Death: A Guide to Pre-Death Dreams and Visions*. Boston, MA: Beacon Press.

Chou, K. L., Moro-De-Casillas, M. L., Amick, M. M., Borek, L. L., & Friedman, J. H. (2007). Testosterone not associated with violent dreams or REM sleep behavior disorder in men with Parkinson's. *Movement Disorders*, 22(3): 411–414.

Dumhoff, G. W., & Schneider, A. (2008). Studying dream content using the archive and search engine on Dream-Bank.net. *Consciousness and Cognition*, 17(4): 1248–1256.

Goll, J. W., & Goll, M. A. (2006). *Dream Language: The Prophetic Power of Dreams*. Shippensburg, PA: Destiny Image Publishers.

Hartmann, E., & Brezler, T. (2008). A systematic change in dreams after 9/11/01. *Sleep*, 31(2): 213–218.

Jung, C. G. (1965). A. Jaffe (ed.), R. Winston & C. Winston (trans.), *Memories, Dreams, Reflections*. New York: Vintage.

Kamphuis, J. H., Tuin, N., Timmermans, M., & Punamaki, R. L. (2008). Extending the Rorschach trauma content index and aggression indexes to dream narratives of children exposed to enduring violence. *Journal of Personality Assessment*, 90(6): 578–584.

Keegan, L. (1994). *The Nurse as Healer*. Albany, NY: Delmar Publishers.

Kramer, M., & Barasch, M. I. (2000). Dreamspeak. *Psychology Today*, 33(5): 56–61.

Marszalek, J. F., & Myers, J. E. (2006). Dream interpretation: A developmental counseling and therapy approach. *Journal of Mental Health Counseling*, 28(1): 18–37.

Mellick, J. (2001). *The Art of Dreaming*. New York: Gramercy Books.

Moss, R. (1996). *Conscious Dreaming: A Spiritual Path for Everyday Life*. New York: Crown Trade Paperbacks.

Moss, R. (2007). *The Three "Only" Things: Tapping the Power of Dreams, Coincidence, and Imagination.* Novato, CA: New World Library.

Mulder, T., Hochstenbach, J., Dijkstra, P. U., & Geertzen, J. H. (2008). Born to adapt, but not in your dreams. *Consciousness and Cognition,* 17(4): 1266–1271.

Nielsen, T. A., & Stenstrom, P. (2005). What are the memory sources of dreaming? *Nature,* 237(27): 1286–1289.

Reiser, M. F. (2001). The dream in contemporary psychiatry. *American Journal of Psychiatry,* 158(3): 351–359.

Rhudy, J. L., Davis, J. L., Williams, A. E., McCabe, K. M., & Byrd, P. M. (2008). Physiological-emotional reactivity to nightmare-related imagery in trauma-exposed persons with chronic nightmares. *Behavioral Sleep Medicine,* 6(3): 158–177.

Rossi, E. (1985). *Dreams and the Growth of Personality,* 2nd ed. New York: Brunner/Mazel.

U. B., Basoglu, C., Ebrinc, S., & Cetin, M. (2008). Nightmare disorder, dream anxiety, and subjective sleep quality in patients with borderline personality disorder. *Psychiatry and Clinical Neurosciences,* 62(1): 48–55.

Stores, G. (2008). Rapid eye movement sleep behavior disorder in children and adolescents. *Developmental Medicine and Child Neurology,* 50(10): 728–732.

Taylor, H. R., Freeman, M. K., & Cates, M. E. (2008). Prazosin for the treatment of nightmares related to posttraumatic stress disorder. *American Journal of Health-System Pharmacy,* 65(8): 716–722.

Zillmer, E. A., Spiers, M. V., & Culbertson, W. (2007). *Principles of Neuropsychology,* 2nd ed. Florence, KY: Wadsworth.

Resources

International Association for the Study of Dreams
  1672 University Ave.
  Berkeley, CA 94703
  209.724.0889
  www.asdreams.org

DreamGate
  www.dreamgate.com

European Association for the Study of Dreams
  58190 Neuffontaines
  France
  33.03.86.24.86.41
  www.oniros.fr/home

The Lucidity Institute
  21555 Spencer St.
  Napa, CA 94559
  209.254.8597
  www.lucidity.com

20

Intuition

It is not the mountain we conquer, but ourselves.

Intuition is behind every diagnosis, formulation, patient contact. If it weren't I'd be an analytic machine.

DR. OLIVER SACKS, NEUROBIOLOGIST

Intuition comes from the Latin word *intueri*, which means to look within. Intuition is described as something people see, hear, or feel rather than think; a powerful form of inner wisdom; an awareness of something without conscious attention or reasoning; or knowledge from an expanded state of awareness. Some people describe it as knowing immediately without thinking. Words and phrases associated with intuition are hunches, instinct, gut feeling, sixth sense, a flash of insight, "It suddenly hit me," "Something just clicked into place," "It just feels right," and "I don't know why, but something tells me I should do this."

BACKGROUND

Intuition is as old as humankind. Scientists, inventors, and artists have credited intuition with their ability to accomplish great things. Archimedes, one of the three greatest mathematicians of all time (born 287 B.C.), was reported to have shouted "Eureka" when he discovered his famous flotation principle. Hippocrates, the father of medicine, wrote about the value of intuition, which he called "instinct." He warned that "cold reason" could obscure one's inner vision. Albert Einstein credited intuition for many of his own inspirations. Thomas Edison used the symbols of his dreams to intuit scientific breakthroughs.

Jonas Salk, who discovered the polio vaccine, wrote an entire book on intuition, maintaining that creativity was the result of the interaction of intuition and reasoning.

The late Edgar Cayce (1877–1945) was one of the most versatile and credible psychics, or medical intuitives, the world has ever known. Cayce, a photographer and devout religious person, was, in a sense, the father of holistic medicine. In the early twentieth century, he emphasized the importance of attitudes, emotions, diet, and exercise in health and illness. He believed the treatment of illness should be physical, mental, and spiritual. Daily, for over 40 years of his adult life, Cayce would lie down on a couch and enter a self-induced meditative state. Then, provided with the name and location of a person anywhere in the world, he would speak in a normal voice and give information about the state of the person's mind and body and prescribe ways to generate physical and mental health. These sessions came to be called "readings," and there are over 14,000 of them on file. A copy of the reading was always sent to the individuals for their own information and use.

Our contemporary times have several well-known medical intuitives. Judith Orloff, MD, is a board-certified psychiatrist, a professor of psychiatry at UCLA, and an author and lecturer on the interrelationship of medicine, intuition, and spirituality. Her book, *Second Sight* (1996), is a memoir about coming to terms with her intuitive abilities. Mona Lisa Schulz, MD, PhD, is a neuropsychiatrist and neuroscientist and has worked for many years as a medical intuitive. Caroline Myss, PhD, is a writer, researcher, and medical intuitive who works closely with Norman Shealy, MD, founder of the American Holistic Medical Association.

PREPARATION

The level of training and abilities varies greatly from one medical intuitive to another. Because the practice of medical intuition is not regulated, anyone can claim the title, and the education and experience vary considerably. Standards are in the process of being developed, but it is difficult to standardize the intangible. Indications that an intuitive is not legitimate include claims of the only true way to heal, resistance to collaboration with primary health care providers, giving advice or telling the client what to do, and/or the charging of exorbitant fees.

CONCEPTS

Right and Left Brain

The cerebrum makes up 80 percent of the weight of the brain. The cerebrum is divided into two hemispheres, right and left. Each of the hemispheres has separate and unique functions. Yet, if one hemisphere is damaged, the other hemisphere seems to be able to take on some of its function. The corpus callosum is composed of 200 million nerve fibers that connect the left and right hemispheres, and it relays sensory information between the two brains.

The *left brain* contains most language functions and interprets, analyzes, sorts, and retrieves information necessary to problem solve and plan ahead. It is rational and focused on the external world. It is often referred to as the masculine half of the brain.

The *right brain* is the emotional, visual, and intuitive part of the brain. The emotional aspect of language is located here. Its focus is on feelings and the state of the internal body. It is often referred to as the feminine half of the brain.

Women have faster and greater access to the right hemisphere because they have a wider corpus callosum than men. As a general rule, most women tend to process information with the right brain, the left brain, and the body all working together. They are also able to communicate their intuition as it comes to them. Most men are more likely to process information with their left brains. The left brain, as the rational, logical, and intellectual part of us, is highly regarded in Western society. The emotional, intuitive right brain is considered inferior. In fact, the left brain often acts as a censor and denies the validity of intuition (Duggan, 2007).

Intuitive healing calls on both hemispheres of the brain. It respects the intelligence of the left brain and calls on the intuitive wisdom of the right brain. Identifying health and illness issues and making decisions are best accomplished when the rational and intuitive brains work together.

Problem Solving

It is important to most people that they make good decisions. Intuition can help people make everyday decisions and improve their problem-solving skills. Sometimes, people simply get a gut feeling about a particular course of action. More often, however, intuition is the result of a four-step process. The first step involves *preparation and analysis*. People use their left brain to collect facts and information and study the situation. The second step is *incubation*. During this phase, the problem is put on the "back burner" by letting the left brain move on to another subject. People often increase right brain activity during this phase by listening to music, meditating, or engaging in movement such as dancing, t'ai chi, or yoga. The third step in *insight*. The intuitive answer may arrive in the form of images, verbal messages, physical sensations, emotions, environmental cues, or just a pervasive sense of knowing. The fourth and last step is *validation*. Once the insight is a conscious thought, the left brain checks to see if the intuitive message answers the question or solves the problem (Nyatanga & de Vocht, 2008; Pretz, 2008).

Intuition and Dreams

Intuition is the language of dreams. The right brain and the body are better able to communicate at night when the left brain is quiet. Dreams offer nightly gauges on the dreamer's physical, emotional, and spiritual health. When disease begins to develop, dreams often provide warnings of specific problems before physical symptoms are apparent. Body cells may send signals through the use of chemicals to a part of the brain. The warning may be in the form of a broken heart, an exploding head, or limbs falling off. Such *early diagnosis dreams* are entirely natural and are reminders of how illness is related to one's entire being. It may be that when people are awake they tune out body messages, and when they are asleep their internal sensations get through more easily to the intuitive mind, which sends a message in a dream. Intuition in the form of dreams may also give advice on preventive measures and ways to provide for one's well-being. Dreams frequently suggest specific courses of treatment for different problems. These suggestions may involve lifestyle changes, conventional medical treatments, alternative therapies, or counseling that addresses the hidden sources of disease. People may neglect the warnings, but intuition is highly inventive in rescripting the message in ways that make it harder and harder to ignore (Orloff, 2009).

TREATMENT

It would be comforting to believe that medical diagnoses and treatment decisions are easily made by primary health care providers. Even with the wonders of science, however, misdiagnoses occur and treatments may cause more problems than the disease itself. Many health care practitioners rely on their intuition to enhance their scientific understanding. More than 5,000 medical tests are currently in use. How would practitioners know which ones to order if they did not use intuition as well as their knowledge and deductive reasoning? Thus, medical intuition is an essential tool for every biomedical and alternative health care provider.

Medical Intuitives

A **medical intuitive** is someone who has skill and/or training in reading the human energy system. Some practitioners are born with this ability, others acquire the skill after a life crisis, and some learn it through training and practice. Medical intuition is not a healing modality, but rather a tool to provide information about what is going on in a person's body, mind, and spirit.

Medical intuitives may or may not meet their clients in person, but they will work only with the client's explicit consent. The intuitive makes it clear that it is not a physician–patient relationship and that there will be no diagnoses or treatment prescriptions. The intuitive will instead tell the person about problematic energetic and emotional factors they detect and may suggest having certain areas checked out by a regular health care provider. Medical intuition is an empowering tool when clients use the information to make changes for the better in their health and lives.

Medical intuition presupposes that body, mind, and spirit are one unified reality. It is based on the belief that the body is animated by an integrated energy called the **life force.** The life force sustains the physical body, but it is also a spiritual entity that is linked to a higher being or infinite source of energy. When the energy flows freely throughout the body, a person experiences optimal health and vitality. When the life force is blocked or weakened, organs, tissues, and cells are deprived of the energy they need to function at their full potential, and illness or disease results.

After quieting or grounding their own energy, medical intuitives tune in to their client's mind–body–spirit energy. They pay attention to the energy without censoring, questioning, or analyzing. Some intuitives are *clairvoyant*. This means that intuition comes to them visually and they see pictures of the inner parts of the body. They are able to see energy or qi as it flows through the body and are able to detect where this energy has become blocked. Some intuitives are *clairsentient*. This means that they are able to feel the energy or emotions in the body. They may experience actual sensations in their own bodies or they may scan clients' bodies seeking out changes in the energy field of the body. Some intuitives are *clairaudient*. They receive intuitive information through sounds. This may be random and dissociated words or may be a sentence or even an in-depth conversation.

In a sense, biomedical health care providers work from the outside in and look at the symptoms of the physical body. Medical intuitives work from the inside out and are more interested in spiritual, emotional, and psychological issues that create the environment for illness and disease to occur. Many medical intuitives work with (or are) medical doctors.

Self-Healing

Some people believe that curing their illness or disease is something that must be done to them or for them. They have lost their intuitive understanding of what is not functioning properly and why, and often ignore symptoms or numb their pain. They have little understanding of how they set the internal scene for their illness or disease.

With this mind-set, people become disconnected from their ability to heal themselves and feel like victims of their own body processes.

People interested in self-healing recognize that dysfunction and disease are ways the body talks. All people have the ability to intuit what their bodies are communicating. They can learn to trust and use their inner intelligence to tell them what is right and wrong, what's good and should be strengthened, and what's unhealthy and needs to be changed. Intuition may tell a person when to exercise, when to rest, or when to see a biomedical health care provider. Self-healers also understand that intuitions do not heal in and of themselves. To heal, they must act on the intuitive information.

Thoughts trigger biochemical responses and biochemical responses trigger thoughts. Thoughts, words, and beliefs are the link between people's inner experiences and the directions their lives take. Many individuals have longstanding negative tapes playing in their heads much of the time. This **negative self-talk** includes statements such as these: I'm bad; I'm fat and ugly; no one likes me; I have no control; I'm no good; it's hopeless; I'm never going to feel better; I'm always sick; I'm all alone in this life; the world is a dangerous place; I might as well give up; and so on. The unconscious mind "hears" these thoughts and words and begins to treat them as reality. Thus, one's expectations become a self-fulfilling prophecy, and people become driven by negativity (Orloff, 2009).

In contrast, **positive attitudes** are a part of self-healing and foster growth and adaptive change. Positive beliefs set the stage for healing to occur. Positive self-talk includes statements such as these: My body is a holy vessel; I have the ability to heal myself; I like and respect my body; my body, emotions, and spirit are all one; I am well loved; I am good to other people; I enjoy being healthy; I listen to my intuition; my body knows what it needs to get well; and so on. The unconscious takes these positive attitudes seriously, and they become a self-fulfilling prophecy for health and well-being (Orloff, 2009). There is an old Navajo saying that illustrates this process: "If you want to see what your body will look like tomorrow, look at your thoughts today."

Another facet of self-healing is **body scanning,** or learning to decode subtle body messages before there is pain or disease. Most people can learn to discern imbalances long before these can be medically verified. Body scanning begins with meditation. When people have a quieter conscious mind they can more easily recognize messages coming from the body, emotions, and subconscious mind. Meditation is the amplifier of intuition. Once the mind is quiet, open, and waiting, the individual scans the entire body.

During this process the person notes any areas that are hot or cold, and sensations of tingling, buzzing, quivering, aching, tightness, or numbness. With practice, people can learn to understand the unique language their bodies use to communicate needs and problems. With this intuitive understanding, people can take steps to create a healthier and happier life (Orloff, 2009).

RESEARCH

While medical intuition has some compelling anecdotes, research into the phenomenon is in its infancy. Within biomedicine there are "master" diagnosticians who can assess a patient's condition and prognosis with extremely subtle cues. Healers in many cultures claim to make assessments by intuition. It will be interesting to see in the future if medical intuition, which is subjective and metaphysical, can be understood from the objective and scientific viewpoint.

There are a number of studies on intuition in nursing practice. These qualitative studies began in the mid-1980s and continue on today. Nursing intuition does not lend itself to randomized, blinded studies. Effken (2007, p. 188) states: "The value of intuition for clinical practice has been well documented; but because it cannot easily be measured, it can be denigrated in today's evidence-based research and practice environment."

INTEGRATED NURSING PRACTICE

Intuition in Patient Care

Nursing practice is based on more than scientific understanding. It is also inspired by intuition. Experienced nurses are able talk about their intuitive sense and give examples of it from their own practice but are often discouraged by a work environment that emphasizes linear deductive reasoning (Banning, 2007).

Mona Lisa Schulz, a physician and medical intuition, states that one of the most intuitive groups of people she knows are nurses in intensive care units. A patient may appear objectively stable but the nurse who is caring for him will insist that he is about to "go bad" or go into a crisis state. When asked how the nurse knows, the reply is usually "I just know." It might be a smell, a slight tinge of color, a touch, or some other subtle cue that alerts the nurse. When science and medical knowledge say one thing and a nurse's gut feeling says something else, it is important to look at the situation again (Schulz, 1998).

Patricia Benner has studied nurses and intuition for some time. She describes the intuitive process of nurses as "skilled pattern recognition." She believes that nursing intuition is based on previously acquired knowledge, memory, and experience. She also found that intuitive nurses do not always trust what they are experiencing when they cannot provide the "proof" that others demand of them. Benner suggests that nurses and others might more readily accept intuition if it is called skilled pattern recognition instead (Benner & Tanner, 1987).

McCutcheon and Pincombe (2001) believe that nursing intuition is based on "a complex interaction of attributes, including experience, expertise and knowledge, along with personality, environment, acceptance of intuition as a valid 'behavior' and the presence or absence of a nurse/client relationship" (p. 345). Their study acknowledges that nurses acting on intuition can positively affect patient care and that ignoring intuition can negatively impact that care.

Nyatanga and de Vocht (2008) and Gobet and Chassy (2008) believe that simple decisions are better processed by the conscious mind while complex decisions are better processed by the unconscious mind. It is thought that the unconscious mind is able to detect familiar patterns since more information is stored as unconscious thought.

Intuitive Leadership

Business executives have understood for some time that intuition is an important part of successful leadership. Just as businesses are doing, nurse managers can turn to experts in the field of intuition to shape decisions, assess professional relationships, and decide on courses of action. Respecting intuition is part of the environment in which innovation and new ideas naturally emerge. Intuitive leaders are able to look past their preconceptions and assumptions long enough to anticipate new possibilities. This creativity can result in new ideas for nursing research, new systems of care, and new health care products. As people are able to broaden their awareness and see new options, they will also see improved professional relationships and teamwork. Greater innovation and workable strategies mean more motivated employees and decreased nursing "burnout."

TRY THIS

Positive Affirmations

Positive affirmations are a way of purposefully changing your inner reality. They are always stated in the present tense as if they have already occurred. For a week think about and jot down changes you would like to see in your life. Formulate several affirmations for each of these changes. For example, if you are struggling and would like your financial situation to improve, you might develop these affirmations: I have all the money I need and want; I am financially secure; money comes in as I need it; I pay my bills easily; I am very comfortable about money. Affirmations about your career might include the following: I am an excellent nurse; I make sound and wise decisions; I care about my clients; my clients respond to my care of them; I am respected by other professionals; I really like being a nurse.

- Write out affirmations in a number of areas such as career, health, parenting, and personal relationships.
- Make a tape recording of your affirmations, pausing several seconds between each one.
- Several times a day, when driving or during some other quiet time, play your affirmation tape. After each taped affirmation, repeat the affirmation aloud.
- Pay attention to how things begin to change in your life. Remember, the thoughts you have become the reality of your life. Make that a positive process.

TRY THIS

Practice Intuition

Intuitive abilities improve with attention and practice. Try the following:

- Think of something specific you would like an answer to.
- Do a relaxation exercise or move into a meditative state.
- Allow any answers to come into your awareness.
- Don't make any judgments about any of the answers or question where they came from.
- Jot down the answers to consider and review when you return to a normal state of consciousness.
- If you received no answers, try a different question or seek an inner guide or teacher to help you find the answer.

References

Banning, M. (2007). A review of clinical decision making: Models and current research. *Journal of Clinical Nursing*, 17: 187–195.

Benner, P., & Tanner, C. (1987). How expert nurses use intuition. *American Journal of Nursing*, 87(1): 23–31.

Duggan, W. (2007). *Strategic Intuition*. New York: Columbia University Press.

Effken, J. A. (2007). The informational basis for nursing intuition: Philosophical underpinnings. *Nursing Philosophy*, 8: 187–200.

Gobet, F., & Chassy, P. (2008). Towards an alternative to Benner's theory of expert intuition in nursing. *International Journal of Nursing Studies*, 45: 129–139.

McCutcheon, H. H. I., & Pincombe, J. (2001). Intuition: An important tool in the practice of nursing. *Journal of Advanced Nursing*, 35(5): 342–348.

Nyatanga, B., & de Vocht, H. (2008). Intuition in clinical decision-making: A psychological penumbra. *International Journal of Palliative Nursing*, 14(10): 492–496.

Orloff, J. (2009). *Emotional Freedom: Liberate Yourself from Negative Emotions and Transform Your Life*. Prospect, KY: Harmony House Publishers.

Pretz, J. E. (2008). Intuition versus analysis: Strategy and experience in complex everyday problem solving. *Memory & Cognition*, 36(3): 554–566.

Schulz, M. L. (1998). *Awakening Intuition*. New York: Three Rivers Press.

Resource

International Association of Medical Intuitives
www.medical-intuitives.net

21

Music Therapy

*Music washes away from the soul the
dust of everyday life.*

BERTHOLD AUERBACH

Music's the medicine of the mind.

JOHN A. LOGAN

Music therapy is the clinical and evidence-based use of music interventions to accomplish individualized goals within a therapeutic relationship by a credentialed professional who has completed an approved music therapy program (American Music Therapy Association, n.d.). It is an established health care profession in which music is used to promote wellness or improve the quality of life for those with disabilities or illness. Specifically, music therapy interventions focus on stress management, pain control, feeling exploration, memory enhancement, and promotion of improved communication and physical rehabilitation (American Music Therapy Association, n.d.).

The Canadian Association for Music Therapy defines music therapy as the skillful use of music and musical elements by an accredited music therapist to promote, maintain, and restore mental, physical, emotional, and spiritual health. Music has nonverbal, creative, structural, and emotional qualities. These are used in the therapeutic relationship to facilitate contact, interaction, self-awareness, learning, self-expression, communication, and personal development (Canadian Association for Music Therapy, n.d.).

BACKGROUND

It is generally believed that the utilization of music for healing goes back to ancient times. The *I Ching, Chinese Book of Wisdom,* one of the oldest books in Chinese culture, references music as a powerful healing force. Thousands of years ago humans were playing primitive instruments and most known primitive societies had some form of music. World Wars I and II were the impetus for the development of music therapy as a profession in the United States. Music was used in the Veterans Administration Hospitals as a way to address traumatic war injuries. Doctors and nurses began to notice the effect music had on veterans' psychological, physiological, cognitive, and emotional state. Consequently, this brought about a call for professionally trained music therapists. Since then, colleges and universities have developed programs to train musicians and others about how to use music for therapeutic purposes. The first music degree therapy program in the world was founded at Michigan State University in 1944. In 1950, a professional organization was formed by a collaboration of music therapists who worked with veterans, psychiatric populations, and persons who were cognitively impaired and hearing or visually impaired. This was the birth of the National Association for Music Therapy (NAMT). In 1998, NAMT joined forces with another music therapy organization to become what is now known as the American Music Therapy Association (AMTA) (American Music Therapy Association, n.d.),

PREPARATION

Music therapists must have a genuine interest in others and wish to establish healing/therapeutic relationships. This relationship would include the characteristics of empathy, caring, nonjudgmental attitudes, and empowerment. Because music therapists are musicians as well as therapists, they should also have a love for and a belief in the healing effects of music.

The education of a music therapist is a baccalaureate degree in music therapy. This program of study includes coursework in general studies, music, music therapy psychology, biological, social, and behavioral sciences. There is also a requirement of practicum and fieldwork experiences. At the completion of an AMTA-approved academic training and internship, students are eligible for admission to the certification exam administered by the Certification Board for Music Therapists, Inc. Upon passing the national examination the student acquires the credential "Music Therapist-Board Certified (MT-BC)." Master's and doctorate degrees in music therapy are also available for those students wishing to pursue advanced studies (American Music Therapy Association, n.d.).

CONCEPTS

Music and the Brain

Ways in which the brain processes music and the effect of music on the brain are of great interest, particularly in the field of neuroscience. The publication of the work *Pourquoi Mozart* (1991) by the French researcher Tomatis piqued interest in something called the Mozart Effect. Tomatis was particularly interested in the physiological effects of music on healing and believed that the music of Mozart had the greatest effect. A seminal study by Rauscher, Shaw, and Ky (1993) demonstrated that 10 minutes of listening to a Mozart Sonata improved the spatial-temporal intelligence or the ability to mentally manipulate objects in three-dimensional space. Results also showed that college student's IQ scores improved by 8 to 9 points. This started a popular notion that listening to music made people smarter. Unfortunately, this was not quite so. The improvement was not permanent (nor did the researchers claim it was) and, in fact, lasted only about 10 to 15 minutes. Despite the controversy surrounding this theory, the term "Mozart Effect" has been popularized to reflect the healing power of music in general.

Although not fully understood, it seems that there is not just one area of the brain that can be called the "music center." More than likely, listening to and perceiving music is a comprehensive experience. Sacks (2007) contends that musical powers are made possible because the brain uses systems that have already been developed for other purposes. He states, "This might go with the fact that there is no single music center in the human brain, but the involvement of a dozen scattered networks throughout the brain" (Sacks, 2007, p. xi). Some scientists believe that the brain is hardwired for music, and others believe that this is not so. Pinker (1997) is one of the neuroscientists who believes that there is no evolutionary basis that music, or any of the arts, is adaptive and hardwired in the brain. Although much too simple an explanation, he bases this belief on the notion that biologically, music could vanish tomorrow, and from an adaptive perspective, nothing would really change. Other scientists such as Levintin (2006) disagree and point to the universality of music in cultures and the apparent ability of infants to perceive music early on.

In considering the role of the brain, Levintin (2006) identifies the cumulative experience of perceiving music. The motor cortex allows for movement such as foot tapping, dancing, and playing an instrument; the sensory cortex allows for tactile feedback; the auditory cortex allows for the perception and analysis of tones and sounds; the prefrontal cortex allows for the creation of expectations and satisfaction of expectations; the visual cortex allows for reading music and looking at other's and one's own movements; the hippocampus allows for memory for music and musical experiences; the amygdala allows for the emotional reaction to music; and lastly, the cerebellum allows for movement and the emotional reaction to music. It is unclear exactly how music affects the brain and healing, but it is fairly certain that it does. Both scientific and anecdotal evidence supports this (Sacks, 2007).

Entrainment

The human brain produces different brain waves during various states of consciousness, attention, and arousal. Beta waves (14–30 hertz) are associated with normal or waking consciousness, and the person feels awake and alert. Alpha waves (8–14 hertz) are produced in an altered or relaxed state of consciousness. Theta waves (4–8 hertz) occur during the first stage of sleep. Delta waves (below 5 hertz) are associated with deep sleep.

The brain's electrical response to rhythmic sensory stimulation is referred to as **entrainment.** When there is an external consistent rhythmic sensory stimulation, the brain produces the rhythm in the form of electrical impulses or brain waves. This synchronization of brain waves to external stimulation is also called Frequency Response (FFR). A drum beat at a steady 200 to 280 beats a minute entrains theta brain waves. Music in the 8- to 14-hertz range entrains alpha brain waves. Throughout history, drumming, chanting, and music have been used to create altered states of consciousness.

Quality of Life

In addition to how music and hence, music therapy, affects the brain, it is also important to recognize how music therapy is capable of affecting individual quality of life. Quality of life is a broad concept that can be defined contextually. This means that quality of life for a person dying of cancer might be defined by that person differently than by a person trying to work on her or his anxiety disorder. Quality of life for people experiencing severe chronic pain might be defined differently by them than by those who are recovering from a hurtful divorce. If quality of life is about a sense of well-being in a particular circumstance, then the definition of quality of life by Victor Frankl (1963) is helpful. He contends that quality of life is tied to a person's perception of meaning. The quest for meaning is fundamental to the human condition, and we are brought in touch with a sense of meaning when we reflect on that which we have created, loved, believed in, or left as a legacy.

TREATMENT

Music therapists are in an excellent position to help people improve their quality of life through exploration of the meaning of life events. Music therapy intervention can also be implemented in a wide variety of clinical circumstances.

The uses for music therapy are wide and varied, ranging from cancer care, chronic pain, autism, and psychiatric disorders to stress reduction and improvement of learning and self-esteem. Under most circumstances, the major contraindication is patient preference. First and foremost, the treatment of individuals with a music therapy modality involves the use of music. How music is used depends on the needs of the patient and the goals of therapy. As with any therapeutic regime, a thorough assessment is necessary in order to determine the goals of treatment, consideration of patient preferences, and determination of appropriate interventions. Creation of a comprehensive treatment plan that is individualized to each patient is vital.

The use of music in therapy is often individualized to the specific treatment needs of the person being treated. For example, **Callirobics**® is a system of using music and handwriting to improve eye–hand coordination and fine motor skills. Children use popular children melodies, whereas teens and adults use music that reflects their personal tastes. The term has been created out of two words: *calli*graphy and a*erobics*. Contact information is provided in the resources section.

The **Listening Program**® has been developed for people with autism, learning disabilities, or those with aphasia following a brain attack. Classical music is psychoacoustically modified to stimulate the auditory processing system. This music is believed to improve reception, processing, utilization, and storing of environmental information. Advanced Brain Technologies, a neurotechnology company, has developed software and music programs used to certify nurses, teachers, therapists, and music professionals in the Listening Program. In May 2008, the Occupational Therapy program at Idaho State University announced a research affiliation with Advanced Brain Technologies to investigate the use of the Listening Program for individuals with autism spectrum disorder and in the reduction of depressive symptoms and improved social interactions in college students. Contact information is provided in the resources section.

Dr. Galina Mindlin, a neuropsychiatrist, introduced music therapy for the brain. **Brain Music Therapy** relies on a person's electroencephalogram of the wave patterns when the person is relaxed and when the person is activated. The results are used to create therapeutic music through the use of a mathematical formula. One composition promotes relaxation, and the other composition promotes activating states in the brain. Contact information is provided in the resources section.

Singing bowls are standing bells that are played by rubbing a wooden, plastic, or leather-wrapped mallet around the rim of the bowl to produce a continuous "singing" sound. A warm bell tone can be produced by striking the bowl with a soft mallet. Singing bowls are used worldwide for meditation, relaxation, and pain reduction. The vibrations lower heart and respiratory rates and relax brain wave patterns.

Therapeutic Techniques

The techniques that a music therapist chooses to use are dependent on the goals of the treatment plan. Although not an exhaustive list, some of the more common are listening, composing, re-creating (playing), and improvising.

In the technique of **listening,** the patient is exposed to live or recorded music and asked to react to the music. Emphasis is often on identification of feelings elicited by the music. The therapist can also focus on particular activities related to the listening of music, such as drawing, story sharing, relaxation exercises, life reminiscence, and meditation. This technique can be used to soothe patients and allows for a nonthreatening way to explore feelings. In **composing,** the person is asked to create some type of musical product. This can be songs, lyrics, music videos, or audio recordings. This technique can help patients build self-esteem, identify ways in which their work is affected by their feelings, and most important, provides a way to express feelings such as joy and fear. **Re-creating** music is when a patient sings or plays previously composed music. This technique can help persons develop gross and fine motor skills and assist in the rehabilitation of physical problems. Playing and/or singing music with a group can also encourage cooperation with others and encourage group cohesiveness and pro-group behavior. **Improvising** is a technique that is used to encourage patients to make up their own music in the moment. Often this is directed by the therapist, who will encourage the patient to improvise music spontaneously to describe a certain feeling or situation. This technique can help develop spontaneity and help persons communicate their thoughts and feelings.

RESEARCH

The research literature is rich on identifying the benefits of music and music therapy in the promotion of health and healing. The following is a summary of some of the systematic reviews and research on the efficacy of music therapy.

Systematic Reviews:

- In a systematic review on music therapy for autistic spectrum disorders, the researchers found that music therapy may help children with autistic spectrum disorder to improve their communicative skills. Music therapy might be helpful because it addresses some of the core problems prevalent in autism. More research is needed (Gold, Wigram, & Elefant, 2006).
- In a systematic review on music therapy for depression, the researchers found that music therapy is an acceptable form of therapy by people with depression and is associated with improvement of mood. More research is needed (Maratos, Gold, Wang, & Crawford, 2008).
- In a systematic review on the effects of music as an intervention on hospitalized patients, it was found that music was effective for the reduction of anxiety during normal care delivery (Evans, 2002).

Research Studies:

- In a study that measured the effects of music therapy on the quality and length of life of people diagnosed with terminal cancer, it was found that quality of life was higher for those people receiving music therapy, and their quality of life improved over time as they received more music therapy (Hilliard, 2003).
- In a controlled study that measured the effects of music therapy on the psychological health of women during pregnancy, it was found that a prescribed 2-week regime of music therapy reduced the intensity of anxiety, depression, and stress in pregnant women (Chang, Chen, & Huang, 2008).
- Preliminary data in a study that measured the effect of long-term interactive music therapy on behavior profile and musical skills in young adults with severe autism found beneficial results on certain core domains of autism (Boso, Emanuel, Minazzi, Abbamonte & Politi, 2007).

- In a study that measured the effect of music therapy on the spirituality of persons in an in-patient hospice unit as measured by self-report, it was found that there was a statistically significant increase in spiritual well-being on the day in which the participants received music therapy (Wlodarczyk, 2007).

INTEGRATED NURSING PRACTICE

Nurses can tap into the healing power of music. Although the practice of music therapy takes specialized credentials, music can be used more generally as a nursing intervention. For instance, teaching stress reduction is a common health promotion activity. Music is a very effective tool for reducing stress. Teaching patients how to do progressive relaxation accompanied by their favorite music often reinforces the relaxation response. Some patients like to meditate, and meditating to music is effective for some people. Relaxation coupled with music helps to decrease the wear and tear that comes from the sympathetic nervous system stimulation from stress. The same is true when people are anxious and angry. Consequently, music can be used to decrease the deleterious effects of any situation that is stressful or anxiety producing.

Music can also be used as a nonpharmacologic intervention for pain management. We know that muscle tension increases the pain response. Helping patients relax to music can decrease muscle tension and, therefore, is helpful for pain reduction. The same principle would hold true for women in labor. Deep breathing, progressive relaxation, and imaging enhanced by music can be very effective in creating a positive birthing experience.

Music can also be used while caring for the older population. Many times music helps people remember positive things about their life. Reminiscence is a developmental exercise that is healthy. The use of music is also very soothing and calming. Doing gentle exercise enhanced by music encourages increased mobility and strength.

Music can also be used in palliative care as playing music can create a peaceful and calm environment. One must be sure that the patient desires this intervention and is not agitated by it. There are many clinical situations in which music can be used to create an atmosphere of healing.

TRY THIS

Music for Stress Reduction

- Keep a "bag of tricks" that you take to work with you. It does not matter what environment you work in. What is in your bag will depend on your job, but always keep a small CD player with an array of CDs that are used for stress reduction and relaxation. Then when you encounter a clinical situation that calls for the use of music, you will be set to intervene and not have to go looking for equipment. Also keep a set of external earphones for situations where the music might disturb others.

- Ask patients who seem anxious if they would like to listen to some relaxation music. Teach them how to deep breathe slowly while listening to the music. The music and the deep breathing decrease sympathetic nervous system stimulation, thereby decreasing the physiological arousal that is prevalent in anxiety.
- Use music to soothe yourself from stress. Choose and play some of your favorite music that comforts or calms you. Find a comfortable position either sitting or lying down. As you listen to the music, focus on your breathing, and let the music lead you to a relaxed state. Focus on how peaceful and calm you feel.
- Experiment with various types of music. You may want to purchase Dr. Andrew Weil's *Mindbody Tool Kit*, which is available at bookstores.

References

American Music Therapy Association (n.d.) Official definition and description of music therapy. www.musictherapy.org. Accesssed November 30, 2008.

Canadian Association for Music Therapy/Association de Musicothérapie du Canada. Definition of music therapy. www.musictherapy.ca. Accessed November 30, 2008.

Boso, M., Emanuel, E., Minazzi, V., Abbamonte, M., & Politi, P. (2007). Effect of long-term interactive music therapy on behavior profile and musical skills in young adults with severe autism. *Journal of Alternative and Complimentary Medicine*, 13(7): 709–712.

Chang, M., Chen, C., & Huang, K. (2008). Effects of music therapy on psychological health of women during pregnancy. *Journal of Clinical Nursing*, 17(19): 2580–2587.

Evans, D. (2002). The effectiveness of music as an intervention for hospital patients: A systematic review. *Journal of Advanced Nursing*, 37(1): 8–18.

Frankl, V. E. (1963). *Man's Search for Meaning*. New York: Pocket Books.

Gold, C., Wigram, T., & Elefant, C. (2006). Music therapy for autistic spectrum disorder. *Cochrane Database of Systematic Reviews* 2006, Issue 2. Art. No. CD004381. DOI: 10.1002/14651858.CD004381.pub2.

Hilliard, R. E. (2003). The effects of music therapy on the quality and length of life of people diagnosed with terminal cancer. *Journal of Music Therapy*, 40(2): 113–137.

Levitin, D. J. (2006). *This Is Your Brain on Music*. New York: Dutton.

Maratos, A. S., Gold, C., Wang, X., & Crawford, M. J. (2008). Music therapy for depression. *Cochrane Database of Systematic Reviews* 2008, Issue 1. Art. No. CD004517. DOI: 10.1002/14651858.CD004517.pub2.

Pinker, S. (1997). *How the Mind Works*. New York: W.W. Norton

Rauscher, F. H., Shaw, G. L., & Ky, K. N. (1993). Music and spatial task performance. *Nature*, 365: 611.

Sacks, O. (2007). *Musicophilia: Tales of Music and the Brain*. New York: Vintage Books, Random House.

Tomatis, A. A. (1991). *Pourquoi Mozart*. Paris: Editions Fixot.

Wlodarczyk, N. (2007). The effect of music therapy on the spirituality of persons in an in-patient hospice unit as measured by self-report. *Journal of Music Therapy*, 44(2): 113–122.

Resources

American Music Therapy Association
   8455 Colesville Rd., Suite 1000
   Silver Spring, MD 20910
   301.589.3300
   www.musictherapy.org

Brain Music Therapy Center
   330 West 58th St., Suite 202
   New York, NY 10019
   212.581.0821
   www.brainmusictreatment.com

Callirobics®
   www.callirobics.com

Healing Music Organization
   P.O. Box 3731
   Santa Cruz, CA 95063
   831.588.7498
   www.healingmusic.org

The Listening Program®
   www.thelisteningprogram.com

Society for the Arts in Healthcare
   2437 15th St., NW
   Washington, DC 20009
   202.299.9770
   www.thesah.org

22

Biofeedback

We all carry within our souls the capacity to heal ourselves. Modern doctors, therefore, must learn to take their patients on spiritual journeys. Those who do not will miss out on some truly incredible healing tools.

LEWIN MEHL-MADRONA

Biofeedback is a method for learned control of physiological responses of the body. It is a relaxation technique that uses electronic equipment to amplify the electrochemical energy produced by body responses. Normally out of conscious awareness, biofeedback provides perceptible information that individuals can use to gain voluntary control over various physiological processes.

BACKGROUND

The experimental data to support the feasibility of learned control first appeared in the 1950s. In 1961, experimental psychologist Neal Miller proposed that the autonomic nervous system was trainable, contrary to beliefs about human physiology at the time. As psychologists and physiologists continued this research, it became clear that dramatic gains could be achieved by using biofeedback information to assist people suffering from specific conditions, including headaches, ulcers, hypertension, and many other stress-related illnesses. The result of this work was the creation of biofeedback therapy, now widely used by both conventional and alternative practitioners. With the advent of computers, the technology has become more powerful (Robbins, 2008).

PREPARATION

Biofeedback does not belong to any particular field of health care but is used in many disciplines, including nursing, psychology, social work, chiropractic, medicine, dentistry, physical therapy, rehabilitation, psychiatry, respiratory therapy, occupational therapy, physician assisting, exercise physiology, and sports medicine. Since 1981, all biofeedback therapists must have certification from the Biofeedback Certification Institute of America (BCIA). Applicants must hold a bachelor's degree or higher in one of the approved health care fields. Certification requires 50 hours in didactic biofeedback education and 100 hours in clinical experience. BCIA also offers specialty certificates in EEG biofeedback (40 hours of didactic information and 220 hours of clinical training) and pelvic muscle dysfunction biofeedback (50 hours of didactic information and 100 hours of clinical training). When applicants meet the requirements, they are allowed to sit for a qualifying examination that consists of both written and practical assessment. The BCIA provides directories of certified practitioners throughout the United States.

CONCEPTS

The nervous system has two major components: voluntary and involuntary or autonomic. In normal circumstances, the voluntary component is under a person's control. If someone decides to stand, the brain sends a message to the appropriate muscle groups, and the person stands. In contrast, the autonomic nervous system functions without conscious thought. Although people may be able to change their rate of respiration, for example, they are not able to consciously stop breathing indefinitely.

People receive biofeedback from their bodies all the time. When they do not eat, they feel hungry. When they run, they get winded. When they experience stress, their muscles tense. Other types of biofeedback are more difficult to discern. With the use of technology, however, people can learn to adjust their thought processes to control body processes such as blood pressure, temperature, muscle tension, bronchial dilation, gastrointestinal functioning, and brain wave activity. The concept is simple: If individuals can develop sensory awareness of an involuntary function, they can learn to sense it. For example, if skin temperature in the hands is converted into an audible signal, the beeps give one's ears and brain feedback. As people learn to dilate the arteries in their hands, thus raising skin temperature, the beeps speed up, providing instant feedback on what is occurring in the body. Biofeedback teaches people what it feels like to be relaxed internally so they can recreate the feeling whenever they choose (Swingle, 2008; West, 2007).

TREATMENT

Biofeedback instruments are highly sensitive electronic devices that monitor physiologic processes. Signals from the body are amplified by the instruments and converted into usable information. The instruments may have meters, tones, or a computer display that presents the information to the trainee.

Temperature or **thermal feedback** is a primary tool for general relaxation training and treatment of specific vascular diseases. Blood flow in the hands responds to stress and relaxation, and clients learn to relax by watching the rise and fall of finger temperature. Thermal feedback may be used to decrease generalized muscle tension in people with temporomandibular joint (TMJ) syndrome. Migraine headaches may be alleviated by simply raising the temperature in the hands.

Electrodermal response (EDR) or **galvanic skin response (GSR)** feedback devices measure sweat gland activity of the fingertips or palm. This response is highly sensitive to emotions and thoughts. It is used in general relaxation training to help people reduce the impact of significant stressors and anxiety and to treat excessive sweating.

Electromyography (EMG) feedback measures muscle tension with sensors placed on the skin over appropriate muscles. EMG feedback is used for general relaxation training and insomnia that is due to overactivation of the autonomic nervous system. Biofeedback readings of the masseter muscle are used to treat TMJ. EMG biofeedback is able to detect muscle imbalances, allowing individuals to reeducate the involved muscles. Some people experiencing muscle spasms and back pain benefit from EMG biofeedback. People with spinal cord injuries may use biofeedback to strengthen muscles and provide the sensation of movement. An EMG device has been developed to treat kyphosis, a curvature of the spine. In addition, this type of biofeedback is the primary tool for treatment of tension headache and pain reduction.

Respiratory resistance [R(os)] biofeedback measures the rate, volume, and rhythm of respiration and is useful in treating both asthma and the hyperventilation of anxiety and panic attacks. **Gastrointestinal biofeedback** is helpful in treating irritable bowel syndrome, colitis, heartburn, functional dyspepsia, and Crohn's disease. **Cardiovascular (EKG) feedback** is available through portable heart rate monitors to augment a person's ability to control heart rate. In addition to being used by persons with cardiac disease, many professional athletes use this system to aid their training.

Pelvic muscle dysfunction biofeedback is used for people with chronic constipation related to pelvic dysfunction. It can also successfully treat incontinence. Sensors measure and report the activity of the internal and external rectal sphincters for the treatment of fecal incontinence and the activity of the detrusor muscle for the treatment of urinary incontinence. Pelvic floor biofeedback is also used to treat sexual problems such as vaginismus or postpartum pelvic changes.

Electroencephalograph (EEG) biofeedback, also called *neurofeedback*, records information about brain wave activity from sensors placed on the scalp. Changes in brain waves reflect changes in attention as well as in states of arousal from sleep to alert wakefulness. This type of feedback is used for mind quieting, attention control, short-term memory improvement, mood swings, posttraumatic stress disorder, and alcohol and drug addiction. Neurofeedback is helpful in cases of insomnia related to mental or emotional problems. People with brain injuries may experience improvement of symptoms with this type of biofeedback.

Tactile and audio biofeedback involves providing information to the brain about body motion. It is primarily used for postural control and improving balance.

After the desired mode of treatment is determined for the specific disorder, electrodes are attached to the person in the area to be monitored. These electrodes feed the information to a computer that registers the results either with a sound tone that varies in pitch or speed or on a visual monitor. EEG measurements produce a kind of video game of brain waves. The human brain produces different brain waves during various states of consciousness. Beta waves are associated with normal or waking consciousness, alpha waves are produced in an altered or relaxed state of consciousness, and theta and delta waves are associated with unconscious and sleeping states. When the client produces waves associated with concentration, the game speeds up. The game slows down when brain waves associated with daydreaming are produced. This type of computer system can make learning control of body processes more interactive and fun, especially for children.

A biofeedback therapist leads the client in mental exercises to help the person reach the desired result such as muscle relaxation or contraction or more alpha brain waves. Through trial and error, trainees eventually learn how to control the inner mechanism involved. Training typically requires eight to ten sessions, although people with long-term or severe disorders may require more sessions. Clients are expected to practice the skill 15 to 20 minutes a day throughout the training period to incorporate what they have learned into their lives.

RESEARCH

Research exists to demonstrate the effectiveness of biofeedback in a number of conditions, of which the following is a small sample.

- A systematic review of biofeedback as a treatment for constipation related to pelvic floor dysfunction found seven randomized controlled trials that met the criteria. Three studies compared electromyography biofeedback (EMG-FB) with non-biofeedback treatments such as laxatives, diazepam, and sham feedback. In these studies, biofeedback was significantly better for symptom improvement. Four trials compared EMG-FB with non-EMG-FB techniques such as balloon training or manometry biofeedback. EMG-FB significantly improved symptoms compared to non-EMG-FB techniques (Koh, Young, Young, & Solomon, 2008).
- A biofeedback device that provided audio and tactile feedback was tested on nine healthy volunteers. The subjects demonstrated improved postural corrections during various trial conditions. It is hoped that this type of feedback may be helpful to the elderly population who experience loss of balance problems and thus an increased risk of falls (Giansanti, Dozza, Chiari, Maccioni, & Cappello, 2009).

- Forty-two women, age 60 and older, suffering from urge urinary incontinence were treated with 8 weeks of biofeedback to the pelvic floor muscles. The frequency of incontinency was reduced by 45 percent. Those who had a concurrent depression experienced the greatest improvement in psychological burden (Tadic et al., 2007).
- A meta-analysis of EMG-FB in the treatment of tension headaches found 53 studies that met the criteria. Twenty-one were pre-post studies and 32 were control group studies, some of which were randomized and a few had single or double-blind designs. EMG-FB was found to reduce the frequency of headaches as well as improve muscle relaxation, anxiety, and depression. The effects were continued up to several years after the EMG-FG training (Nestoriuc, Rief, & Martin, 2008).
- Twenty-five people, ages 20 to 55 years, who experienced intractable seizures, received 17 to 82 sessions of neurofeedback treatment. The seizures of all of these individuals went into remission, and 19 people no longer needed an anticonvulsant to control their seizures (Walker, 2008).

INTEGRATED NURSING PRACTICE

Certified biofeedback therapists, many of whom are nurses, help interpret signals from monitoring devices while leading the client through physical and mental exercises to achieve the desired change in the body function being measured. As a nurse without specific training, your primary intervention is to provide information about biofeedback to appropriate clients. You can explain the types of monitoring devices and the conditions for which they are typically effective. In addition, you can help individuals find certified therapists. Explain that biofeedback creates a greater awareness of specific body parts and their functions. With training, clients can regulate these functions. Biofeedback helps people to relieve or eliminate symptoms, provides an internal locus of control, and helps them reduce their own health care costs.

TRY THIS
Mind Control of Muscular Strength

- Face your partner. Put your right hand on your partner's shoulder, palm up.
- Clench your right fist, and hold your arm straight.
- Have your partner grasp your elbow with both hands and pull down while you resist. The pull needs to be gradual until you both get a sense of how much force is needed to bend your arm.
- Then imagine you are a fire engine or pump. You are rooted to the earth and are drawing water up and it is pushing through your arm and out of your fingers at high speed with tremendous force. Such force that nothing can bend your arm.

(continued)

- Then place your arm again on your partner's shoulder, this time with the fingers outstretched, holding onto the feeling and the image of the pump pushing water through your arm with great force.
- Ask your partner once more to apply gradual force to bend your arm. You will need to apply a little muscle power, but will find you can relax and hold steady with much less effort than before.

Source: Rutherford, L. (1996). *Principles of Shamanism*. San Francisco: Thorsons.

References

Giansanti, D., Dozza, M., Chiari, L., Maccioni, G., & Cappello, A. (2009). Energetic assessment of trunk postural modifications induced by a wearable audio-biofeedback system. *Medical Engineering & Physics*, 31: 48–54.

Koh, C. E., Young, C. J., Young, J. M., & Solomon, M. J. (2008). Systematic review of randomized controlled trials of the effectiveness of biofeedback for pelvic floor dysfunction. *British Journal of Surgery*, 95: 1079–1087.

Nestoriuc, Y., Rief, W., & Martin, A. (2008). Meta-analysis of biofeedback for tension-type headache: Efficacy, specificity, and treatment moderators. *Journal of Consulting and Clinical Psychology*, 76(3): 379–396.

Robbins, J. (2008). *A Symphony in the Brain*. New York: Grove Press.

Swingle, P. G. (2008). *Biofeedback for the Brain*. Piscataway, NJ: Rutgers University Press.

Tadic, S. D., Zdaniuk, B., Griffiths, D., Rosenberg, L., Schafer, W., & Resnick, N. M. (2007). Effect of biofeedback on psychological burden and symptoms in older women with urge urinary incontinence. *Journal of the American Geriatric Society*, 55(12): 2010–2015.

Walker, J. E. (2008). Power spectral frequency and coherence abnormalities in patients with intractable epilepsy and their usefulness in long-term remediation of seizures using nuerofeedback. *Clinical EEG and Neuroscience*, 39(4): 203–205.

West, K. (2007). *Biofeedback*. New York: Chelsea House Publications.

Resources

Association for Applied Psychophysiology and Biofeedback
10200 West 44th Ave., Suite 304
Wheat Ridge, CO 80033–2840
303.422.8436
www.aapb.org/

Biofeedback Certification Institute of America
10200 West 44th Ave., Suite 310
Wheat Ridge, CO 80033-2840
866.908.8713
www.bcia.org/

Biofeedback Foundation of Europe
P.O. Box 555
3800 AN Amersfoort, The Netherlands
31.84.83.84.696
www.bfe.org/

EEG Spectrum International
21601 Vanowen St., Suite 100
Canoga Park, CA 91303
818.789.3456
www.eegspectrum.com

23

Movement-Oriented Therapies

Stop a minute, right where you are. Relax your shoulders, shake your head and spine like a dog shaking off cold water. Tell that imperious voice in your head to be still.

BARBARA KINGSOLVER

A number of therapies focus on movement, body awareness, and breathing, and their purpose is to maintain health as well as to correct specific problems. This chapter presents two Eastern movement-oriented therapies—qigong and t'ai chi—and three Western movement-oriented therapies—the Alexander Technique, the Feldenkrais Method, and the Trager® Approach. Common to these various approaches is the retraining of one's body to improve coordination and balance, to release and change postural faults, and to relieve structural and functional stress. A major principle is that awareness has to be experienced rather than taught verbally, which may then lead to more effective use of one's whole self.

Qigong, also spelled *Chi Kung, Chi Gong,* and *Chi Gung,* is pronounced "chee goong." Qigong is a Chinese discipline consisting of breathing and mental exercises that may be combined with modest arm movements. Qigong is one of the four pillars of Traditional Chinese Medicine; the others being acupuncture, massage, and herbal medicine (see Chapter 4). *Qi* is the term for "vital energy" and "life force," and *gong* means "work" or "discipline." Qigong can be translated as "mastery of qi," "cultivation of energy," "air energy," "breath work," and "energy work." People discover how to generate more energy and conserve what they have in order to maintain health or treat illness (Zhang, 2008).

T'ai chi, sometimes spelled as *taiji,* is pronounced "teye chee." T'ai chi arose out of qigong and is a discipline that combines physical fitness, meditation, and self-defense. Literally translated, it means "great ultimate fist" and is sometimes translated as "supreme boxing" or "root of all motion." Although it is considered a martial art, t'ai chi is mainly practiced today as a health discipline (Wayne & Kaptchuk, 2008).

The **Alexander Technique** is a method to improve postural and movement dysfunction that can lead to pain and disease. It is designed to reduce and eliminate body misuse in daily activities, especially with respect to the head, neck, and shoulders. The **Feldenkrais Method** uses gentle movement and directed attention to improve movement and enhance functioning. The physics of body movement are combined with an awareness of the way people learn to move, behave, and interact. The **Trager Approach** uses light, rhythmic rocking and shaking movements that loosen joints, ease movement, and release chronic patterns of tension. All three of these Western approaches are considered to be educational in nature as opposed to medical interventions.

BACKGROUND

Written records on qigong go back 4,000 years. For almost all of that time, this practice remained a closely guarded family secret, available only to the elite classes in China. This discipline was handed down covertly and was not revealed until the beginning of the twentieth century. In the late 1970s, the Chinese government funded several scientific studies of qigong, which had been banned during the Cultural Revolution as superstitious practice. When a scientific basis was established, the government added qigong to the list of treatment methods offered in Traditional Chinese Medicine hospitals. T'ai chi, a modern offshoot of qigong, began in the fourteenth century, only 600 years ago, created by a Taoist priest. T'ai chi gained popularity in the United States in the 1960s as people explored alternatives to conventional medicine. Some experts estimate that more than 800 million people practice qigong or t'ai chi internationally—nearly 20 percent of the world's population (Wayne & Kaptchuk, 2008).

The Alexander Technique was developed more than a century ago by F. M. Alexander, an Australian actor who had lost his voice while performing. He carefully watched himself while speaking and observed that undue muscular tension accounted for his vocal problem. He sought a way to eliminate that restriction, and the technique he developed focused on correcting the misuse of the neuromuscular activity of the head, neck, and spine. The Alexander Technique is taught in the curriculum of music conservatories, theater schools, and universities throughout the world as a foundation for improved health and creative exploration. It is also a useful tool to help able-bodied people and those with disabilities maximize their movement potential (Brennan, 2007).

The Feldenkrais Method was developed by Moshe Feldenkrais (1904–1984), a Russian-born Israeli physicist, mechanical engineer, and judo expert. After suffering crippling knee injuries, Feldenkrais used his own body as his laboratory and taught himself to walk again. In the process, he developed a system for accessing the power of the central nervous system to improve human functioning (Wildman, 2006).

The Trager Approach was developed by Milton Trager, in the early 1930s, on the basis of his experience as a boxing trainer. He spent the next 50 years—first as a lay practitioner and later as a physician—expanding and refining his discovery. It is a method of movement reeducation designed to produce positive, pleasurable feelings and tissue changes by means of sensorimotor feedback loops between the mind and the muscles (Mairi, 2006).

PREPARATION

For most people, qigong and t'ai chi are personal disciplines. Most practitioners spend 30 to 60 minutes a day doing the exercises. With more intensive practice over many years, some become masters. A t'ai chi master is generally one who has exceptional skill in doing the form or in using the principles in boxing and in life. A qigong master is one who has developed the ability to emit healing energy and has achieved proven success in healing with qi. Masters may also have qualities that are generally considered supernatural in the areas of special insight and spiritual transcendence. Rarely, if ever, will a true master call herself or himself a master. Rather, they say that "the practice is the teacher" and that "the qi is the teacher."

It is difficult to learn qigong or t'ai chi from a book, audio recording, or video. While simple forms may be grasped this way, the more complex forms are nearly impossible to learn without a teacher's guidance. In the Chinese tradition, one chooses and remains devoted to a teacher. The teacher–disciple relationship is revered as the only path to advanced skill. The honor and reverence that is bestowed on the teacher is part of the belief system that empowers the disciple.

The North American Society of Teachers of the Alexander Technique (NASTAT) is the certifying body for practitioners. A NASTAT-certified teacher must complete a 1,600-hour training program over a minimum of 3 years. The emphasis of the training is on observation and modification of human movement patterns to identify and eliminate sources of movement dysfunction.

All Feldenkrais practitioners must complete 800 to 1,000 hours of training over a period of 3 to 4 years. The main purpose of the training is for practitioners to develop a deep understanding of movement, to become aware of their own movement, to become skillful observers of movement in others, and to be able to teach other people to increase their awareness and improve their skills of movement.

The Trager Institute provides training and certifies Trager practitioners. The practitioner training program consists of 226 supervised hours while the senior practitioner program is 500 supervised hours. Students learn the relationship between various groups of muscles and organs that produce patterns of posture and movement. The focus is on the mechanics of movement, the kinesthetic interaction, and principles of neuropatterning underlying movement.

CONCEPTS

Wide Applicability

Almost anyone can participate in movement-oriented therapies. These therapies can be learned by the young and old, by people physically challenged or physically fit, and by those in good health and those recovering from long-term injury or illness. In China, 80-, 90-, and 100-year-old people get up every morning before dawn and go out to the parks to practice qigong or t'ai chi, (Figure 23.1), even in the middle of winter. These Eastern practices can be done alone, in pairs, or in large groups.

Qi

Qi is the invisible flow of energy that maintains physiologic function and the health and well-being of individuals. Imbalance of the flow of energy can be treated in a variety of ways, including practicing qigong and t'ai chi. The principles underlying these movement-oriented therapies are the same as those used in acupuncture (see Chapter 13). The "forms," or sequences of movements, are specifically designed to stimulate pressure points all along the body and to encourage deep, rhythmic breathing, which fills the body with life-giving qi. The ultimate goal is to strengthen the flow of qi through the body to promote health

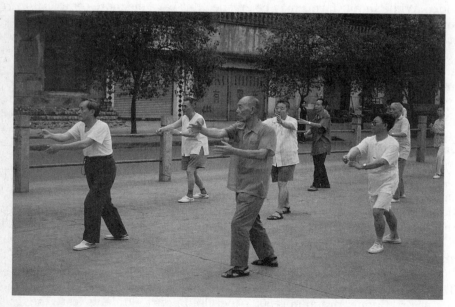

FIGURE 23.1   Men and Women Practicing T'ai Chi Outdoors in Leshan, China.

Source: Dorling Kindersley Media Library/Ken Robertson

and well-being. When qi is flowing in balance, the body stays healthy, resistant to disease, and can activate its own healing efforts.

Qigong and t'ai chi consist of soft, slow, continuous movements that are circular in nature. When practiced by a master, the movements are so slow and fluid that they look like swimming in air. The softness of movements develops energy without nervousness. The slowness of movements requires attentive control that quiets the mind and develops one's powers of awareness and concentration. The continuous circular nature of the movements develops strength and endurance. Yin and yang refer to the balance of forces in the universe. T'ai chi movements are designed to express these forces in balanced form by pairs of opposites. For example, a motion that ultimately involves turning to the right often begins with a small movement to the left. In qigong, students learn to sense their qi and follow it as it moves around the body. As they become more skillful, they learn to strengthen their qi and direct it to specific areas of the body that are weak or ailing (Wilson, 2007).

Movement Patterns

The human body is viewed as a remarkable instrument, capable of responding with flexibility and resilience. But as the years pass, people often develop habitual reactions, beliefs, and movement patterns that cause physical and mental strain. These habits are typically expressed by tight muscles, collapsed posture, or lack of mobility. When muscles are working overtime, people eventually feel tight, tense, heavy, or tired. The sources of these problems are many—injury, illness, or stress. Lifelong misuse of muscles arises from sitting, standing, or walking incorrectly or too much sitting and too little walking. For example, after years of walking incorrectly, back or knee problems can occur. A knee replacement is a temporary solution only, because the real problem lies not in the knee, but in the way the person moves from the hip. Movement-oriented practitioners believe the only lasting remedy is in reeducating the body to walk correctly to avoid injuring the knee. Likewise, back problems can be eliminated by learning appropriate ways of moving (Wilson, 2007),

Sensory-movement activities are used to increase people's sense of postural awareness, free them from habitual patterns, and restore the proper use of muscles. Practitioners lead students through movements to enable them to discover a more fluid range of motion. As people develop new, alternative ways of moving, they experience positive sensory feelings and learn what it is like to be freer and lighter. The goal is to teach people how to move with minimum effort and maximum efficiency through increased consciousness of how their bodies work.

TREATMENT

Qigong is an easy and nontiring exercise that contains sets of moves designed to gather qi. Most people spend 30 minutes a day doing the exercises and another 30 minutes in meditation. Some forms are quite complex. For example,

Wild Goose Qigong has two sections with 64 movements in each section. Although it is difficult to learn, Wild Goose Qigong is exceptionally beautiful. In China, the goose is considered to be a marvelous creature who flies high into the clouds to gather cosmic energy and information and bring it to earth. Guo Lin Gong, a walking form of qigong, is practiced in China particularly by people with cancer. Improvements have been documented in a wide range of conditions such as stroke, hypertension, spinal cord injuries, multiple sclerosis, joint disease, cerebral palsy, headaches, and many forms of cancer (Zhang, 2008).

Yang is the most popular form of t'ai chi and was developed in the early twentieth century by Yang Cheng Fu. It is composed of 108 separate motions that can take 6 to 12 months to learn. When they are strung together, the result is a cross between slow-motion shadow boxing and dancing. Each movement has a name, such as "repulse the monkey," "the snake creeps down," "the white crane spreads its wings," or "parting the wild horse's mane," which describes what it looks like or what purpose it serves. For example, when one is trying to concentrate, monkey thoughts are distractions. As the monkey is pushed away, the person is not allowing distractions to take attention away from the process of the moment. T'ai chi also incorporates breathing exercises for the purpose of improving and strengthening the flow of qi. One form involves reversed breathing, which is contracting the stomach with the in-breath and expanding the stomach with the out-breath. The benefits of t'ai chi are seen in conditions such as hypertension, osteoporosis, and arthritis. T'ai chi can decrease stress and fatigue, improve mood, and increase energy. It is beneficial to cardiorespiratory function, balance, and flexibility (Ho et al., 2007).

Water t'ai chi is a combination of the principles of water exercise using t'ai chi movements. It is performed upright in chest-deep water, which allows for total submergence of arms and provides adequate stabilization of the body. Water provides about 12 times the resistance of air, so the body naturally moves more slowly in the water. The exercises improve strength, flexibility, balance, coordination, and posture.

The Alexander Technique includes simple movements that improve balance, posture, and coordination and relieve pain. During a session, the client goes through a series of standing and seated exercises while the practitioner applies light pressure to points of contraction in the body. The techniques help people learn how to use their bodies with less tension and more awareness. The recommended course is 30 lessons, depending on the client's participation and initial level of functioning (Brennan, 2007).

The Feldenkrais Method consists of two parts: awareness through movement and functional integration. They are convenient labels for doing essentially the same thing in different ways. Awareness through movement is more like conventional exercises in format, with the teacher guiding a group class with words rather than by personal manipulation. The lessons consist of comfortable, easy movements that gradually increase in range and complexity designed for all levels of movement ability. Functional integration is a hands-on lesson that usually lasts 45 minutes to an hour and is performed with the client fully clothed and standing, sitting, or lying on a table. The practitioner touches and moves the client in gentle, noninvasive ways. The intent of this touch is to explore the person's responses to touch and movement and then suggest alternative ways of moving.

Feldenkrais exercises are small, gentle movements, such as pelvic tilts—slowly and deliberately lifting the spine from the coccyx to the waist, one vertebra at a time. To be effective, the movements must be effortless. If exercise becomes painful, no learning takes place, because the brain is too focused on how to stop doing the painful activity. Feldenkrais exercises are said to improve flexibility, posture, range of motion, relaxation, ease of movement, physical performance, vitality, and well-being. They are also said to relieve joint pain, stress, muscle tension, low back pain, neck and shoulder pain, jaw pain, and headaches.

The Trager Approach is a process of using motion in muscles and joints to produce particular sensory feelings. These feelings are relayed to the central nervous system and then, through the process of feedback loops, they trigger changes in the tissues. A Trager session takes 60 to 90 minutes with the client wearing a swimming suit and lying on a well-padded table. The practitioner touches in such a gentle rhythmic way that the person actually experiences the possibility of being able to move each part of the body freely and effortlessly. Because active participation of the client is discouraged, the passive body can freely learn new movements. Trager practitioners work in a meditative state they call "hook-up." This state allows the practitioner to connect deeply with the client in an unforced way, to remain continually aware of the slightest responses, and to work efficiently without fatigue (Mairi, 2006).

Following this session, the student is given instruction in the use of *mentastics*, a system of simple, effortless movement sequences designed to maintain and even enhance the sense of lightness, freedom, and flexibility that was instilled during the treatment session. Mentastics, Dr. Trager's coined term for "mental gymnastics," is a powerful means of reinforcing positive changes. The Trager Approach is said to decrease various types of chronic pain, headaches, and TMJ pain, improve muscle spasms, and aid in recovery from stroke and spinal cord injuries.

RESEARCH

The National Institutes of Health is currently funding studies on t'ai chi, Alexander technique, Feldenkrais, and animal qigong. Research in the medical effects of qigong has been a subject of interest in China in recent years and has been the topic of nine international conferences since 1986. More than 4,000 abstracts have been translated into English, and copies are available from the Qigong Institute. Research exists to demonstrate the effectiveness of t'ai chi or qigong in a number of conditions, of which the following is a small sample:

- A nursing study looked at older adults with dementia who are at high risk for falls and injuries, a group that is typically excluded from t'ai chi studies. A program was developed using simple t'ai chi movements with clients and paired family members/staff. Clients were able to mirror their partners and with repetition were able to engage in the exercise (Yao, Giordani, & Alexander, 2008).

- A meta-analysis of randomized controlled trials of the effect of qigong on persons with essential hypertension compared qigong with controls of no treatment, drugs and exercise, and drugs and muscle relaxation techniques. The qigong was better than the no-treatment controls but was not significantly better than the other control. One reason may be that 2 months of qigong practice was not long enough to master the technique in order to derive the benefits (Guo, Zhou, Nishimura, Teramukai, & Fukushima, 2008).
- A study was conducted with a control group of 17 people and an experimental group of 22 people with lower limb disability who either used wheelchairs or crutches. The experimental group received 30 sessions of t'ai chi over 15 weeks. There was no intervention for the control group. The experimental group demonstrated significant improvement in muscle strength and shoulder range of motion. There was no significant improvement in cardiovascular or pulmonary function (Cheung, Tsai, Fung, & Ng, 2007).
- Men with osteopenia or osteoporosis were randomly assigned to an 18-week t'ai chi balance training program or to a no-intervention control group. The t'ai chi group demonstrated a significant improvement in balance at the end of the study while the control group demonstrated no balance improvement (Maciaszek, Osinski, Szeklicki, & Stemplewski, 2007).

Recent studies on Alexander technique have focused on chronic back pain. In one study, 579 individuals with chronic back pain were followed for 12 months. 144 people were randomized to normal care, 147 to massage, 144 to six Alexander technique lessons, and 144 to twenty-four Alexander technique lessons. Compared to normal care and massage therapy, those receiving Alexander technique experienced significant reduction in back pain and improved quality of life (Little et al., 2008).

INTEGRATED NURSING PRACTICE

Like most moderate physical activities practiced on a daily basis, t'ai chi and qigong can improve balance, stability, agility, flexibility, stamina, and muscle tone. They are good exercise for people who are already in shape. But they can also be adapted for older adults, children, or people with injury or illness. The movements are gentle and put less stress on the body than do other exercises. The breathing exercises are a form of meditation that quiets the mind and reduces the negative effects of stress.

If you or others you know are healthy and wish to maintain your health, learning t'ai chi or qigong is highly recommended. Experienced practitioners spend at least 20 and up to 60 minutes in daily practice. As a nurse, you can encourage your clients to consider practicing one of these forms. To increase health, it is important that clients build up stamina over a period of time. Clients who are seriously ill may only be able to do the simple breath practice as they focus on absorbing healing qi from the environment. When they can manage it, they add simple hand gestures to the breathing. As they continue to improve, they sit in a chair and do the hand motions, moving to a standing position when they feel able. Finally, they do the walking form.

When starting t'ai chi and qigong, it is best to begin with simple exercises. You can teach people a few basic principles of standing and moving so they can begin to feel what it is like to inhabit their body with awareness. Getting the body into alignment is a most important part of these movement therapies. Instruct people to stand with their feet at shoulder-width apart, buttocks tucked in, spine straight, shoulder relaxed, knees unlocked, and the head straight and resting lightly on top of the spine as if a string from the top of the head were gently suspending the body from above. Standing in this position, have them pay attention to their own breathing, inhaling deeply and exhaling all the way. Standing in this position, have people locate their *tan t'ien* (pronounced don-tee-en), which is the body's center of gravity and stability, located about one-and-a-half inches below the navel and into the center of the body. T'ai chi and qigong teach people to find and maintain their center through movement, whereas in meditation and yoga, centering is found in stillness. The tan t'ien is considered to be the source of energy and, as they practice, people will find that all the movements begin to flow more easily as they learn to move from the tan t'ien.

Two common movements in t'ai chi that are part of various sequences are the t'ai chi fist and the t'ai chi ball. The fist is formed by imagining a robin's egg in the center of each palm and then slowly curling one finger at a time around the egg, beginning with the little finger and ending with the thumb resting lightly on top. Throughout all the forms, frequent references are made to "picking up the ball." Have people visualize forming a ball out of the air and picking it up and moving with it. The ball is designed to help movements flow more easily.

Standing like a tree or the horse-riding stance contributes to a sense of rootedness and stability in the body. For this posture, instruct people to separate their legs wider than the shoulders and bend their knees, thus lowering the center of gravity closer to the earth. The top part of the body feels light while the lower half feels heavy. At first, the position may feel strenuous because the muscles in the legs have not been used in this way. With practice, people enjoy the feeling of stability it gives them. Next, direct people to bring their arms up as if embracing an invisible person, joining their fingertips in front of them. Direct them to slowly turn from side to side, letting their waist initiate the movement. Their legs should feel "soft," so that they follow the movement led by the waist. Their gaze should travel slowly across an imagined horizon.

T'ai chi and qigong are popular, and lessons are available in most towns and cities. They are taught in health clubs, schools, YMCAs, community centers, hospitals, clinics, and other facilities. Explain to your clients that it is useful, in most cases, to begin with a teacher. They can ask around to find a teacher whom others like, or they can observe a class or participate in a trial class. Some people try several teachers or forms before they find the one that meets their personal preferences. Encourage people to find general forms that they like and will do regularly. If possible, they should try to find a place to learn that is convenient. If it is too far, it may become difficult for people to continue in the practice. As t'ai chi and qigong have become more popular, people can be found practicing in parks. In some cases, individuals prefer to have time alone in nature. Often, however, people are happy to have others join them, and frequently informal groups form. These groups may develop socially as people get to know one another and socialize after the practice.

The claims for the Alexander Technique, the Feldenkrais Method, and the Trager Approach focus more on enhancing well-being than on healing illness. They are designed to relieve muscle tension, increase relaxation, reduce stress, and alter poor habits of posture and movement in those who are healthy. You can refer clients to the appropriate associations to locate certified teachers of these techniques.

TRY THIS

Feel Your Qi

- Stand with your feet shoulder-width apart, your knees slightly bent, your spine upright, and your shoulders relaxed. Breathe easily.
- Start to flex or bounce gently at the knees.
- Still bouncing, shift your weight back and forth from your right to your left leg.
- Keep your breathing relaxed and deep.
- Begin to snap all of your fingers, flipping each one past your thumb.
- Then, still bouncing and finger-snapping, twist at your waist, to the right, then to the left.
- While you are doing all of this, make your exhale a sigh of relief. Do five of these sighs in a slow, relaxed manner.
- Now stop and close your eyes and turn your attention inward. Feel the buzzing, humming, or tingling sensation that is in your hands, legs, and body. This is qi. You are literally feeling the activity of the profound medicine you have produced within yourself.

Source: Jahnke, R. Health Action, 243 Pebble Beach, Santa Barbara, CA 93117.

TRY THIS
Wave Hands Like Clouds (Water T'ai Chi)

- Stand in chest-deep water with your feet several inches apart.
- Lift your arms to shoulder level.
- Step laterally with the right foot.
- Circle both arms under and out of the water. The right arm circles clockwise and the left arm counter-clockwise.
- Repeat four times.
- Step laterally with the left foot.
- Repeat the arm sequence four times.

References

Brennan, R. (2007). *The Alexander Technique Manual: Take Control of Your Posture and Your Life.* Courtenay, BC, CA: Connections Publishing.

Cheung, S. Y., Tsai, E., Fung, L., & Ng J. (2007). Physical benefits of tai chi chuan for individuals with lower-limb disabilities. *Occupational Therapy International,* 14(1): 1–10.

Guo, X., Zhou, B., Nishimura, T., Teramukai, S., & Fukushima, M. (2008). Clinical effect of qigong practice on essential hypertension: A meta-analysis of randomized controlled trials. Journal of Alternative and Complementary Medicine, 14(1): 27–37.

Ho, T. J., Wen-Miin, L., Lien, C. H., Chiang, T., Kuo, H. W., Chu, B. C., et al. (2007). Health-related quality of life in the elderly practicing T'ai Chi Chuan. *Journal of Alternative and Complementary Medicine,* 13(10): 1077–1083.

Little, P., Lewith, G., Webley, F., Evans, M., Beattie, A., Middleton, K., et al. (2008). Randomized controlled trial of Alexander technique lessons. Exercise and massage (ATEAM) for chronic and recurrent back pain. *British Journal of Sports Medicine,* 42(12): 965–968.

Maciaszek, J., Osinski, W., Szeklicki, R., & Stemplewski, R. (2007). Effect of tai chi on body balance: Randomized controlled trial in men with osteopenia or osteoporosis. *American Journal of Chinese Medicine,* 35(10): 1–9.

Mairi, A. (2006). *Trager for Self-Healing.* Novato, CA: New World Library.

Wayne, P. M., & Kaptchuk, T. J. (2008). Qigong: Where did it come from? Where does it fit in science? What are the advances? *Journal of Alternative and Complementary Medicine,* 12(4): 351–353.

Wildman, F. (2006). *Feldenkrais: The Busy Person's Guide to Easier Movement,* 3rd ed. Berkeley, CA: The Intelligent Body Press.

Wilson, S. D. (2007). *Qi Gong for Beginners.* New York: Sterling Publishing Company.

Yao, L., Giordani, B., & Alexander, N. B. (2008). Developing a positive emotion-motivated Tai Chi (PEM-TC) exercise program for older adults with dementia. *Research and Theory for Nursing Practice,* 22(4): 241–255.

Zhang, T. C. (2008). *Earth Qi Gong for Women.* Berkeley, CA: BlueSnake Books.

Resources

American Society for the Alexander
    Technique
  Box 60008
  Florence, MA 01062
  800.473.0620
  www.Alexandertech.com

East-West Academy of Healing Arts
  117 Topaz Way
  San Francisco, CA 94131
  415.285.9400
  www.eastwestqi.com

Feldenkrais Guild of North America
  5436 N. Albina Ave.
  Portland, OR 97217
  800.775.2118
  www.feldenkrais.com

Taoist Tai Chi Society of Canada
  588 East 15th Ave.
  Vancouver BC V5T 2R5, Canada
  604.681.6609
  http://taoist.bc.ca

The Trager Institute
  21 Locust Ave.
  Mill Valley, CA 94941–2806
  415.388.2688
  www.trager.com

Spiritual Therapies

*And if you would know God be not therefore a
solver of riddles.*

*Rather look about you and you shall see Him
playing with your children.*

*And look into space; you shall see Him walking in
the cloud, outstretching His arms in the
lightning and descending in rain.*

*You shall see Him smiling in flowers, then rising
and waving His hands in trees.*

KAHLIL GIBRAN

24

Shamans

*Few people even scratch the surface, much
less exhaust the contemplation of their
own experience.*

RANDOLPH BOURNE

*We choose our joys and sorrows long
before we experience them.*

KAHLIL GIBRAN

Shaman (pronounced "SHAH-min") is a word from the
Tungus people of Siberia. This term has been adopted
widely by anthropologists to refer to those known in the
West as "medicine men," "witch doctors," "witches," "magicians,"
and "seers." Not every kind of medicine person or witch doctor,
however, is a shaman. A shaman is a woman or man who enters
an altered state of consciousness, at will, to contact and utilize another type of reality to acquire knowledge and power and to help
other people. Shamans use ancient techniques to achieve and
maintain well-being and healing for themselves and members of
their communities, serving as a link between the worlds of matter
and spirit. Shamanism is not a belief system. Rather, it is a broad
umbrella covering ancient, indigenous, and holistic healing practices worldwide (Madden, 2002). For further information on Native American healers, see Chapter 6.

BACKGROUND

The origins of shamanism go back at least 40,000 to 50,000 years
to Stone Age times, making it the oldest of all healing therapies.
All over the world, evidence from ancient cave drawings and
similar records supports the conclusions that indigenous peoples

shared a similar understanding of how the universe works, how to maintain health and strength, how to cope with serious illness, and how to deal with the trauma of death. One of the most remarkable aspects of shamanism is that concepts and treatment methods are similar in widely separated and remote parts of the planet among peoples isolated from one another. Anthropologists have studied shamanism in North, Central, and South America, Africa, Australia, Indonesia, Malaysia, Bali, Tibet, Korea, Siberia, and across Europe, and found that shamans functioned fundamentally in much the same way and with similar techniques worldwide. The basic uniformity suggests that, through trial and error, people arrived at the same conclusions (Walsh, 2007).

Today, shamanism survives in less "developed" regions of the world in spite of the advent of Western scientific medicine. There is no equivalent health professional in Western medicine, and the scope of the shaman as a healer extends beyond the capacities and expertise of physicians. The field of holistic medicine is reclaiming many techniques long practiced in shamanism, such as visualization, altered state of consciousness, hypnotherapy, meditation, positive attitude, and stress reduction. Shamanic healing is rapidly gaining popularity among urban Americans as people turn back to the old cultures for help and guidance in finding a better balance with nature and with themselves. Shamanic practice and biomedical treatment are not in conflict. Contemporary shamans are perfectly willing to have their patients see a conventional physician because the primary goal is wellness. Any kind of technological treatment or medication that will contribute to the strength of the patient is welcomed (Weatherup, 2006).

PREPARATION

People discover in a wide variety of ways that their purpose in life is to become a shaman. Often potential healers have prophetic dreams about their future calling. The dream may even include details about locating a teacher and how long the training period will be. In some cases, people are led to shamanism through personal and private mystical experiences, while in others, they are drawn from the ranks of cured patients.

The journey from apprentice to shaman is illustrated in the following example of Native American shamans. The first step is "embracing personal history." This process includes working through old traumas, fears, anger, hate, abandonment, betrayals, and wounds. The purpose is to heal the emotions so that one is no longer controlled by them but rather, consciously guided by feelings. The second step is "facing death and making death an ally." This step means examining one's attitudes and beliefs to "put to death" any that are inaccurate or outdated. It includes remembering that bodies are temporary and will one day be claimed by death. It is moving beyond personal history and recognizing that all people are part of a family, village, tribe, city, country, and ultimately all humanity. The third step is "stopping the world," which involves clearing the mind of its mental garbage. The fourth step is "controlling the dream and finding new vision and purpose." It is the time to quest for vision and seek direct connection with the dream world and its spiritual teachers. The *Vision Quest* is part of many old-world cultures and is a time when one fasts and prays in a sacred place, often a mountaintop, for up to 4 days and nights. The person prays for a vision and thus a reconnection with the Creator and Creation. Following the Vision Quest, the person is expected to make life changes that were called for. The fifth and final step is taking full responsibility for all of one's actions without guilt or shame. Apprentice shamans go through this path of transformation as they become healers and helpers in service to other people (Buhner, 2006; McGaa, 2002).

Shamanic initiation is experiential and often gradual. Shamans must learn how to achieve the shamanic state of consciousness, must become familiar with their own guardian spirits, and must successfully help others as a shaman. After learning the basic principles and methods, new shamans extend their knowledge and power by shamanic journeying. Many years of shamanic experience are necessary for the few shamans who become true masters of knowledge, power, and healing.

CONCEPTS

Environment

For the shaman, everything exists as part of an infinite web of life. Plants, stones, and the earth herself are all perceptive beings; they are all consciously aware and have a story to tell. In the shamanistic tradition, people communicate intimately and lovingly with "all their relations," as the Lakota would say, talking not just with other people, but also with animals, plants, and all the elements of the environment, including rocks and water. From the shaman's viewpoint, one's surroundings are not "environment," but family. A deep respect for all forms of life is present, with a great awareness of one's dependence on the environment. Shamans believe their powers are the powers of the animals, of the plants, of the sun, of the basic energies of the universe. They are expected to live in harmony with nature and to provide strength in daily life and help save others from illness and death (Shimer, 2004).

Power

In shamanism, the preservation of one's personal power is fundamental to well-being. Specific shamanic methods restore and maintain personal power and use it to help others who are weak, ill, or injured. In shamanism, the word *medicine* means "vital force" or "energy." People's medicine is their power, their knowledge, and their expression of their life energy.

Many shamans keep power objects—their medicine—in a medicine bundle. This bundle is normally kept wrapped up and is unrolled publicly only on ritual occasions. The objects inside are highly personal and, as with other matters of power, one does not boast of them because to do so might result in power loss. Almost any small object can be included, but the quartz crystal is highly prized among the shamans of North and South America, Australia,

Southeast Asia, and elsewhere. Quartz crystals are six-sided stones that are usually transparent to milky white and in a sense, appear to be "solidified light." The quartz crystal is considered the strongest power object and is viewed as a spirit helper. For thousands of years, shamans have used their quartz crystals for power in seeing and divination. Interestingly, in modern physics, the quartz crystal is also involved in the manipulation of power. Its remarkable electronic properties made it a basic component in early radio transmitters and receivers. Later, quartz crystals became basic components for modern electronic hardware such as computers and timepieces (Cohen, 2007).

State of Consciousness

The **ordinary state of consciousness (OSC)** is an agreed-on consensus of what reality is. This OSC, also called "ordinary reality" or simply "reality," is determined by every society and learned by individuals from childhood. Reality, then, is composed of predetermined expectations. For example, in Western societies, people are not surprised when they put a card in a machine and money comes out. Another characteristic of Western ordinary reality is that it can be measured and quantified. As Candace Pert (1997) states, "Measurement! It is the very foundation of the modern scientific method, the means by which the material world is admitted into existence. Unless we can measure something, science won't concede it exists, which is why science refuses to deal with such 'nonthings' as the emotions, the mind, the soul, or the spirit" (p. 21).

Nonordinary realities are other levels of consciousness. They can be experienced during dreaming or induced by drugs, fasting, sleep deprivation, or environmental factors. In Western society, this level of consciousness is often viewed as psychosis rather than another legitimate reality.

Shamans move, at will and with serious intention, between an ordinary state of consciousness and a **shamanic state of consciousness (SSC).** The SSC is an altered state of consciousness that may vary from a light to a deep trance. Shamans journey back and forth between these realities for the specific purpose of healing or aiding the community in some manner. Shamans operate in nonordinary reality or SSC only a small portion of the time and then only as needed to perform shamanic tasks. During this trance state, shamans' souls are believed to leave their bodies and ascend to either the upper world or lower world. Unlike the altered state of consciousness during dreaming, the SSC is a conscious waking state, and at any time, shamans can will themselves out of it, back into the OSC. The experience is like a waking dream in which shamans can control their actions and direct their adventures. Unlike a mind-altering drug experience, the SSC experience is not dependent on a chemically determined length of time, nor does it risk the possibility of being locked into a "bad trip" (Walsh, 2007).

Shamanic Cosmology

Shamanic cultures throughout the world have a three-tiered cosmology or way of viewing the universe. The *middle world* is the world of OSC or ordinary reality. It is the world of matter and the world in which people live their daily lives. The lower world and the upper world are SSC worlds, nonordinary reality, or worlds of the spirit, not to be confused with heaven and hell. These worlds are just as real as the ordinary reality of the middle world.

The *lower world* is the world of power animals. These archetypical energies take the form of animal guides who have knowledge and wisdom to share and help people navigate through life. *Power animals* tend to provide practical help and guidance. The capability of power animals to speak to humans is an indication of their power. The belief that shamans can shape-shift into the form of their power animal is common to many cultures. Sharing the identity of one's power animal varies among shamans. Some speak publicly about them while others fear that disclosing the animal's identity may cause it to leave the person. Many cultures believe that every person is born with a particular animal spirit that is to be their guide throughout life. A similar belief in Western cultures is that of guardian angels watching over people, especially children (Ingerman, 2008; Rutherford, 2008).

The *upper world* is the world of spirit guides. *Spirit guides* are beings that look more like people and are more familiar to most individuals. It is in the upper world that people meet their guardian angels. The help from spirit guides tends to be more general and philosophical in comparison to the practical help from the lower world. These worlds are complementary and equal, and neither is superior to the other.

Power animals and spirit guides teach people how to empower themselves, improve their lives, and even heal themselves. One does not have to be a shaman to make contact with one's personal power animal and spirit guide. The most traditional method of accessing this nonordinary reality is the shamanic journey.

Imagination

Most indigenous people make little distinction between what Westerners call imagination and reality. Imagination is just as real and just as concrete as ordinary reality. In fact, most of the material things of the "real" world were someone's imagination first. Automobiles, televisions, and computers have come from the imaginary realm. In fact, logic and reason have always been preceded by imagination. Western people often ask whether the power animals and guardian spirits are real or imagined. If the information that is received from power animals and guardian spirits empowers people, improves their lives, and helps them heal, the question does not apply. It is real because people's lives are changed (Sandore, 1997).

VIEW OF HEALTH AND ILLNESS

In the shamanic worldview, the ability to maintain good health is a matter of power. If the body is power-full, it resists the intrusion of external, harmful forces. No room is available for disease and illness in a power-filled body.

Being power-full is like having a protective force field surrounding the body. Possession of guardian spirit power is also fundamental to health. From a shamanic point of view, illnesses usually are intrusions that break the force field of power-fullness. In some ways, this concept is not too different from the biomedical concept of infection. Serious illness and other misfortunes are usually only possible when people are dis-spirited, meaning they have lost their power and their guardian spirits. This loss results in an inability to fight off unwanted intrusions. Illness is viewed as a separation—from one's power, from one's guardians, from nature, from community, and from the Great Spirit. Even Western everyday language reflects this view when people say, "I'm having a low-energy day" or "I wasn't myself last night."

Severe trauma can result in soul loss, a natural survival mechanism. It is believed that a part of one's self or soul goes into hiding to ensure that the individual will survive the extreme stress. Western psychiatrists refer to this phenomenon as *dissociation*. Some people believe that soul loss occurs when people stop being generous and become selfish and dishonest. Sometimes, people's souls remain lost until they go through a process of soul retrieval. Symptoms of soul loss are an inability to focus and concentrate, a lack of connection to one's emotions, a feeling of being "spaced out" and not really present, a feeling of being an observer of life, or chronic depression. Soul retrieval brings buried memories and emotions back to the surface, much like the process of psychotherapy (Walsh, 2007).

The Hmong believe there are two treatments of illness. Natural causes of illness are treated with herbs and massage. Supernatural causes of illness are more serious, and treatment consists of a shaman journeying to the spirit world (Helsel, Mochel, & Bauer, 2005).

TREATMENT

More detailed information on treatment modalities utilized by Native American shamans is found in Chapter 6. Shamans may be called on to help those who have become ill or those who have lost their power, their spirit guides, or even their souls. In such cases, shamans use the shamanic journey to recover that which was lost. Shamans also journey to gather information to help and guide individuals or groups, solve problems, and answer questions. Shamans, by offering their total commitment to a patient for as long as several days, develop intense relationships that underscore the importance of caring as well as curing in the shamanic healing tradition. In old cultures, shamans would do the journeying for patients, but in today's world, anyone can experience a shamanic journey. It is through this process that people meet and talk with their power animals and spirit guides and restore their own power and self-healing (Ingerman, 2008).

Basic tools for entering the SSC prior to the shamanic journey are the drum, providing lower vibrations, and the rattle, providing higher vibrations. A drumbeat at a steady 200 to 280 beats a minute serves as a focus for concentration and quiets the chattering mind. The pace of the drumbeat corresponds to theta brain waves associated with the hypnotic state, facilitating the move into nonordinary reality. It is a remarkably safe practice for most people, because one can return to an ordinary state of consciousness at any time. Some people add dancing or chanting to the drumbeat as another way to reach this altered state of consciousness (Ingerman, 2008).

Some shamans use teacher plants as a catalyst to the shamanic journey. Throughout the world are many teacher plants. Peyote, San Pedro cactus, ayahuasca, psilocybin, and red-and-white mushrooms are some examples. Shamans consider these plants to be gifts to be used with care and awareness. The use is never intended to be recreational, but rather as part of a sacred ceremony (Cohen, 2007).

Sometimes communities share in a group healing ceremony. An example is found among the indigenous people of Hawaii, who come together as a group and experience a forgiveness ritual before the shaman begins the healing work. Family and community members convey concern for the patient by their participation in the ritual. This process underscores the belief that no one lives in isolation but is connected to and affected by other people. When people join in a show of community support, new levels of healing are possible (Walsh, 2007).

Hawaiian medical practices are experiencing a resurgence, and researchers are studying the healing modalities, training patterns, cultural attributes, and the use of Hawaiian medicines. The three significant modalities are massage (ho'olomilomi), herbal medicine (la'au lapa'au), and conflict resolution (ho'oponopono). The majority of the practitioners are skilled in more than one healing modality. All treatment sessions begin and end with spiritual blessings to initiate the healing process. Health is considered to be a state of harmony between people, nature, and the gods (Chang, 2001).

RESEARCH

Clinical evidence of results from shamanic healing is anecdotal, and most published studies have been done by social scientists, folklorists, and historians. In another sense, the ancient methods of shamanism have been tested immeasurably longer than those of biomedicine. The similarities between shamans and scientists include an awareness of the complexity of the universe and the vast array of knowledge still to be uncovered and understood. As Harner (1990) describes the similarity:

> Both shamans and scientists personally pursue research into the mysteries of the universe, and both believe that the underlying causal processes of that universe are hidden from ordinary view. And neither master shamans nor master scientists allow the dogma of ecclesiastical and political authorities to interfere with their explorations. It was no accident that Galileo was accused of witchcraft [shamanism]. (p. 45)

Research has demonstrated that drumming produces changes in the brain. The beat of the drum contains many sound frequencies that transmit impulses along the nerve pathways in the central nervous system. Shamanic drumming produces frequencies in the theta wave range of four to seven cycles per second. Studies have found that the rhythmic auditory stimulation of drumming increases the production of theta waves, the brain waves of the trance state (Walsh, 2007).

INTEGRATED NURSING PRACTICE

Albert Schweitzer reportedly once observed, "The witch doctor succeeds for the same reason all the rest of us [doctors] succeed. Each patient carries his own doctor inside him. They come to us not knowing this truth. We are at our best when we give the doctor who resides within each patient a chance to go to work" (Harner, 1990, p. 135). This belief is almost identical to Florence Nightingale's basic premise that healing is a function of nature that comes from within the individual.

A current example of a combination of the techniques of shamanism with biomedicine is the well-known work of Dr. O. Carl Simonton and Stephanie Matthews-Simonton in treating people with cancer. As part of their treatment, clients are taught to relax and visualize themselves on a walking journey until they meet an "inner guide," which is a person or animal. The client then asks the guide for help in getting well. The process is similar to a shamanic journey and the meeting of a power animal.

Contemporary shamans work among today's Native American, Hmong, and other indigenous cultures. Their repertoire of curative powers now includes some modern and biomedical practices, and they may collaborate with conventional health care practitioners. Today, many shamans share their knowledge about healing with others, which has contributed to a recent renewal of interest in this oldest of healing therapies. Lectures, retreats, and weekend meetings, where shamans teach the principles of living in balance with nature, are now available to the general public (Helsel et al., 2005; Villoldo, 2008).

As nurses, we must remember that we all have our own world view. Until we recognize this ethnocentrism (our way is the best way), we are likely to impose our view of the world on our clients. We must not only raise our awareness of other worldviews but also respect and honor worldviews that are different from ours.

In sharing information with clients, you can explain that shamanism offers a chance for contemplation. Guides offer more in the way of introspection and insight than physical cure. A shamanic journey may increase self-understanding, guidance for living, and a spiritual rejuvenation—all of which are important for the healing process.

In the old cultures, shamans would do the journeying while an apprentice or helper drummed. In today's world, it is more appropriate for each of us to learn to journey for ourselves and restore our own power. Personal power is believed to be basic to health and well-being. Some of your clients may wish to meet in drumming circles every 1 or 2 weeks while others will prefer to work alone. Drumming tapes have been designed and produced for shamanic journeying. As in any other field of learning, it may be more effective to work firsthand with a professional during a workshop or retreat.

The shamanic journey begins with the drum. Among all the instruments used in healing, the drum produces some of the most powerful effects. Drumming has been used in organizations, ranging from therapy groups and 12-step programs to rehabilitation centers. Human bodies are multidimensional rhythm machines with everything pulsing in synchrony. Drumming can influence how strongly and harmoniously life moves within and around us. The *Try This* exercise that follows presents an overview of the shamanic journey that you may want to experience for yourself.

In the shamanic tradition, healing is not just for the individual but also for the community. In shamanism, ultimately no distinction is made between helping others and helping yourself. By helping others, one becomes more powerful, self-fulfilled, and joyful. The broader purpose is the helping of humankind. The desire to help others is what draws many people into the profession of nursing.

The North American Nursing Diagnosis Association identifies the diagnoses of potential for enhanced community coping and ineffective community coping. It is expected that nurses apply the nursing process with individual clients, families, groups, and communities. Perhaps someday we will see a modern version of the shaman working side by side with us. This cooperation is already starting to take place where native shamans live, as on some North American Indian reservations and in some places in Australia. Equally exciting is the idea of nurses being trained in shamanic techniques and health maintenance so they can combine both approaches in their practice.

TRY THIS

Shamanic Journey

- Find a private, secure place where you will not be disturbed.
- Assume a comfortable position, either sitting or lying down. You may want to cover your eyes to block out room light.
- Set the intent of your journey: Decide if you want to go to the upper world or lower, and form the intent to meet your guardian spirit or your power animal.
- Turn on a drumming tape. Let your body relax, let it sink down into Mother Earth. Take a few deep, slow breaths. Let the drumbeat become part of you; feel it resonate through your body.
- In your mind, bring yourself to a place in nature that is special for you, one that holds personal meaning. It might be a tree you climbed as a child, the lake you

(continued)

swam in on summer vacations, the place you now walk your dog. Imagine that place and go there in your mind. Feel the energy of that place.

- If you are going to the lower world, find a place where you can enter the earth such as a hollowed out tree stump, an animal den, a cave, or whatever you want to imagine. When you enter the earth, you will be in a long cave. Take your time and follow it. Eventually it will open up into the lower world. Walk around and enjoy the beauty of the lower world. Explore. Soon you will come in contact with power animals. Introduce yourself. Dialogue with the animal, and ask what information the animal has for you.
- If you are going to the upper world, find a way to get up into the sky. You may climb a mountain or a tall beanstalk, use a hot air balloon, or even shape-shift into the form of an eagle and fly up. Eventually, you will come to the interface between the middle world and the upper world. Find a way through this interface, which is something like a membrane. The upper world is an ethereal, light, crystalline place. Explore. Soon you will meet your guardian spirit. Introduce yourself. Dialogue with the spirit, and ask what information the spirit has for you.
- Eventually, the journey has to end. It can end when you decide to end it, when no more information remains to be gained, or when the drumbeat changes, signaling an end. Return home by the same path you took to get there.
- Allow the information to sink into your consciousness. It is best if you write the information down in a notebook, in a concrete form you will remember. The shamanic journey is much like a dream—it will leave you quickly. Writing it down is a method to keep the information you gained during the journey.

Source: Richard Sandore, MD, personal communication, 1998.

References

Buhner, S. H. (2006). *Sacred Plant Medicine.* Rochester, VT: Bear & Company.

Chang, H. K. (2001). Hawaiian health practitioners in contemporary society. *Pacific Health Dialog,* 8(2): 260–273.

Cohen, K. (2007). *Honoring the Medicine: The Essential Guide to Native American Healing.* New York: Random House.

Harner, M. (1990). *The Way of the Shaman.* San Francisco: Harper.

Helsel, D. G., Mochel, M., & Bauer, R. (2005). Chronic illness and Hmong shamans. *Journal of Transcultural Nursing,* 16(2): 150–154.

Ingerman, S. (2008). *Shamanic Journeying: A Beginner's Guide.* Boulder, CO: Sounds True, Incorporated.

Madden, K. (2002). *The Book of Shamanic Healing.* St. Paul, MN: Llewellyn Publisher.

McGaa, E. (Eagle Man). (2002). *Native Wisdom.* San Francisco: Council Oak Books.

Pert, C. (1997). *Molecules of Emotion.* New York: Scribner.

Rutherford, L. (2008). *The View Through the Medicine Wheel.* Winchester, UK: O Books.

Sandore, R. (1997). *Introduction to the Shamanic Journey.* Prone Stone Recording. Soaring Spirit.

Shimer, P. (2004). *Healing Secrets of the Native Americans.* New York: Black Dog & Leventhal Publishers.

Villoldo, A. (2008). *Courageous Dreaming: How Shamans Dream the World into Being*. Carlsbad, CA: Hay House, Incorporated.

Walsh, R. (2007). *The World of Shamanism: New Views of an Ancient Tradition*. Woodbury, MN: Llewellyn Publications.

Weatherup, K. (2006). *Practical Shamanism: A Guide for Walking in Both Worlds*. La Mesa, CA: Hands Over Heart Publishing.

Resources

Dance of the Deer Foundation
Center for Shamanic Studies
P.O. Box 699
Soquel, CA 95073
831.475.9560
www.shamanism.com

Eagle's Wing Center for Contemporary
Shamanism
BM Box 7475
London WCIN 3XX, UK
01435.810233
www.shamanism.co.uk

The Foundation for Shamanic Studies
P.O. Box 1939
Mill Valley, CA 94942
415.380.8282
www.shamanism.org

Institute for Contemporary Shamanic
Studies
125-720 King St. W
Box 438
Toronto, ON M5V 3S5
416.603.4912
www.icss.org

25

Faith and Prayer

Faith can give us courage to face the uncertainties of the future.

MARTIN LUTHER KING, JR.

Faith is not something to grasp, it is a state to grow into.

MAHATMA GANDHI

You're being religious when you believe in Jesus or Buddha or any other truly holy being, but wow, you're being spiritual when you become the loving compassionate, caring being they all inspire you to be.

ROBERT THURMAN

Health care sciences have begun to demonstrate that spirituality, faith, and religious commitment may play a role in promoting health and reducing illness. Nurse clinicians and researchers, as well as others, are becoming more interested in the connection between religious faith and survival. Increasingly, people are beginning to recognize that faith is good medicine.

Spirituality is that part of us that deals with relationships and values and addresses questions of purpose and meaning in life. Spirituality unites people and is inclusive in nature, not exclusive. It is not loyal to one group, continent, or religion. Although spirituality is not a religion, being involved in a particular religion is a way some people enhance their spirituality. Yet people can be very spiritual and not religious. Spirituality involves individuals, family, friends, and community. *Individual* aspects are the development of moral values and beliefs about the meaning and purpose of life and death. The development of our spirituality provides a grounding sense of identity and contributes to our self-esteem. Spiritual aspects relating to *family* and *friends* include the search for meaning through relationships and the feeling of being connected with others and with an external power, often identified as God or a Supreme Being. *Community* aspects of spirituality can be understood as a common humanity and a belief in the fundamental sacredness and unity of all life. It is that which motivates people toward truth and a sense of fairness and justice to all members of society. Our spiritual health is expressed through humor, compassion, faith, forgiveness, courage, and creativity. Spirituality enables us to develop healthy relationships based on acceptance, respect, and compassion.

Religion can be described in a number of ways. The definition chosen for this text is one developed by Mickley, Carson, and Soeken (1995), three nursing researchers. They believe that religion develops and changes over time and is composed of people's beliefs, attitudes, and patterns of behavior that relate to the supernatural—God, the Divine One, the Great Spirit, Creator, and so forth. Religion usually includes a group of people who hold similar beliefs, have sacred texts, share religious symbols, and participate in shared traditions or rituals. Many people may say they are spiritual but not religious, while most religious people also identify themselves as spiritual (Carson & Koenig, 2008; Koenig, 2008).

Faith refers to our beliefs and expectations about life, our selves, and others. In a religious context, faith refers to a belief in a Supreme Being who listens and responds to people and who cares about their well-being. In a spiritual context, faith is thought of as the power to accept the nature of life as it is and live in the present moment. It is a sense of letting go of the need to control while trusting and waiting for the moment when answers come (Carson & Koenig, 2008).

Prayer is most often defined simply as a form of communication and fellowship with the Deity or Creator. The universality of prayer is evidenced in all cultures having some form of prayer. The Hindus speak of the thousand names of God, and surely there are a hundred ways to pray. Imagine a circle or wheel with many spokes leading to the center or Supreme Being. Each spoke is a different religion with different prayers, but they all lead to the center. Prayer has been and continues to be used in times of difficulty and illness even in the most secular societies. Prayer for self and prayer for others are the most frequently used forms of alternative therapies (Masters & Spielmans, 2007).

A common image of prayer in the United States is something like this: "Prayer is talking aloud to yourself, to a white, male, cosmic parent figure, who prefers to be addressed in English" (Dossey, 1997, p. 10). This cultural view of prayer fails to encompass how prayer is regarded by many people throughout the world. For some, prayer is more a state of being than of doing; for others, prayer is silence rather than words; for some, prayer is a thought or a desire of the heart; others pray to a female Goddess or a Divine Being who looks like they do. Buddhists do not believe in a personal God as creator and ruler of the world. Yet prayers, offered to the universe, are central to the Buddhist tradition. Prayer may be simply being still and knowing that God is God. Prayer is part of many religious traditions and rituals and may be individual or communal, public or private (Wachholtz & Pearce, 2009). Larry Dossey (1997) provides a broad definition of prayer: "Prayer is communication with the Absolute. This definition is inclusive, not exclusive; it affirms religious tolerance; and it invites people to define for themselves what 'communication' is, and who or what 'the Absolute' may be" (p. 11). According to a Sufi saying, prayer is when you talk to God, and meditation is when God talks to you. In this definition, meditation is thought of as passive and receptive and prayer as active and engaging. The boundaries between meditation and prayer, however, are often blurred.

BACKGROUND

Until the last 200 years, medicine and religion were so thoroughly united that healers and priests were often the same individuals. The first hospitals were founded in monasteries by physicians who were usually monks. Today, many cultures throughout the world continue to regard their healers as a source for guidance in matters of faith and wellness. In the West, religion and medicine were fused until the end of the Middle Ages in the mid-1400s. Philosophers such as Descartes (1596–1650), Locke (1632–1704), and Hume (1711–1776) promoted the scientific basis of knowledge, believing that truth could only be realized through the examination of empirical data and the rational, scientific method. Centuries later, Western societies continue to experience the consequences of this split between religion and medicine. Western physicians are educated to think primarily in terms of what can be empirically proven in the laboratory. Discussions of spirituality and religion are considered by many physicians to be "off limits" with such discussion belonging to spiritual or religious leaders. In the past, when arguments arose between religion and medicine, religion usually did not fare well. Thus, many religious leaders today are cautious about what science is beginning to say about their faith. As nurses such as M. Dossey, Carson, Burkhardt, Nagai-Jacobson, Taylor, Winslow, Treloar, Koerner, Goertz, and Holt-Ashley and physicians such as B. M. Dossey, Matthews, Koenig, and Benson research and write more about the blending of religion and health care, the practice of these professions will evolve to, once again, include the forgotten "faith factor" in health care.

Research has shown that religious practices such as worship attendance and prayer have significant health and survival implications. Religiosity/spirituality is associated with longer life in healthy populations but not in people suffering from disease (Chida, Steptoe, & Powell, 2009).

In some situations, religion may have a negative impact on people's lives. Religious participation can lead to more, not fewer, problems when unscrupulous leaders coerce or manipulate others to give up all personal autonomy. Problems also occur when religion fosters excessive guilt or shame or encourages people to avoid dealing with life's problems. Some religious groups urge their members to avoid all conventional medical care, which can lead to life-threatening situations (Wachholtz & Pearce, 2009).

CONCEPTS

Universality of Faith

Throughout history and around the world, people have called upon a Divine Being to sustain them. People are nourished by life-affirming beliefs and philosophies. They meditate and say prayers that elicit physiologic calm and a sense of peacefulness, both of which contribute to longer survival. Benson (1997) believes that a genetic blueprint makes believing in the Great Mystery part of people's nature. Through the process of natural selection, mutating genes retain the impulses of faith, hope, and love, and faith is a natural physiologic reaction to the threats to mortality that everyone faces. Benson (1997) goes on to say that "according to my investigations, it does not matter which God you worship, nor which theology you adopt as your own. Spiritual life, in general, is very healthy" (p. 212).

Crises

Serious illness presents a spiritual crisis. As long as people are well, they maintain their autonomy and their ability to function at home, work, or school. Their feelings of self-worth are supported as they find meaning and purpose in their many activities. Once serious illness occurs, some of these things change. Ill people may have to depend on others for personal care and experience other radical lifestyle changes. Body concept changes may threaten self-esteem. In these situations, most people are forced to reevaluate life's meaning and purpose. Religious people draw heavily on their resources of faith to see them through difficult situations like serious illness. Positive religious coping involves such beliefs as "God will care for me." One research study asked 345 patients with advanced cancer which of the two interventions they would prefer: (1) interventions to extend life even though that would mean more pain or (2) interventions to relieve pain even though it would mean that they would not live as long. The greater the use of positive religious coping, the more individuals wanted more aggressive end-of-life care near the time of death (Phelps et al., 2009).

Twelve Remedies

Numerous studies demonstrate that religious involvement promotes health. It appears at this time that a number of religious "ingredients" promote health and well-being. Although some may be found in nonreligious settings, they are more commonly found operating together in religious organizations. Matthews and Clark (1998) have termed these "religious remedies," a listing of which appears in Box 25.1.

BOX 25.1

Religious Remedies

1. Relaxation response
2. Healthful living
3. Aesthetics of worship
4. Whole-being worship
5. Confession and absolution
6. Support network
7. Shared beliefs
8. Ritual
9. Purpose in life
10. Turning over to a Higher Power
11. Positive expectations
12. Love for self and others

Source: Matthews, D. A., & Clark, C. (1998). *The Faith Factor.* New York: Viking.

The first remedy is the **relaxation response,** which can be evoked with meditation and prayer (Matthews & Clark, 1998). The relaxation response buffers stress by clearing the mind and freeing the body from everyday tension. Practiced regularly, the relaxation response decreases heart rate, lowers metabolic rate, decreases respirations, and slows brain waves. In addition, it enhances measures of immunity. Benson (1997) found that when religious beliefs were added to relaxation response activities, worries and fears were significantly reduced when compared to the relaxation response alone. Most worship services provide time for silent prayer or meditation and help people take time out from busy schedules. With regular practice of the relaxation response, people report experiencing an increase in spirituality. They often describe the presence of an energy, a power, or God, that is beyond themselves. Those who feel this presence often experience the greatest medical benefits (Benson, 1997).

The second remedy is one of **healthful living** (Matthews & Clark, 1998). Some religious groups actively promote a healthy lifestyle as part of their doctrine. Religious prescriptions may include dietary moderation, rules about sexual behavior, and regulations regarding hygiene as well as avoidance of tobacco, alcohol, and drugs.

Remedy number three is the **aesthetics of worship,** which taps into a universal appreciation for beauty. Visual symbols of faith are reassuring and calming images. Stained-glass windows, beautiful architecture, and floral arrangements all provide an experience of harmony and balance. Sacred music uses audible beauty to communicate the splendor of God. The smell of incense may evoke a deep sense of peace and quietude (Matthews & Clark, 1998).

The fourth remedy is **whole-being worship.** Christians who sing familiar hymns, Jews who sing "Torah Ora" when the Torah scroll is presented, and Buddhists who chant their prayers—all participate in whole-being worship through music. This combination of physical activity (singing), cognitive activity (reading the words), and spiritual activity (prayer through song) evokes a sense of peace. Movements such as kneeling, standing, bowing heads, folding hands, or even dancing engage people on all levels of being. As people worship with body, mind, and spirit, they go through a unifying experience that is as good for them as it feels (Matthews & Clark, 1998).

Remedy number five is **confession and absolution.** Harboring guilty feelings can literally make people sick. In many religions, people are encouraged to confess their sins, repent, and are given assurance of forgiveness and absolution. This process allows individuals to review their mistakes, share their personal pain, and learn from and move on rather than becoming preoccupied with personal shortcomings (Matthews & Clark, 1998).

The sixth remedy is one's **support network**—those family members and friends who offer practical help, emotional support, and spiritual encouragement in times of need. People are social beings whose health often deteriorates when they become isolated and lonely. Lack of human companionship has been linked to depression of the immune system and a lowered production of endorphins, the neurotransmitter that produces the feeling of well-being. Religious organizations often provide many opportunities for social interaction from religious services to sacred study groups, to youth, women's, and men's groups, and to community outreach groups. Koenig (2008) describes some of the benefits from group interaction, which offers a sense of partnership, helps with coping, creates a sense of community and safety, encourages a cooperative approach to problem solving, helps to change behaviors and thoughts, supports taking control, and encourages personal action.

Remedy number seven is **shared beliefs.** Most people prefer to associate with individuals who share similar beliefs and points of view. Great things can be achieved when groups are unified around common values. Religious traditions are opportunities for people to share common beliefs. Individuals who feel they are part of a group find they are not alone and gain strength from the power of shared beliefs. Participation in regular worship not only helps people feel connected and helps them rise above their differences, but it also is an antidote to the alienation often prevalent in Western society (Matthews & Clark, 1998).

The eighth remedy is **ritual.** Ceremony and ritual are ways of creating sacred space and time, when normal ways of relating are put aside, and people can listen and pray with an open heart to their Divine Being. Religious ritual is a powerful healing mechanism that has soothing and calming effects. As Benson (1997) states:

> There is something very influential about invoking a ritual that you may first have practiced in childhood, about regenerating the neural pathways that were formed in your youthful experience of

faith. . . . Even if you experience the ritual from an entirely different perspective of maturity and life history, the words you read,
the songs you sing, and the prayers you invoke will soothe you in
the same way they did in what was perhaps a simpler time in your
life. (p. 177)

Rituals provide people a link with tradition and give them a sense of security (Matthews & Clark, 1998).

The ninth remedy is that of finding a **purpose in life** (Matthews & Clark,
1998). Victor Frankl (1984) describes people's search for meaning as being the
primary motivation in their lives. This search for meaning becomes more intense during periods of illness as people struggle with age-old questions such
as "Why me?" "Why now?" "Did I do something to deserve this?" Religion
and worship attendance provide a framework of meaning, a sense of purpose
in life, and a meaningful interpretation for difficult times. People who are dying often seem to arrive at a sense of what life's purpose is. As they tell it, the
purpose of life is to grow in wisdom and to learn to love better. They discover
that health is not an end but rather a means. In other words, health enables
people to serve a purpose in life, but health is not the purpose in life.

Remedy number ten is **turning one's life over** to the Great Mystery or
God. It is an acknowledgment that no one has total control over her or his
life. Religion provides an avenue for asking for guidance, intervention, and
strength. Faith in a God who is loving and caring provides comfort for
those going through difficult times. Worship services often leave people
feeling less burdened and anxious, as well as more peaceful (Matthews &
Clark, 1998).

The eleventh remedy is that of **positive expectations.** During a time of
illness or distress, religion often provides a sense of hope and the strength to
endure that which has happened. The expectancy of help from the Divine
Source works in the same way as does the expectancy of help from a medication, procedure, or caregiver. Various holy writings promise health and healing to the faithful, and researchers are beginning to document the effect of this
expectation on the outcome of disease (Matthews & Clark, 1998). Gregg
Braden (2008) writes about the role of belief in both creating illness and healing from illness on personal, community, and worldwide levels.

The twelfth, and last, remedy is **love for self and others.** All religions focus on loving God and other people. This love includes helping others,
strangers, as well as family and friends (Matthews & Clark, 1998). When people love and help others, they often experience better health than those who
do not.

These 12 religious remedies can be found outside of religious organizations. Frequent religious participation, however, provides many of these
remedies in one context. Research is demonstrating that religious participation is an important factor in the prevention of disease, achievement of
well-being, healing from illness, and extension of life span. One mystery
that remains, however, is why some people are cured and others are not.

One can be very spiritual and still get sick and die. It must be remembered that religious participation and spirituality are no guarantee for physical health. Failure to recognize this basic reality can result in inappropriate self-blame (Matthews & Clark, 1998).

How Prayer Works

No one knows how praying for others works. Skeptics say it cannot happen, because no accepted scientific theory explains it. In the development of theories, however, empirical facts often lead to the development of an explanatory theory. For example, it was well known that penicillin worked before anyone discovered how it worked. The debate has now shifted from whether prayer works to how prayer works.

Larry Dossey (1993), Joellen Goertz Koerner (2007), and Gregg Braden (2008) have proposed that prayer is "nonlocal," an idea derived from the field of quantum physics. The word *local* means that something is present in the here and now; each of us exists here and not somewhere else and now and not at some other time. The word *nonlocal* means that something is not confined by place or time. All the major theistic (belief in a personal God as creator) religions agree on the nonlocal nature of God; that (S)He is everywhere, is not confined by space and location, and exists throughout time. According to the concept of nonlocality, consciousness cannot be localized or confined to one's brain or body, nor can it be confined to the present moment. Consciousness is basic to the universe, perhaps similar to matter and energy. According to this theory, neither energy nor information travels from one mind to another, because the two minds are not separate but rather interconnected and omniscient. Dossey, Koerner, and Braden have proposed that consciousness-mediated events such as prayer, telepathy, precognition, and clairvoyance may be explainable as developments continue in quantum physics. As in any new theory, the nonlocal theory raises more questions than it answers. Evidence exists that prayer works, even though the exact mechanism is unknown at this time.

TREATMENT

Some people seek nurses, doctors, counselors, and therapists who focus on spiritual concerns as well as physical and emotional concerns. This focus is especially helpful for those who are dealing with issues related to meaning and purpose in life. Alternatively, people may seek the help of religious leaders who include healing practices in their religious practice. Faith healing has not been scientifically proven but remains a popular option for many. Some people go to specific places for healing. The Catholic Church has documented 36 "miracles" at Lourdes, for example. A variety of spiritually focused healing groups are also available. People with addictive disorders benefit from 12-step programs, which rely on both group support and the specific invocation of a Higher Power.

Two different types of prayer are directed and nondirected. In **directed prayer,** the praying person asks for a specific outcome, such as for the cancer to go away or for the baby to be born healthy. In contrast, in **nondirected prayer,** no specific outcome is asked. The praying person simply asks for the best thing to occur in a given situation. Studies show that both approaches are effective in promoting health.

Prayer can also be described according to form. **Colloquial prayer** is an informal talk with God, as if one were talking to a good friend. **Petitional prayer** or intercessory prayer is asking God for things for oneself or others. The focus is on what God can provide. **Intercessory prayer** is simply praying for someone else. **Ritual prayer** is the use of formal prayers or rituals such as prayers from a prayer book or in the Jewish siddur, or the Catholic practice of saying the rosary. **Meditative prayer,** also known as contemplative prayer, is similar to meditation and is a process of focusing the mind on an aspect of God for a period of time.

RESEARCH

It is difficult to compare studies on faith and prayer, when researchers do not agree on conceptual models with operational definitions. Different opinions exist on what should be included in the research studies. This is a hurdle that must be overcome before a systematic review is possible.

The following is a small sampling of studies related to spirituality, religious practice, and prayer:

- A meta-analysis of prayer and health found (1) no significant effect for distant intercessory prayer on health; (2) the studies were too widely varied to determine a relationship between frequency of prayer and changes in health; (3) individual's subjective experience of the prayer was a greater predictor of the person's well-being than was the type of prayer utilized; and (4) the content of the prayer may be a factor in health outcomes (Masters & Spielmans, 2007).
- 71 HIV-infected adults were randomized into a treatment group (Mantram repetition—repeating a spiritual word or phrase as much as possible throughout waking hours) and a control group (videotapes on HIV and group discussion). Both groups met for five weekly classes. Measurements of faith and saliva cortisol levels were done three times: preintervention, postintervention, and 5-week follow-up. Individuals in both groups, who had a high sense of faith, demonstrated lower levels of salivary cortiosl at all three times of measurement. Faith levels increased in the mantram individuals compared to the control individuals (Bormann, Aschbacher, Wetherell, Roesch, & Redwine, 2009).
- 83 individuals who had frequent migraine headaches were randomized into four groups: spiritual meditation (God is good, God is joy), internal secular meditation (I am good, I am joyful), external secular meditation (grass is green, cotton is fluffy), and progressive relaxation. The spiritual

meditation groups had a significant difference in the following: decrease in the number of headaches, a greater increase in pain tolerance, a greater decrease in trait anxiety, and headache self-efficacy. The findings were not significant for an improvement in positive effect, a lessening of depression, or general spiritual well-being (Wachholtz & Pargament, 2008).

- 87 individuals, who were post-solid organ transplant, participated in the validation of a brief serenity scale. Serenity is considered to be a dimension of one's spirituality. The tool measured three factors of serenity (1) acceptance—accept what is happening and attempt to deal with it, (2) inner haven—a sense of comfort or peace of mind, and (3) trust—that some good will come out of all that is happening. Those individuals who scored high on the serenity scale had a more positive effect and a better quality of life. Those who scored low on the serenity scale experienced more anxiety and depression (Kreitzer, Gross, Waleekhachonloet, Reilly-Spong, & Byrd, 2009).

- Beuscher and Beck (2008) reviewed studies examining the role of faith and spirituality in people in the early stage of Alzheimer's disease. As these individuals looked for meaning in their distress, the studies found that prayer and attendance at religious services seemed to bring some sense of peace and an improved quality of life.

- A community sample of 120 Christian and 234 Jewish people were asked about their religiousness (importance of religion) and religious practices (e.g., prayer frequency) and levels of personal distress. Those individuals with higher religious core beliefs experienced less worry, anxiety, and depression compared to those with negative religious core beliefs (Rosmarin, Krumrei, & Andersson, 2009).

USING RESEARCH TO HEAL

Bormann, J. E., Thorp, S., Wetherell, J. E., & Golshan, S. (2008). A spiritually based group intervention for combat veterans with posttraumatic stress disorder. *Journal of Holistic Nursing*, 26(2): 109–116.

What Is This Study About?

There are a growing number of U.S. veterans living with posttraumatic stress disorder (PTSD) as a result of the involvement of the United States in wars in Iraq and Afghanistan. To date, very little consideration has been given to spiritually based interventions for managing symptoms related to PTSD. Therefore, the purpose of this study was to assess the feasibility, effect sizes and satisfaction of mantram repetition (the spiritual practice of repeating a sacred word/phrase throughout the day) for the specific purpose of managing symptoms related to PTSD.

(continued)

How Was the Study Done?

This study was a two group (intervention and a usual care delayed-treatment control) by two time (preintervention and postintervention) experimental design. Twenty-nine veterans, all diagnosed with PTSD, were randomly assigned to the intervention (n=14) or the delayed-treatment control (n=15) for 6 weeks. Veterans ranged in age from 40 to 76 years with a mean age of 56. The majority of the participants (66%) were White. All had served in the Korean, Vietnam, or first Gulf War. There were no statistical differences related to participants who described themselves as religious or spiritual compared to the control group. Both groups experienced an equivalent number of months in combat. This study was approved by a Human Research Protections Program and the Veteran's Administration Healthcare System's Research and Development Committee. The mantram intervention was for 6 weeks (90 min/week). In this group, the veteran silently repeated a specific mantram selected from a provided list through-out the day as often as possible. Participants were asked to choose a mantram that they were comfortable with, positive and fit with their beliefs or philosophy. In addition, participants in this group were taught the principles of "slowing down" and "one-pointed attention." The veterans in the usual care group and mantram group continued with their prescribed medical care in either a weekly or monthly visit to their primary care provider. The usual care group did not interact in any group meetings during the 6-week intervention. All participants were assessed by various measures for PTSD and psychological distress. In addition, quality of life measures, spirituality, and mindfulness attention were evaluated. Program satisfaction was evaluated postintervention.

What Were the Results of the Study?

The specific focus on determining feasibility of the study found that combat veterans from the Korean, Vietnam, and first Gulf wars volunteered to participate in the study. However, veterans returning from Iraq and Afghanistan did not participate in the study. The second objective of evaluating the effect size for PTSD symptom severity and other psychological outcomes revealed medium-to-large effect sizes on most variables, especially self-reporting of PTSD. Lastly, participant satisfaction of the program indicated that the intervention and control group (control group was offered the intervention after the 6-week program) evaluated the program with moderate to high satisfaction.

What Additional Questions Might I Have?

Would the findings be significantly different with a larger population enrolled in the research? What complementary and alternative therapies would be beneficial for veterans experiencing more recent war-related PTSD?

How Can I Use This Study?

Nurses can use the findings of this study in assisting postwar veterans to explore alternative methods in overcoming PTSD. Including spirituality as an intervention for some veterans may provide a safe and cost effective method in providing holistic care.

Source: Contributed by Dolores M. Huffman, PhD, RN, Associate Professor of Nursing, Purdue University Calumet.

INTEGRATED NURSING PRACTICE

Every serious illness is a spiritual crisis because it is a confrontation with one's own mortality. Every nurse, regardless of personal belief, must recognize that religion and/or spirituality is often an essential part of the life of those entrusted to her or his care. To avoid these issues is to fail to truly be a nurse healer because our task is to address the physical, psychological, and spiritual needs of clients. You can, as a nurse, incorporate faith and prayer issues in your care of clients, regardless of your own personal religious beliefs or worldviews. When you remember that people are spiritual beings, you will be more alert to spiritual concerns. It is important that you promote an atmosphere that accepts and encourages many forms of spiritual expression.

The International Code of Ethics for Nurses, the ANA Code of Ethics, and the Joint Commission on Accreditation of Healthcare Organizations all state that nurses must assess clients' spiritual needs. Why is it, then, that some nurses do not incorporate faith and prayer into their professional practice? Some nurses are unaware of the research data regarding the faith factor. That situation is beginning to change as schools of nursing develop courses to teach students about the faith–health connection. Some nurses have been told specifically that they are not to mix nursing and faith. This recommendation was made out of a concern that we might blur the professional–personal boundaries and cause harm to our clients. Some believe they do not have enough time while others are unfamiliar with spiritual assessment tools. As more research is being documented, nurses are reexamining the relationship between nursing and faith (Dunn, Handley, & Dunkin, 2009). Taylor, Mamier, Bahjri, Anton, and Petersen (2009) examined a self-study program designed to help nurses learn to talk with patients regarding religion and spirituality. They found significant differences in pre- and post-test responses.

Faith and prayer can be explored effectively with people of most age groups. The depth and focus of the conversation will vary based on the cognitive and developmental ability of the individual or family. Health maintenance visits provide an opportunity to explore spiritual beliefs and practices in the context of an overall assessment of lifestyle, risks, and resources. Doors can be opened in a nonthreatening, nonurgent fashion, and the topic can be validated for future discussion. See Chapter 2 for a list of nursing spirituality assessment tools. In the face of major illness, terminal disease, or dying, the discussion of faith and prayer is even more relevant. Clearly though, discussion of this topic should not be restricted to these types of client encounters. Box 25.2 provides an example of a nursing assessment regarding faith and prayer.

Respecting people's beliefs and experiences also means that nurses do not force spiritual issues on clients, push religion on them, or attempt to convert them to a particular faith. Prayer should never be imposed on patients or used as a substitute for high-quality nursing care. Nor should prayer be used as an invocation of magic. Doing so violates the trust that is basic to the nurse–client relationship. Promoting the benefits of faith and prayer includes respecting clients' choices about doctrine, denomination, beliefs, and traditions (Carson & Koenig, 2008).

BOX 25.2

Faith and Prayer Assessment

Do you consider yourself a spiritual or religious person?

What does your faith mean to you? Has it changed during your illness?

What is the importance of this faith in your daily life?

Do your beliefs influence the way you think about your health or look at your illness?

How important is your religious identification? Do you belong to an organized group?

Tell me about your religious practices, such as worship, prayer, or meditation.

How important is prayer for you now?

What type of prayer would feel comfortable to you now?

What aspects of your faith would you like me to keep in mind as I care for you?

Would you like to discuss religious implications of your care?

Sources: Burkhardt, M. A., & Nagai-Jacobson, M. G. (2002). *Spirituality: Living Our Connections.* Albany, NY: Delmar; Taylor, E. J. (2003). Prayer's clinical issues and implications. *Holistic Nursing Practice,* 17(4): 179–188; and Winslow, G. R., & Winslow, B. W. (2003). Examining the ethics of praying with patients. *Holistic Nursing Practice,* 17(4): 170–177.

Of course, some nurses and physicians do incorporate faith and prayer into their care. Dr. Alijani, a faculty member at Georgetown University Medical School and a well-known surgeon, believes that faith plays a significant role in his patient's well-being. He sees prayer as the literal lifeline between health and spirituality: "Just as my body needs water, carbohydrates, protein, and lipids, my mind needs Allah, and the only way to receive Allah is to pray" (Matthews & Clark, 1998, p. 73).

Health care practitioners are not meant to replace clergy. The roles are distinct. Although many clients may want their spiritual needs addressed by nurses and physicians, others do not, preferring to have these issues addressed by clergy. The practitioner needs to take into account, however, where and how the client's belief enters into the healing process. Nor should health care practitioners be forced against their wishes into participating in clients' religious practices. In the best of worlds, health care professionals and clergy work closely together to provide meaningful holistic care.

Although intercessory prayer is guided by beliefs, experiences, and faith traditions, you can provide some basic guidelines on how clients can incorporate the benefits of intercessory prayer into their lives (Matthews & Clark, 1998):

- If you are ill, ask specifically for people's prayers for healing. It may involve clergy, members of a congregation, adding your name to a prayer list, or asking family and friends to pray for you on a regular basis.

- Pray for your own healing.
- Seek out healing services. Many churches and synagogues offer opportunities to participate in a prayer service or healing service.
- Pray persistently. Keep praying regardless of apparent results. Continuing prayer is an expression of faith and hope.
- Pray for others who are suffering.

As a nurse, you can also teach yourself and others to take time out to count blessings and say "thanks" for the good things in life. Paying attention to what you already have and what is going right helps alleviate stress, anxiety, and depression. An act of gratitude often restores a sense of balance and perspective. You can make the following suggestions:

- Remember to say "thank you." Make it a habit whenever someone helps you out, gives you a compliment, or gives you a gift.
- Create rituals of thanks, for example, saying grace before meals or daily prayers. Practice them until they become a habit.
- Every night before you go to bed, make a list of five things for which you are grateful. It will help take the focus off the stresses in your life.
- Take the time to give back. Look for opportunities to help others and recycle the good fortune you have in your life.
- Once a day, strike a grateful pose. It could be kneeling in prayer or standing with your arms extended joyfully to the sky.
- Take 10 minutes each day to be grateful. Go outside into nature, meditate, or pray. Whatever you do, take the time to appreciate all that you have right now.

As nurses, we must educate ourselves about the clinical relevance of faith and prayer for our clients. The time has come to give more than lip service to the spiritual aspects of our nursing care. It is important that we let our clients know that we will do everything we can do scientifically but that science and technology have their limitations. Perhaps it is appropriate also to let them know that we may pray for guidance in providing competent and compassionate care.

TRY THIS

Projecting Love

1. Visualize someone for whom you have loving feelings. Let the love you feel surround your whole body inside and out. Concentrate on these feelings and project them to this person.
2. Next, visualize someone toward whom you have warm feelings that are not as strong as for the first person. As you focus, send these feelings of love and appreciation to that person.

(continued)

3. Next, visualize someone toward whom you have neutral feelings, nothing strong either way. As you focus on the person, bring the same intensity of love and appreciation you felt for the first two people to the third. Send these feelings to that person.

4. Now visualize someone you have some difficulty with, perhaps whom you dislike but not very intensely. Bring to this person the same feelings of love and appreciation.

5. Finally, visualize someone you have a strong dislike for, and again, as you focus on this person, bring the same degree of love and appreciation you felt for the others. It may be helpful to focus on the person's heart as you do this exercise. Send these feelings to that person.

Source: Collinge, W. (1998). *Subtle Energy.* New York: Warner Books.

References

Benson, H. (1997). *Timeless Healing.* New York: Fireside Book.

Beuscher, L., & Beck, C. (2008). A literature review of spirituality in coping with early-stage Alzheimer's disease. *Journal of Nursing and Healthcare of Chronic Illness* in association with *Journal of Clinical Nursing,* 17(5a): 88–97.

Bormann, J. E., Aschbacher, K., Wetherell, J. L., Roesch, S., & Redwine, L. (2009). Effects of faith/assurance on cortisol levels are enhanced by a spiritual mantram intervention in adults with HIV: A randomized trial. *Journal of Psychosomatic Research,* 66: 161–171.

Braden, G. (2008). *The Spontaneous Healing of Belief.* Carlsbad, CA: Hay House, Inc.

Carson, V. B., & Koenig, H. G. (2008). *Spiritual Dimensions of Nursing Practice.* West Conshohocken, PA: Templeton Foundation Press.

Chida, Y., Steptoe, A., & Powell, L. H. (2009). Religiosity/spirituality and mortality. A systematic quantitative review. *Psychotherapy and Psychosomatics,* 78(2): 81–90.

Dossey, L. (1993). *Healing Words: The Power of Prayer and the Practice of Medicine.* San Francisco: Harper.

Dossey, L. (1997). The return of prayer. *Alternative Therapies,* 3(6): 10–17, 113–120.

Dunn, L. L., Handley, M. C., & Dunkin, J. W. (2009). The provision of spiritual care by registered nurses on a maternal—infant unit. *Journal of Holistic Nursing,* 27(1): 19–28.

Frankl, V. (1984). *Man's Search for Meaning.* New York: Simon & Schuster.

Koenig, H. G. (2008). *Medicine, Religion, and Health.* West Conshohocken, PA: Templeton Foundation Press.

Koerner, J. G. (2007). *Healing Presence: The Essence of Nursing.* New York: Springer Publishing.

Kreitzer, M. J., Gross, C. R., Waleekhachonloet, O. A., Reilly-Spong, M., & Byrd, M. (2009). The brief serenity scale: A psychometric analysis of a measure of spirituality and well-being. *Journal of Holistic Nursing,* 27(1): 7–16.

Masters, K. S., & Spielmans, G. I. (2007). Prayer and health: Review, meta-analysis, and research agenda. *Journal of Behavioral Medicine,* 30(4): 329–338.

Matthews, D. A., & Clark, C. (1998). *The Faith Factor: Proof of the Healing Power of Prayer.* New York: Viking.

Mickley, J. R., Carson, V., & Soeken, K. L. (1995). Religion and adult mental health. *Issues in Mental Health Nursing,* 16: 345–360.

Phelps, A. C., Maciejewski, P. K., Nilsson, M., Balboni, T. A., Wright, A. A., Paulk, M. E., et al. (2009). Religious coping and use of intensive life-prolonging care near death in patients with advanced cancer. *JAMA,* 301(11): 1140–1147.

Rosmarin, D. H., Krumrei, E. J., & Andersson, G. (2009) Religion as a predictor of psychological distress in two religious communities. *Cognitive Behaviour Therapy,* 38(1): 54–64.

Taylor, E. J., Mamier, I., Bahjri, K., Anton, T., & Petersen, F. (2009). Efficacy of a self-study program to teach spiritual care. *Journal of Clinical Nursing,* 18(8): 1131–1140.

Wachholtz, A. B., & Pargament, K. I. (2008). Migraines and meditation: Does spirituality matter? *Journal of Behavioral Medicine,* 31(4): 351–366.

Wachholtz, A. B., & Pearce, M. J. (2009). Does spirituality as a coping mechanism help or hinder coping with chronic pain? *Current Pain and Headache Reports,* 13(2): 127–132.

Resources

Anglican Fellowship in Prayer
1106 Mansfield Ave.
Indiana, PA 15701
724.463.6436
www.afp.org

Buddhist Association of Canada
1330 Bloor St. W
Toronto ON M6H 1P2, Canada
416.537.1342
www.buddhismcanada.com

The Interface Between Medicine and Religion
John Templeton Foundation
300 Conshohocken State Rd., Suite 500
West Conshohocken, PA 19428
610.941.2828
www.templeton.org

Islamic Health and Human Services
Book Tower Building, Suite 2040–41
1249 Washington Blvd.
Detroit, MI 48226
313.961.0678
www.hammoude.com

National Center for Jewish Healing
120 West 57th St.
New York, NY 10019
212.399.2320

National Federation of Spiritual Healers
Old Manor Farm Studio
Church St., Sunbury-on-Thames
Middlesex TW16 6RG, UK
0845.1232.777
www.nfsh.org.uk

Shalem Institute for Spiritual Formation
5430 Grosvenor Rd.
Bethesda, MD 20814
301.897.7334

Other Therapies

The old gods are dead or dying
and people everywhere are searching,
asking: What is the new mythology to be,
the mythology of this unified earth
as one harmonious being?

JOSEPH CAMPBELL

26

Bioelectromagnetics

*You, yourself, as much as anybody in the
entire universe, deserve your love and
affection.*

BUDDHA

Bioelectromagnetics is the emerging science that studies how
living organisms interact with electromagnetic fields. What
underlies all of biochemistry is *electromagnetism*, a form of
energy. Quantum physics has demonstrated that what people see
as solid matter—be that a person or an object—is actually 99.9999
percent empty space filled with energy. Everything is, in fact, energy vibrating at different rates (Braden, 2008).

The earth is 85 percent crystal. Its crust is largely silicon and
oxygen, combined with aluminum, iron, calcium, sodium, potassium, and magnesium. From these chemicals comes a wide variety of crystal colors, shapes, sizes, and hardness. Different
crystals are formed under varying conditions of temperature,
pressure, space, and time. Diamonds, for example, are found only
at a few locations in the world because the exact conditions for
their formation are relatively rare (Kliegel, 2009).

Crystals are solid minerals with a symmetrical internal
atomic structure and can be classified according to their external appearance: cubic, tetragonal, hexagonal, trigonal, or-
thorhombic, monoclinic, and triclinic. The most desirable
crystals are called precious or semiprecious gemstones such as
diamonds, amethyst, aquamarine, rose quartz, opal, topaz, and
turquoise. Imitation or synthetic gemstones are made of materi-
als that look like gems but have a different chemical structure
and physical properties. An example would be blue glass cut to
imitate a sapphire.

BACKGROUND

In the eighteenth century, Guigi Galvani, an Italian physician, conducted experiments on frog muscle to demonstrate that bioelectricity exists within living tissue. Shortly after that, Alessandro Volta, a physicist, found that animal tissue was not needed to produce a current and went on to invent the electric battery in 1800. Michael Faraday, a British chemist, became the greatest experimentalist in electricity and magnetism of the nineteenth century; he produced the first electric motor and succeeded in showing that a magnet could induce electricity. From this early work came many devices for the diagnosis and treatment of disease, including many that are in use today.

In the late 1950s in Japan, doctors began to see a new syndrome of low energy, insomnia, and generalized aches and pains. After extensive research it was discovered that these complaints came from people who spent large amounts of time in metal buildings and were thus shielded from the earth's natural magnetic field. The disorder was labeled "magnetic field deficiency syndrome," and symptoms were alleviated by the external application of magnetic fields to the patients' bodies. Today, magnetic healing continues to be a significant part of mainstream medicine in Japan. Similarly, early Russian cosmonauts who spent more than a year in space were amazed to find that they had lost nearly 80 percent of their bone density. As a result, spacecrafts were designed to include strong artificial magnetic fields on board to avoid this problem. Both of these examples illustrate how magnetic fields are essential to good health and well-being (Collinge, 1998; Trivieri, 2002).

Throughout the ages, crystals have been a part of cultural development. Early people used crystals to make tools and weapons and to generate a spark with which to make fire. Crystals, or gemstones, were also portable forms of wealth and status. The oldest examples of jewelry made of gold, silver, and semiprecious stones were found in the tomb of Queen Pu-abi at Ur, which dates back to 3000 B.C. Early Egyptians, the first to develop cosmetics, highlighted their eyes with powdered malachite (green) and lapis lazuli (blue). Gemstones were worn as amulets, objects believed to bring good luck, protect against evil, and ensure safe travel after death into the next life. The contemporary custom of wearing birthstones is a reflection of this history. Native Americans believed quartz crystals to be the home of supernatural forces that would bring good luck to their hunting trips. The first-known reference to the healing power of certain crystals comes from an Egyptian papyrus from 1600 B.C. It gave directions for curative use, such as placing crystals on various areas of the body and grinding them up and mixing with a liquid for internal consumption (Kircher, 2006).

CONCEPTS

Geomagnetic Field

Every atom and cell of the body is a small magnetic field that radiates out into space, decreasing in strength with distance and ultimately becoming lost in the jumble of other magnetic fields. Like the human body, the earth radiates an energy field outwardly, called the **geomagnetic field.** This energy originates in the earth's core and radiates out beyond the atmosphere, stimulating and protecting all life on earth. Migrating birds or fish returning to their spawning grounds navigate over great distances with the help of magnetic field receptors in their brains. It is believed that they tune in to the magnetic field of the earth to determine location and direction. Animals are attuned to the geomagnetic field and can sense subtle changes in it. For example, dogs, horses, and cattle often become agitated just before an earthquake (Smith, 2008).

Every few years, the sun becomes hyperactive and releases a high-speed cloud of charged particles, called a **coronal mass ejection (CME).** Energy is dumped into the earth's magnetic field, creating a geomagnetic storm that may last a few hours up to a few days. This geomagnetic storm creates havoc with power grids, mobile phone signals, navigational systems, and satellite systems.

A magnetic field is like a generator, generating internal energy that can penetrate the body as if it were air. A strong magnet held on one side of the hand can easily deflect a compass needle on the other side of the same hand. As the magnetic field penetrates the body, it causes one's atomic particles to fly around faster and interact with more force.

Subtle changes occur in the strength of the geomagnetic field with the time of day. The day side of the planet—that side facing the sun—always has a slightly weaker field, because the energy coming out of the earth is being "pushed" back and compressed by the radiation from the sun. Thus, the magnetic field passing through the human body is stronger on the nighttime side, away from the sun. Chemical reactions, the healing process, and other cellular activities accelerate in the presence of a stronger field, and, thus, they are improved slightly at night because of the stronger field (Collinge, 1998).

Like a giant mirror, the moon reflects radiation from the sun toward the earth, thus affecting the earth's energy field. The full moon and the new moon are opposite in their effect on the geomagnetic field. The greatest amount of solar radiation is reflected toward the earth during a full moon, which pushes back and compresses the earth's energy, resulting in a weaker magnetic field than during a new moon.

A stronger magnetic field is more conducive to sleep, which makes sleep at night more refreshing and healing than sleep in the daytime, and sleep in the full moon phase is longer and more restful than sleep in the new moon phase. In addition, the sun "agitates" the earth's field with sunspot activity. These intense magnetic explosions on the sun spray additional radiation on the earth, in turn disturbing the geomagnetic field. During these periods of geomagnetic disturbance, higher admission rates to psychiatric facilities and higher rates of violence are characteristic. On the other hand, when the earth's magnetic field is most quiet, more paranormal experiences like mental telepathy, clairvoyance, and precognition take place (Terra-Bustamante et al., 2009).

Endogenous Magnetic Fields

Endogenous magnetic fields are those produced within the body. This electrical activity demonstrates patterns that provide medically useful information. EKGs and EEGs, for example, provide information about the endogenous magnetic fields of the heart and brain and are diagnostic in any number of conditions. New technologies in developing instruments that are extremely sensitive have opened new lines of research.

Like other kinds of magnetic fields, the human energy field is the strongest at its source and fades with distance. Another name for this energy field is **aura** and it is the field that surrounds the body as far as the outstretched arms and from head to toe. See Chapter 2 for more detailed information on auras. The human energy field is both an information center and a highly sensitive perceptual system that transmits and receives messages as people interact with their surrounding environment. Patterns of circulation of energy within the body include the meridian system and the chakras. Virtually every alternative healing therapy has a way of interpreting these subtle energy fields (Braden, 2008).

Recent research has uncovered a form of endogenous radiation, an extremely low-level light known as **biophoton emission.** It is believed that biophoton emission may be important in gene expression, membrane transport, and bioregulation. Externally applied energy fields may alter biophoton emission to the benefit or detriment of the organism. This, as well as other endogenous fields of the body, may prove to be involved in energetic therapies such as Therapeutic Touch (Hossu & Rupert, 2006).

Exogenous Magnetic Fields

Exogenous magnetic fields are those produced by sources outside the body and can be classified as either artificial or natural. **Artificial exogenous fields** are created by such things as power lines, transformers, appliances, radio transmitters, and medical devices. Artificial electromagnetic fields are unpolarized. Their behavior is chaotic and disordered as they pass through the body's cells. This chaotic nature disturbs the endogenous magnetic fields, resulting in damage to the body's tissues. A number of studies have found an association between these fields and an increase in brain tumors, childhood leukemia, depression, suicide, chromosomal abnormalities, and learning difficulties. The frequency at which some of these exogenous fields pulse can also create problems for people. For example, the household current in the United States is pulsed at 60 cycles per second compared to brain frequencies of 8 to 22 cycles per second while awake and as low as 2 cycles per second while sleeping. The more electrical devices in the bedroom, the more likely the interference with the brain's natural frequencies resulting in disturbed sleep and fatigue. As long as televisions and computers are plugged in, they emit electrical impulses even when turned off. It would be the best, therefore, to unplug all electrical devices in the bedroom prior to sleep (Yang et al., 2008).

The earth's geomagnetic field is one example of a **natural exogenous field.** Another example is moving water. When people are at beaches, on river banks, beside waterfalls, or even walking outside after a powerful rainstorm, they often experience feelings of relaxation and peace. While these feelings may be attributed to the psychological cues from these environments, they also have an energetic basis. When water moves or flows, it releases negative ions into the air. When people are surrounded by negative ions, they seem to balance their energy fields. As Collinge (1998) states, "It is as if the metaphors of 'cleansing' and 'washing away' that we associate with moving waters have a real basis in their impact on the field of emotional energy that surrounds and penetrates our body" (p. 93).

Ionizing/Nonionizing Fields

Electromagnetic fields can also be classified as ionizing or nonionizing. A field is an **ionizing electromagnetic field** if its energy is high enough to dislodge electrons from an atom or molecule such as gamma rays or X-rays. Because these rays are strongly ionizing in biological matter, prolonged exposure is harmful. **Nonionizing electromagnetic fields** may have nonharmful and even beneficial effects on biological tissue. This effect is the basis for bioelectromagnetic (BEM) field application and research.

The actual mechanism by which BEM produces biological effects is under intense study. It is likely that BEM affects the cell membrane, perhaps at the receptors where neurotransmitters and neurohormones bind. Alteration in the binding process then alters the cell's internal processes. Interestingly, some specific frequencies of BEM affect specific target tissues, just as drugs affect specific tissues. Magnetic fields are also believed to stimulate cellular metabolism and oxygenate tissues, which relieves inflammation and facilitates cellular repair.

Resonance

Another principle related to electromagnetics is **resonance,** which is simply defined as sympathetic vibration. For example, when a tuning fork, turned to note A, is sounded near a piano or guitar, any string that is tuned to that same tone will pick up the vibration and begin to move, while the other strings will not. Crystals possess electromagnetic properties and are capable of resonating in harmony with another form. It is believed that when the body's natural frequencies become unbalanced, people experience disease. The resonance of crystals is believed to harmonize and balance the body's frequencies back to optimum, healthy levels. The disrupted field (the ill person) receives energy from the stronger field (the crystal) until the two find their own balance and resonate in harmony. At the current time, however, no explanations for crystal healing fit within known scientific facts (Kircher, 2006; Smith, 2008)

TREATMENT

Magnetic field therapy and crystal healing work on the principle that every animal, plant, and mineral has an electromagnetic field that enables organic beings and inorganic objects, such as crystals, to communicate and interact as part of a single, unified energy system. There are **static magnetic fields** produced by natural or artificial magnets and **pulsating magnetic fields** produced by electrical devices. These magnetic fields are able to penetrate the body and affect the functioning of cells, tissues, organs, and systems. These therapies work best in combination with other healing modalities and are considered to be adjunct treatments to conventional medicine. They should not be used by themselves for any major disease or medical condition (Eden, 2008).

Nonionizing BEM medical applications are classified into two types, thermal or nonthermal. *Thermal* or heat applications include radio-frequency (RF) hyperthermia, laser and RF surgery, and RF diathermy. The most important BEM modalities in alternative medicine are the nonthermal applications. The term *nonthermal* means that it causes no significant gross tissue heating. An example is microwave resonance therapy where the mechanism of action is thought to be in the modification of the cell membrane. The major alternative healing applications of nonthermal, nonionizing electromagnetic fields are bone repair, nerve stimulation, wound healing, the treatment of osteoarthritis, electroacupuncture, tissue regeneration, immune system stimulation, and neuroendocrine modulations (Robitaille & Berliner, 2006). Box 26.1 describes these applications.

Being immersed in a field of negative ions seems to balance people's energy and relieve pain. Physicians specializing in orthopedics and sports medicine have been recommending *magnets* since 1993. Athletic performance is enhanced and risk of serious injury is decreased when magnets are used to warm up muscles and joints. People wear magnets on their wrists, elbows, and knees for joint pain or on their heads for headaches. Magnets are used to speed the healing of wounds. Though not recognized as medical devices by the Food and Drug Administration, magnets have been widely used in Asia for years. Blood cells, believed to have tiny positive charges at one end and negative charges at the other end, respond to the pull of magnets, thus increasing blood flow to the area. The increased blood flow brings in more healing nutrients and carries off toxins. Magnets appear to block pain by altering the electromagnetic balance between negatively charged and positively charged ions in the nerve pathways that carry pain messages. The magnets used are about five to ten times as strong as refrigerator door magnets and cost between $15 and $35 a pair depending on the size.

A few *contraindications* for magnetic therapy need to be observed. Until further research is conducted, pregnant women should not wear magnets over the abdominal area. Magnets should not be used by persons wearing pacemakers, defibrillators, aneurysm clips in the brain, cochlear (inner ear) implants, or other implanted electrical devices. Magnets decrease the stickiness of platelets, which contributes to increased bleeding. For that reason,

BOX 26.1

Applications of Nonthermal, Nonionizing Electromagnetic Fields

Transcutaneous electrical nerve stimulation (TENS)	Used for pain relief
Transcranial electrostimulation (TCES)	Used to reduce symptoms of depression, anxiety, and insomnia; may be effective in drug dependence
Repetitive transcranial magnetic stimulation (rTMS)	Used in place of electroconvulsive therapy in certain types of mood disorders; used in diagnostic nerve conduction studies
Pulsed electromagnetic fields (PEMFs)	Used to stimulate bone growth; fractures
Electromyography	Used to diagnose and treat carpal tunnel syndrome and other movement disorders
Magnetoencephalography (MEG)	More accurate and precise than EEG. Used in psychiatry and in development of new medications
Electroretinography	Noninvasive monitoring of rapid eye movement sleep
Magnetic resonance imaging (MRI)	Identifies structural abnormalities in three dimensions
Magnetic molecular energizing (MME)	Improves oxygen carrying capacity, assimilation of nutrients, manufacture of enzymes, metabolic waste removal, and reduction of free radicals
Vagus nerve stimulation (VNS)	Used for hard-to-treat seizure disorders; depression
Power spectral analysis (PSA)	Monitors the amplitude and latency of brain electrical discharges

they should not be used by people on anticoagulants or who have an actively bleeding or open wound. Magnets should not be used with a freshly torn muscle that is still bleeding internally. In this situation, it is best to wait 3 to 5 days after the injury, or 10 to 14 days if the tear is severe, before using magnets to aid the healing process.

Crystal healing is based on tuning in to the natural vibrations of a mineral from the earth, which has infused it with its energies. For this reason, neither imitation nor synthetic crystals are suitable for healing. In **electrocrystal therapy,**

the body is initially scanned with a specially adapted video camera that relays a colored picture of the auric field to a computer screen. The therapist marks those areas where the color of the aura is inappropriate, indicating stress or dysfunction. Electrocrystal therapy uses quartz crystals in saline solution that are enclosed in a sealed, glass electrode connected to a battery. Up to five electrodes are placed against the affected area or over a chakra point. The crystals are electrically stimulated, which amplifies their natural healing vibrations until they vibrate and resonate at a desired frequency. This treatment is thought to bring the endogenous fields back to a harmonious state (Kliegel, 2009).

Crystal cards, meant to be worn on the body, were developed as a result of the NASA space program. Astronauts travel into space with a number of pyramid-shaped quartz crystals, electronically charged to vibrate at the frequency of the earth's geomagnetic field, to combat the negative effects of spending time outside the earth's magnetic field. The crystal cards sold in stores contain a number of tiny corundum crystals that are electrochemically etched with hydrochloric acid. The acid changes the form of the crystals, which produces beneficial negative ions and harmonizes cellular activity.

Electronic gem therapy blends modern technology with traditional Ayurvedic medicine by combining gemstones or crystals, colored light, and electronic amplification. Depending on the condition, patients either require cooling gems such as emerald, topaz, or carnelian or warming gems such as ruby, chrysoberyl, or citrine. During treatment, the gemstone is electronically vibrated at a frequency set for a specific condition. The energy from the gemstone is focused by special colored lamps called gem transducers onto the part of the body requiring treatment. It is believed the treatment provides additional energy needed to bring about self-healing. The seven chakras are assigned different gemstones corresponding to their vibratory rates. In crystal bodywork, people place crystals on the chakras as they meditate (Kircher, 2006). Box 26.2 lists the gemstones or crystals associated with each chakra. See Chapter 2 for more detailed information on chakras.

RESEARCH

No known published articles demonstrate the effectiveness of crystal healing via clinical trials. Little research has been conducted in the United States regarding the clinical effects of magnets. In Europe and Russia, however, where magnetism is well regarded, hundreds of scientific studies have been documented. One study investigated the use of implanted magnets in esophageal–gastric hog specimens. This study demonstrated that it was possible to reinforce the esophageal sphincter to prevent gastroesophageal reflux (Bortolotti, Grandis, & Mazzero, 2009).

Extensive research in the United States regarding BEM applications is illustrated in the following examples:

- Six people with focal hand dystonia, which interferes with functional use of hands, were given rTMS to their premotor cortex. After 5 days of

BOX 26.2

Crystals, Gemstones, and Chakras

Root Chakra

Agate, bloodstone, tiger's eye, hematite

Sexual Chakra

Moonstone, tiger's eye, citrine, carnelian

Solar Plexus Chakra

Citrine, rose quartz, aventurine quartz, malachite

Heart Chakra

Jade, aventurine quartz, watermelon tourmaline, rose quartz

Throat Chakra

Aquamarine, lapis lazuli, turquoise, celestite

Third Eye Chakra

Amethyst, fluorite, lapis lazuli, sodalite

Crown Chakra

Amethyst, celestite, jade, rock crystal (clear quartz)

treatment, they experienced decreased cortical excitability and improved handwriting (Borich, Arora, & Kimberley, 2009).
- Forty-eight people who were chronic smokers participated in a randomized, double-blind, sham-controlled study using rTMS on the left dorsolateral prefrontal cortex. Ten daily sessions reduced both cigarette use and craving for cigarettes (Amiaz, Levy, Vainiger, Grunhaus, & Zangen, 2009).
- Forty people with schizophrenia were randomized to the control group (received antipsychotics) or experimental group (received antipsychotics and rTMS). The study demonstrated a significant improvement in auditory hallucination in the experimental group compared to the control group (Bagati, Nizamie, & Prakash, 2009).

The following is a small sample of studies related to electromagnetic fields:
- Out of 835 children studies between 2000 and 2008, there were 10 sudden unexplained deaths in epilepsy (SUDEP). These deaths were investigated

in terms of the phase of the moon. Seventy percent of these deaths occurred during the full moon phase. This may be related to the sleep disturbance that occurs during a full moon that may increase seizure frequency (Terra-Bustamante et al., 2009).

- In the past, some studies have related suicide to the full moon phase. This study looked at 65,206 suicides in Austria between 1970 and 2006. They found that there was no lunar effect on the suicide rate (Voracek et al., 2008).

- Medically unexplained stroke is thought to be a psychosomatic disorder. In this disorder, people exhibit stroke symptoms, but there is no medical evidence of a stroke. While stroke admissions are not related to lunar phases, medically unexplained stroke symptoms are significantly increased during full moon phases (Ahmad, Quinn, Dawson, & Walters, 2008).

INTEGRATED NURSING PRACTICE

Awareness of magnetic healing is gaining credibility in the United States and is being applied by increasing numbers of conventional as well as alternative health care practitioners as an adjunctive therapy. Increasing numbers of people are sleeping on magnetic beds at night and wearing small magnets during the day for pain relief, greater energy, and healing. Treatments can last from just a few minutes to overnight and, depending on the situation and severity, may be applied several times a day for days or weeks at a time.

Some controversy surrounds the issue of when to use the north, or negative pole, and when to use the south, or positive pole. Some people believe that the north pole of a magnet enhances healing and health, while the south pole exacerbates disease. Practitioners in Japan and Russia believe no strong evidence supports the use of one pole over the other, but rather that the entirety of the magnet is doing the healing.

Explain to clients that the effectiveness of magnetic treatment depends on the number of magnets used and their strength, thickness, and spacing. Magnets vary in strength and those used for healing purposes are generally between 1,000 and 5,000 gauss. The Tesla is another measurement: one Tesla equals 10,000 gauss. In general, healing magnets are unipolar and are either circular or rectangular. Several can be stacked for increased gauss strength and, therefore, greater effectiveness. The thicker the magnet, the greater the depth of penetration. The problem with this is that, with increasing thickness, the magnet becomes more uncomfortable to wear. Most people wear magnets between one-fourth- and three-eighth-inch thick. In general, the magnet should be larger than the size of the area being treated. Clients who are treating finger joints for arthritis will use a small magnet, while those who are treating the lower back will apply a much larger magnet.

When teaching clients about magnetic therapy, you can explain that the most common use is in the treatment of pain, with reports of successful treatment in arthritis, rheumatism, fibromyalgia, back pain, headaches, muscle sprains and strains, joint pain, tendonitis, shoulder pain, carpal tunnel syndrome, and torn ligaments. A magnetic field can also function like an antibiotic by lowering acidity, which is a hostile environment for microorganisms. A magnetic field applied to the head has a sedating effect by stimulating the hormone melatonin. Biomagnetic therapy increases general well-being by enhancing energy through the repolarization of cells. Many professional athletes revitalize their bodies by sleeping on a magnetic mattress pad. Some even participate in their sport with dozens of magnets taped to their bodies (Eden, 2008).

Magnetic therapy may be one of the most effective methods for achieving relief from arthritis, especially in the hands and feet. People with carpal tunnel syndrome can apply magnets to the front and back of the wrist to help control symptoms. Individuals diagnosed with fibromyalgia can sleep on a magnetic mattress pad and use a magnetic pillow. They may also use magnets over the painful areas during the day. Magnetic insoles increase circulation and help conditions such as numbness, burning, aches, restlessness, and leg cramps. If you have a client with phantom pain following an amputation, you may suggest the use of magnets that improve the flow of blood in the stump and cause the phantom pain to disappear. People with asthma and bronchitis may find that wearing a strong neodymium magnet over the chest and at an equal level on the back will help return breathing to a normal state. For minor burns, people can place a magnet over the site of injury to speed the healing and reduce the pain (Keet & Keet, 2007).

It is unclear at this time whether you should suggest that clients wear the magnets full time or intermittently. This recommendation will need to be determined through further research. At this time, you can encourage clients to experiment with time periods that seem most effective. As our scientific and clinical understanding increases, we will be able to provide greater knowledge about how to manipulate magnets for the best effects.

TRY THIS

Absorbing Earth Energy

Find a grassy, open area that is in its relatively natural state. You may or may not choose to use a blanket. Lie face down with your arms and legs extended in a spread-out fashion. Notice that all your chakras are in direct contact with the earth. Visualize an exchange of energy as you release to the earth, with each out-breath, any stress or negativity you have been carrying. With each in-breath, imagine that your chakras are receiving fresh, balanced, healing energy from the earth. Do this relaxation breathing for at least 20 minutes. You should feel yourself in a pleasant and refreshed state.

Many people use crystals in combination with other healing modalities. Some people choose crystals intuitively while others select crystals on the basis of therapeutic qualities. You can help individuals determine which crystal is "right" for them by asking the following questions (Chase & Pawlik, 2002):

- What do you want the crystal for—healing, meditation, energizing your environment, as a focus for visualization, or for decoration?
- Which crystals are most appealing—geometrically shaped, such as clear quartz, or "massive," such as rose quartz?
- Which colors are appealing to you—pale or deep shades? Do you prefer clear or opaque?
- What size crystal are you looking for?
- Do you prefer cut and polished crystals or ones that are completely natural?
- How much are you prepared to spend?

Members of the quartz family, such as clear quartz, amethyst, and rose quartz, are the crystals used most frequently in healing. Amethyst is the "stone of meditation," creating a state of enhanced spirituality and contentment. Clear quartz represents the clarity of mind that people hope to achieve through meditation. Chapter 17 provides general guidelines for meditation. Building on this process, you can encourage clients to try a crystal for focus in meditation. Maintaining a focus on a crystal helps quiet one's thoughts during meditation. Instruct clients to hold the crystal or place it in front of them on the floor or on a small table. Some people take three similar crystals and position them in an equilateral triangle, forming a charged energy field in which to sit. Explain that they are to half-close their eyes and gaze at the crystal, concentrating on its color, shape, and size during their meditation. As they come out of the meditative state, they should continue to focus on the crystal and open their eyes gradually.

People who are experiencing illness or disease may find that crystal imagery improves the healing process. Explain imagery to clients as described in Chapter 18 and add the following steps (Lilly, 2002):

- Assume your meditative position and focus on the crystal in front of you.
- Close your eyes, while continuing to visualize the crystal.
- Allow this image of the crystal to become bigger and bigger until it completely surrounds you.
- Imagine that you are at the center of the crystal.
- Notice that you have become one with the crystal.
- Image the illness or disease leaving your body as you become one with the crystal.
- Consider how it feels to share the same perfection and clarity as the crystal. Be aware that you are whole and complete as you are one with the crystal.
- Contemplate how the crystal forms a protective shield around you so that you are totally safe and secure.

TRY THIS

Going to the Mountains

If you live near hills or mountains, go to the highest natural point you can reach. High places are concentrations of energy and seem to lift us above our normal conflicting energies. Looking down below, get a sense of the differences in the two energetic environments. The higher point you are on may feel like clear, focused energy while the area below may feel like a mixture of many different energies. After a while you should experience clearer thinking and a sense of inspiration.

Source: Collinge, W. (1998). *Subtle Energy*. New York: Warner Books.

- When you sense that your inner journey is completed, begin to separate yourself from the crystal.
- Reduce the crystal to its normal size.
- Fade this picture from your mind, open your eyes, and take a few deep breaths to bring yourself back into the here and now.
- Be aware of any thoughts, feelings, or emotions that come to you.

When people begin to use crystals, they should keep them on their bodies at all times for a least 3 weeks, to ensure removal of blockages of energy. They can be worn as jewelry, kept in pockets, or worn in medicine bags around the neck. Crystals are used in meditation, spiritual ceremonies, laid on the body during types of massage or bodywork, or when a person is resting. They are believed to strengthen the body, increase energy, and provide a sense of calmness. Red, yellow, and orange stones boost energy; clear and aquamarine stones are used for healing; and lavender and blue-violet stones have calming effects.

References

Ahmad, F., Quinn, T. J., Dawson, J., & Walters, M. (2008). A link between lunar phase and medically unexplained stroke symptoms: An unearthly influence? *Journal of Psychosomatic Research*, 65(2): 131–133.

Amiaz, R., Levy, D., Vainiger, K. D., Grunhaus, L., & Zangen, A. (2009). Repeated high-frequency transcranial magnetic stimulation over the dorso-lateral prefrontal cortex reduces cigarette craving and consumption. *Addiction*, 104(4): 653–660.

Bagati, D., Nizamie, S. H., & Prakash, R. (2009). Effect of augmentatory repetitive transcranial magnetic stimulation on auditory hallucinations in schizophrenia: Randomized controlled study. *The Australian & New Zealand Journal of Psychiatry*, 43(4): 386–392.

Borich, M., Arora, S., & Kimberley, T. J. (2009). Lasting effects of repeated rTMS application in focal hand dystonia. *Restorative Neurology and Neuroscience*, 27(1): 55–65.

Bortolotti, M., Grandis, A., & Mazzero, G. (2009). A novel endoesophageal magnetic device to prevent gastroesophageal reflux. *Surgical Endoscopy*, 23(4): 885–889.

Braden, G. (2008). *The Spontaneous Healing of Belief*. Carlsbad, CA: Hay House.

Chase, P. L., & Pawlik, J. (2002). *Healing with Gemstones*. Franklin Lakes, NJ: New Page Books.

Collinge, W. (1998). *Subtle Energy*. New York: Warner Books.

Eden, D. (2008). *Energy Medicine for Women*. London: Penguin Group.

Hossu, M., & Rupert, R. (2006). Quantum events of biophoton emission associated with complementary and alternative medicine therapies. *Journal of Alternative and Complementary Medicine*, 12(2): 119–124.

Keet, L., & Keet, M. (2007). *Hand Reflexology*, London: Hamlyn.

Kircher, N. (2006). *Gemstone Reflexology*. Rochester, VT: Healing Arts Press.

Kliegel, E. (2009). *Crystal Wands: For Healing, Massage Therapy, and Reflexology*. Findhorn, Forres, Great Britain: Findhorn Press.

Lilly, S. (2002). *Crystal Healing*. London: Element.

Robitaille, P. M., & Berliner, L. (2006). *Ultra High Field Magnetic Resonance Imaging*. New York: Springer.

Smith, K. (2008). *Awakening the Energy Body*. Rochester, VT: Bear & Company.

Terra-Bustamante, V. C., Scorza, C. A., de Albuquerque, M., Sakamoto, A. C., Machado, H. R., Arida, R. M., et al. (2009). Does the lunar phase have an effect on sudden unexpected death in epilepsy? *Epilepsy & Behavior*, 14(2): 404–406.

Trivieri, L. (2002). *Alternative Medicine: The Definitive Guide*. Berkeley, CA: Celestial Arts.

Voracek, M., Loibl, L. M., Kapusta, N. D., Niederkrotenthaler, T., Dervic, K., & Sonneck, G. (2008). Not carried away by a moon light shadow. *Wiener Klinische Wochenschrift*, 120(11–12): 343–349.

Yang, Y., Jin, X., Yan, C., Tian, Y., Tang, J., & Shen, X. (2008). Case-only study of interactions between DNA repair genes (hMLH1, APEX1, MGMT, XRCC1 and XPD) and low-frequency electromagnetic fields in childhood acute leukemia. *Leukemia & Lymphoma*, 49(12): 2344–2350.

Resources

Advanced Magnetic Research Institute
    International
#109, 5421 11th St. NE
Calgary, AL T2E 6M4 CA
1.800.265.1119
www.amri-intl.com

Affiliation of Crystal Healing
    Organisations
P.O. Box 530
Dorking, Surrey RH4 9FG UK
07.837.696.301
www.crystal-healing.org

Bio-Electro-Magnetics Institute
5 Mark Twain Ave.
Reno, NV 89509
775.560.7800
www.bemi.org

27

Animal-Assisted Therapy

There are two means of refuge from the miseries of life: music and cats.

ALBERT SCHWEITZER

A dog wags its tail with its heart.

MARTIN BUXBAUM

Living with a dog is one way to retain something of a child's spirit.

MICHAEL ROSEN

Animal-assisted therapy (AAT) is defined as the use of specifically selected animals as a treatment modality in health and human service settings. AAT has been steadily gaining in popularity in the United States and has been shown to be a successful intervention for people with a variety of physical or psychological conditions. Despite reluctance and skepticism on the part of many administrators of health care facilities, nurses have often advocated the use of animals as a therapeutic intervention. One of the earliest recorded observations of a connection between animals and health was made by Florence Nightingale (1969) in 1860 when she noted "a small pet is often an excellent companion for the sick, for long chronic cases especially" (p. 103). She further suggested that when possible, patients should participate in the care of the animal because this activity was helpful to their recovery. Long banned from health care facilities, dogs, cats, and other pets are gradually being welcomed with open arms.

BACKGROUND

In 900 B.C., Homer wrote about Asklepios, the Greek god of healing whose healing power was transmitted through sacred dogs. In the ninth century, people in Gheel, Belgium, began using animals to care for people with disabilities. Theirs was the first recorded therapeutic farm animal program for patients. The York Retreat in England, founded in 1792 for the treatment of people with mental illness, used small animals such as rabbits and poultry in their treatment plan. The goal was to decrease the use of restraints and medications by helping residents learn self-control through animals that relied on them for care. Bethel, a residential treatment center for people with epilepsy, founded in 1867 in Germany, utilized pets as an important part of the treatment program. This pet program is still in place today and has expanded to include farm animals and a wild game park. In the United States in the 1940s, injured World War II soldiers were encouraged to work with the hogs, cattle, and horses on the farm of the Army Air Corps Convalescent Hospital in New York. Since that time, animals have been used in many U.S. clinical settings from pediatrics to geriatrics, acute care facilities, and chronic care homes, from group accommodations to private homes, from prevention to healing, and even from schools to correctional facilities nationwide (Fine, 2006).

PREPARATION

In the 1990s, the Delta Society developed the first comprehensive standards of practice for animal-assisted therapy. *Standards of Practice for Animal-Assisted Activities and Animal-Assisted Therapy* (1996) defines the role of animals in therapeutic programs.

Therapy dogs and cats are specifically selected for temperament, companionability, and interaction. Temperament is the animal's natural or instinctive behavior and is important in terms of the way the animal will react when stressed. A good therapy pet is calm, tolerant, and friendly. The second major criterion is that the animal has a person who is willing to volunteer time and energy in order to share the pet with others. Dogs must be obedience trained prior to participating in the program. A dog or cat must be at least one year of age before enrolling in the training and visiting program to better ensure that the pet has been effectively socialized and is comfortable interacting with numerous people in a crowded setting. In addition, the animal's immune system is more stabilized by this age. A veterinarian must verify the animal's health and all inoculations must be current. AAT-registering organizations require that a dog and its handler pass several tests prior to registration. In general, dogs have to demonstrate basic obedience skills and must be indifferent to crowds and distractions and unfazed by exuberant or clumsy handling, including ear tugging and "bear hugging." In addition, they must have a high tolerance for unfamiliar or loud noises and peculiar smells. Therapeutic riding horses must have a gentle, tolerant temperament, be well balanced and well muscled, and move with even strides. In addition to the familiar dogs and cats in pet therapy, other animals may include parrots, cockatoos, guinea pigs, rabbits, pot-bellied pigs, dwarf goats, llamas, donkeys, and horses. In recent years, dolphin-assisted therapy has become very popular and a number of these programs exist worldwide. The cost is significantly higher for dolphins than for other AAT programs.

Animal handler volunteers are trained in workshops or through home study courses. The handlers must pass a written test and their animals must pass a skills test. Participation in continuing education is required. Nurses, physical and occupational therapists, psychotherapists, and other health care professionals must receive training before they can direct animal-assisted therapy programs. This educational process is still in the beginning stages and at this time is primarily accomplished through in-service training and seminars and workshops at national and international professional meetings (King, 2007).

Many countries, including the United States and Canada, offer formalized educational programs for registration, certification, or licensure of therapists. These programs offer intermittent sessions that may span one to two years. Most frequently this specialized training is offered to physical therapists, occupational therapists, psychotherapists, and special education teachers.

CONCEPTS

Companion Animals

Many people think of their animals as surrogate children. But one big exception is that these are children who rarely, if ever, disappoint their parents. Pets, especially dogs, often seem to understand what their owners are feeling. For some people, a pet is a reason to get up in the morning. It is something to nurture, touch, and stroke. For stress relief, it apparently does not matter much whether the pet is a Labrador, a tomcat, or a canary. What is most important is the person's relationship with the pet.

The contributions companion animals make to the emotional well-being of people include providing unconditional love and opportunities for affection; functioning as a confidant, playmate, and companion; and assisting in the achievement of trust, responsibility, and empathy toward others. Studies of children with pets indicate that the unconditional love and acceptance conveyed in the child–animal relationship may validate a child's sense of self-worth. In addition, older school-age children often turn to companion animals in times of stress for reassurance. Children often perceive their companion animals as play partners, most often during middle childhood than during adolescence or early childhood (Sockalingam et al., 2008).

Children with interactive pets such as dogs and cats are more attached to their companion animals than are children with other types of pets such as hamsters, fish, and turtles. Emotional bonds are more likely to be formed with animals that are able to respond in an outwardly loving and affectionate way. Behaviors such as tail wagging, barking, and purring often elicit affectionate responses in human caregivers. In North America and Europe, pets are found in the majority of homes with children. Families with children, especially school-age children, are more likely to own companion animals than are families without children. Multiple-pet ownership is also common. Pet ownership remains higher in rural versus urban areas, and in houses versus apartments. Still, across a variety of settings, the majority of children in Western countries are living with companion animals.

Therapy Animals

The characteristics that make many pets cherished family members—unconditional affection, responsiveness, and companionability—also make pets effective in therapy. In this age of high technological health care, it is sometimes easy to forget the importance of unconditional affection. Animals pay little attention to age or physical ability, but accept people as they are. It is insignificant if the person has no hair, is in a wheelchair, or is hallucinating. The underlying concept that supports the use of animals for therapeutic reasons is the bonding experience it provides. Frail or depressed older adults often brighten up and adopt a more positive outlook when they are in the presence of an animal "therapist."

Many health care professionals are finding that loneliness may be as serious as cancer and heart disease for older adults. Older people who stay active, find substitutes for work, and build new relationships as partners and friends die have been found to be the most satisfied with life. Not all older adults, however, have options for remaining active and forming new friendships. Visiting with animals can help people feel less lonely and less depressed. Animals can provide a welcome change from routine or a distraction from disability or pain. People often talk to the animals and share with them their thoughts, feelings, and memories. When people talk to people, their blood pressure tends to go up because of questions of how one is being evaluated or judged. With animals, who are always eager to please and unconditionally accepting, people's blood pressure levels tend to go down (King, 2007).

Animals also make it easier for two strangers to talk. They give people a common interest, provide a focus for conversation, and broaden the circle of friends. When animals visit long-term care facilities, residents laugh and mingle more than when the animals are not around. Animals also help stimulate socialization by providing an opportunity to share stories of animals the residents may have had in the past. Many people like to stroke the animal while talking about the pets that shared their lives.

TREATMENT

Animal-Assisted Therapy

Animal-assisted therapy is the use of specifically selected animals as a treatment modality in health and human service settings. In AAT, an accredited professional guides the human–animal interaction toward specific, individualized therapeutic goals. In one treatment session, a variety of goals can be addressed: *physical goals* such as range of motion, balance, and mobility; *cognitive goals* such as improved memory or verbal expression; *emotional goals* such as increased self-esteem and motivation; and *social goals* such as building rapport and improved socialization skills. Linda Hume, LPN, AAT specialist, has developed a program of animal facilitation in occupational and physical therapy at Northeast Rehabilitation Hospital in Salem, New Hampshire. The following are a few of the goals and activities she has identified for AAT in her clinical setting (Hume, 2002):

- *Increased upper extremity range of motion:* Throw an object for dog to retrieve; use leash to maneuver dog; pet, stroke, brush animal.
- *Mobility:* Ambulate with dog.
- *Improved coordination:* Throw an object for dog to retrieve (releasing); reach for object dog has retrieved.
- *Improved memory:* Ask client to recall dog's name, breed, age, and so forth; command dog to sit and remember to release dog from command.
- *Increased language production:* Use commands with dog; simply converse to or about animal.
- *Object identification:* Direct dog to retrieve specific familiar items by appropriate name—ball, spoon, pen, cup.
- *Attention/concentration:* Attend to dog, task, and therapist.

Therapeutic horseback riding, or hippotherapy, is defined as all rehabilitative uses of horses. The term derives from the Greek word *hippo* meaning "horse." In *hippopsychotherapy*, the riding is designed to support the psychotherapeutic treatment plan. Goals include increased self-confidence, improved self-esteem, refined social competence, the experience of pleasure, and the ability to establish a relationship with the horse. *Remedial educational riding* is used to further the educational and behavioral goals for school-age children with learning problems. The horse is used as a strong motivator for accomplishing specific treatment goals. *Physical hippotherapy* is the use of the rhythmic movement of the horse to increase sensory processing and improve posture, balance, and mobility in people with movement dysfunctions. The transfer of movement from the horse to the client is designed primarily to achieve physical goals, but may also affect psychological, cognitive, behavioral, and communication outcomes. Clients benefiting from hippotherapy include, but are not limited to, adults and children with cerebral palsy, multiple sclerosis, orthopedic problems, posttraumatic spasticity, strokes, scoliosis, genetic syndromes, autism, and developmental delays (Hakanson, Moller, Lindstrom, & Mattsson, 2009).

There are *Dolphin Assisted Therapy* (DAT) programs throughout the world. They are used to lessen symptoms of a wide range of conditions such as depression, Down syndrome, autistic spectrum disorders, speech disorders, cerebral palsy, and traumatic brain injury. There is no evidence at the present time that DAT provides greater benefit than other animal assisted therapies (Phillips, 2008).

The National Animal Assisted Crisis Response organization provides dog and handler teams to help victims of crisis or disaster situations. They have been sent to many situations, including Hurricane Katrina, the Virginia Tech massacre, and the Northern Illinois University massacre. Some victims talk to the comfort dogs while others just want to pet or hug the dogs.

Animal-Assisted Activities

A less formal approach, **animal-assisted activities (AAAs),** includes motivational, educational, and recreational approaches. The goal is to provide "meeting and greeting" human–animal interactions to enhance the quality of life, rather than a specific treatment plan. AAA is used in many types of facilities with a wide variety of animals. AAA visits to sheltered homeless families has been effective. Most shelters do not allow families to bring their pets, and seeing the visiting animal can be therapeutic, especially for children. AAA visits give homeless children a chance to participate in everyday experiences they may not have had recently, such as walking a dog or playing fetch.

Pet Visits

A family **pet visit** is an arrangement for a pet to visit the owner in the health care setting. The concept of pet visits, as therapy for hospitalized people, is not new, especially in facilities with rehabilitation and mental health units. The pet that visits may belong to a pet therapy program or may be the client's own pet. It is believed that allowing a pet to visit can be a healing experience for patients, family members, and even the pet. Pets are even allowed to visit in ICU settings, with the approval of the nurses, provided no medical contraindications are present.

Resident Animals

Resident animals live at health care facilities. Species include fish, birds, hamsters, gerbils, guinea pigs, rabbits, cats, and dogs. The staff is responsible for the complete health and well-being of the animals, and residents are included in providing routine daily care. Grooming and brushing a resident dog, for example, are good therapies for the hands. Some staff report that full-time pets become so perceptive that they actually gravitate to the rooms of people who are the most isolated or depressed. Those residents who have regular visits are more receptive to treatment, have a greater incentive to recover, and have an increased will to live (Friedmann & Son, 2009).

Eden Alternative

Three significant problems that manifest within traditional long-term care facilities are loneliness, helplessness, and boredom. They often have not served as homes for people, but rather as institutions in which to store them. Residents may be intensely lonely, with long stretches of empty time. The basic concept of the **Eden Alternative,** a new approach to long-term care, is quite simple: Long-term care facilities are viewed as habitats for human beings rather than institutions for the frail and elderly.

In the Eden Alternative, nursing homes are places where the residents give as well as receive care and where many diverse species create a natural habitat. Administrators recognize that the care a resident receives is usually completed in 3 to 4 hours of the day, leaving 20 hours to live a life. The approach uses animals, plants, and children to interact with residents of long-term care centers, creating a "human habitat" that makes the residents feel more *at* home—and not so much *in* one. Resident animals are part of the total environment. Children and teenagers from schools and youth volunteer programs frequently visit the home. They come in and interact and build relationships with residents, as opposed to the usual pattern of coming in, putting on a program, and leaving (Thomas, 1996, 1998).

The Eden Alternative empowers residents and the staff members who come into daily contact with them. Residents have more say in their activities, menus, and daily routines; caregivers, maintenance workers, and other employees can set their own work schedules, within given parameters. Supporters of the program believe that employees frequently seem happier in Eden homes as evidenced by fewer sick days and lower staff turnover. The Eden Alternative is really about liberating the spirit of the people who are living and working in long-term care facilities (Thomas, 1996, 1998).

North Carolina and Missouri have declared unofficially that they are Eden Alternative states. Eden programs are also popular in New York, where Dr. William Thomas, MD, founded the approach. Eden Alternative got its start in nursing homes but has grown to include adult day care services and assisted-living facilities. There are Eden homes in Australia and New Zealand. Dr. Thomas' books have been translated into German and Japanese as the movement spreads worldwide.

Green Care

Green care is a total environmental approach using plants, gardens, and animals as therapeutic tools for individuals with physical or emotional problems. The intervention takes place on farms where clients assist in the care of animals and participate in other types of farm work. The program has been implemented in several European countries with positive results (Berget, Ekeberg, & Braastad, 2008).

Service Animals

Service animals are individually trained to do work or perform tasks for a person with a physical or emotional disability. Because they are not considered a "pet," they may legally go anywhere that a person with disabilities goes. Some service animals are trained to "alert" the person that a specific event is going to occur in the near future and is able to notify the human partner of this impending event. Other service animals are trained to "respond," that is, to act in a predetermined manner when a specific event occurs (Fine, 2006).

Most people are familiar with *guide dogs* for those with visual impairment. Other *disability service animals* can be trained to pull a wheelchair, open doors, retrieve dropped objects as small as a dime, turn light switches on and off, carry items in a backpack, and bark to alert for help. *Hearing animals* alert owners to important sounds that need a response such as smoke/fire/clock alarms, telephones, baby crying, sirens, knocks at the door, and so forth. *Seizure response animals*, usually dogs or cats, are able to alert people to the onset of their owner's seizures and can be trained to stay with the person or get help. They also help the person become reoriented and mobile after the seizures. *Diabetic service animals* alert their owners to episodes of hypoglycemia before there are symptoms, giving those persons time to monitor and correct their glucose level. When breathing machines malfunction, *respiratory service dogs* can be trained to nose the phone receiver out of its cradle and hit the speed-dial buttons, all of which are programmed to 911. *Psychiatric service animals* alert and/or respond to human partners experiencing panic attacks, social phobias, agoraphobia, posttraumatic stress disorder, dissociative amnesia, and depersonalizaion disorder. Any person who has a physical or mental impairment that substantially limits a major life activity might be a candidate for a service dog (Fine, 2006; King, 2007).

Training service dogs is an expensive and time-consuming project. The dog spends the first year of life with a foster family who is responsible for socialization and basic obedience training. Next comes 5 to 6 months of intensive training followed by 6 months of in-home training with the new owner. The expense of training an animal usually costs more than $10,000. The benefit, of course, is that people can lead more independent and fulfilling lives.

Screening Dogs

Researchers at Cambridge University hope to receive funding to test their theory that a dog's sense of smell could provide a better early warning system for some cancers than modern science. While people have about 5 million smell-sensing cells, dogs have about 220 million smell-sensing cells. It is estimated that dogs are 1,000 to 100,000 times more sensitive to smells than humans. **Screening dogs** are being trained to detect prostate cancer by smelling urine, lung cancer by smelling breath, and skin cancer by smelling the entire body. It is thought that cancer patients have a different odor that is detectable to trained dogs. It will be interesting to follow the development of this canine diagnosis or "dognosis" in the future (Balseiro & Correia, 2006).

Dogs in the Correctional Setting

Canine Assistants, an organization that trains service dogs, has an at-risk youth program for juvenile male offenders, ages 13 to 18 years. The program is jointly sponsored with the West Florida Wilderness Institute and Camp Sierra Blanca in New Mexico. It is a residential program with an average stay of 6 months. The young men work with service puppies and dogs under the supervision of experienced trainers. The goal is to learn responsibility, patience, and goal setting. Statistics demonstrate increased self-esteem, improved school grades, and a decreased recidivism rate for those involved in the program.

In correctional institutes all across Ohio, puppies and prisoners are teaming up in an unusual program. A nonprofit organization called Pilot

Dogs, Inc., places service puppies under the care of prisoners until the pups are ready for formal training as service dogs. Since the inception of the program in 1992, hundreds of dogs have been placed in prisons. Inmates are chosen based on their records of good behavior and experience with dogs. No violent offenders are permitted to raise the dogs. The puppies sleep in crates in the cells with their partners and accompany them on their daily activities, including trips to the dining hall where the puppies learn to be well behaved around people and become accustomed to the noise and crowds they will be faced with later. The prisoner is responsible for the care and well-being of the dog and for housebreaking, leash-training, and putting the dog through a basic obedience course. After spending about 12 months at the correctional facility, the puppies are removed and placed in an intensive training program.

A major advantage for the dogs is having human contact 24 hours a day, which is less likely to occur in regular foster homes. The chosen prisoners have the pleasure and delight of having a puppy to give love to and get love from. They also have the satisfaction of seeing the benefits of their training as the puppy progresses. At the Purdy Treatment Center, a maximum security prison for women in Gig Harbor, Washington, selected inmates learn to train and groom dogs from the local Humane Society. They socialize the stray dogs for home adoption. In addition they run a grooming and boarding service for dogs in the community. Many other states have adopted the Ohio model, as well as prisons in Australia, England, and Scotland (Furst, 2006; Turner, 2007).

USING RESEARCH TO HEAL

Cole, K. M., Gawlinski, A., Steers, N., & Kotlerman, J. (2007). Animal-assisted therapy in patients hospitalized with heart failure. *American Journal of Critical Care*, 16(6): 575–588.

What Is This Study About?

Heart failure is one of the prevalent diagnoses in adults hospitalized in the United States. Patients hospitalized for heart failure experience a poor prognosis and frequent readmissions for this chronic health problem. Although disease management has improved through the use of polypharmacy, little is known about the effects of complementary and alternative therapies for management of advanced heart failure. Therefore, the purpose of this study was to examine the effects of a 12-minute hospital visit with a therapy dog on improving hemodynamic measures, lowering eurohormone levels, and decreasing state anxiety in patients with advanced heart failure.

How Was This Study Done?

This study used a randomized repeated-measures experimental design with 76 adults living with advanced heart failure. Seventy-five percent of the participants were men, and the majority experienced advanced heart failure due to nonischemic cardiomyopathy (n = 44).

(continued)

This study was approved by the institutional review board. The participants were randomized into one of three groups (n = 19 volunteer-dog team visits, n = 15 volunteer visits only, and n = 11 control group). The group receiving the volunteer-dog team intervention was visited for 12 minutes. At the conclusion of the visit, the participant was provided an instant self-developing photograph of the patient with the dog. The volunteer-only group received a 12-minute visit with usual conversation. The control group was asked to lie quietly for 12 minutes without talking unless they had a specific need or request. Nursing personnel was requested not to interrupt the visits except for an emergency problem. Persons volunteering to visit with or without a dog were kept with the same patients as much as possible. For all groups, the following baseline data (before visit) was collected: blood pressure, heart rate, cardiac index, epinephrine level, norepinephrine level, pulmonary artery pressure (PAP), pulmonary capillary wedge pressure (PCWP), right atrial pressure (RAP), and systemic vascular resistance (SVR). This data was also collected 8 minutes after the intervention started and 4 minutes after the visit concluded. Participants were all in the recumbent position with the head of the bed elevated at 45°. The Spielberger State-Trait Inventory was used to measure state anxiety.

What Were the Results of This Study?

There were several differences noted between the volunteer-dog group and the control group. The participants in the volunteer-dog group had significantly greater decreases in systolic PAP and PCWP than the control group. The volunteer-dog team group had significantly greater decreases in epinephrine levels during and after the visit than the volunteer-only group. Following the intervention, the volunteer-dog team group had the greatest decrease from baseline in state anxiety sum score compared with the other two groups. Decreases in RAP and diastolic PAP in the volunteer-dog team group were significantly greater than those in the volunteer visit only group. In summary, participants who received a visit from the volunteer-dog team had decreased cardiopulmonary pressures, neurohormones levels, and anxiety levels than did the volunteer-visit-only group and the control group. Heart rate, blood pressure, cardiac index, and SVR did not report statistical significance for the intervention.

What Additional Questions Might I Have?

Would animal-assisted therapy (AAT) have the same effect on other cardiac-related health problems? Were there differences noted in persons currently owning a dog and those that did not own a dog? Was there a difference in hospital stay or readmission for those receiving the volunteer-dog team visit?

How Can I Use This Study?

Nurses can support the integration of animal-assisted therapy with traditional Western medicine practices in caring for patients living with advanced heart failure. While this health problem suggests a poor prognosis, introducing AAT may enhance a person's quality of life during a very stressful time and serve as a positive memory for both the individual and family members. AAT could start a positive chain of effects benefitting the individual's self-image beyond just pure symptom reduction.

Source: Contributed by Dolores M. Huffman, PhD, RN, Associate Professor of Nursing, Purdue University Calumet.

RESEARCH

To date, much of the literature on the therapeutic use of animals in health care is anecdotal, but scientific research is beginning to appear. Most of the studies recommend further investigations because they show associations but not causal relationships. A small sample of the literature shows:

- Two hundred and forty-six freshman college students participated in an orientation program that included pet therapy dogs. Ninety-six percent of the participants voiced interest in the university introducing a pet therapy program (Adamle, Riley, & Carlson, 2009).
- Twenty-four individuals with neck or back pain severe enough to interfere with activities of daily living participated in an equine-assisted therapy program under the supervision of a physical therapist and a riding instructor. All the participants experienced some pain relief, increased mobility, and an improved sense of well-being (Hakanson et al., 2009).
- Nine studies regarding dog therapy for individuals with dementia were reviewed. These studies indicated that there was an improvement in social behavior and a lessening of agitation during the dog therapy sessions (Perkins, Bartlett, Travers, & Rand, 2008).
- Thirty adults who were beginning their first radiation therapy for cancer were randomly assigned to one of three groups: a group that received 12 dog visits, a group that received 12 friendly human visits, and a group that had 12 quiet reading periods. The individuals in all three groups described the activities as beneficial. No statistically significant differences were found, which may be related to the small sample size (Johnson, Meadows, Haubner, & Sevedge, 2008).
- Seventy-six patients hospitalized with heart failure were randomized into one of three groups: a 12-minute dog visit group, a 12-minute friendly human visit group, or a usual care group. There was a significant improvement in cardiopulmonary pressures, neurohormone levels, and anxiety for the dog visit group (Cole, Gawlinski, Steers, & Kotlerman, 2007).

One of the largest organizations devoted to animal-assisted therapy is the Delta Society, composed of 1,500 members, 20 percent of whom are health care professionals. The objectives of the Delta Society are to promote study and research relating to human–animal interactions, increase the awareness of the significance of these interactions among health care professionals, and assess the role of the effect of human–pet bonds on the mental and physical well-being of people. Pets and People, a nonprofit volunteer agency founded in 1994, supports the research endeavors of graduate nursing students from the University of Southern Mississippi and Louisiana State University.

INTEGRATED NURSING PRACTICE

An important nursing role is that of advocate. Nurse advocates serve as links between clients and other health care professionals of the community. It is in that role that nurses in a wide variety of clinical settings can explore and encourage the therapeutic use of animals. The benefits of human–animal interaction are many and include such things as attachment, bonding, caring, pain management, stress management, motivation, communication, improved self-esteem, cardiovascular benefits, and improved coordination and balance. Disinterest on the part of health care professionals has been the major obstacle to growth in the field of animal-assisted therapy.

To set up an animal-assisted therapy program, you must begin by approaching the facility's administration with a well-organized plan. This plan should include the following aspects:

- Theory and research background
- Goals and outcomes
- Clearly written policy and procedures
- Staff education about the proposed program
- A plan for volunteer recruitment and training
- A plan for testing and training of potential therapy animals
- A plan for implementation of the program
- A plan for evaluation of the program

You can anticipate some opposition to the initiation of an animal-assisted therapy program. One of the biggest concerns is the potential for transmission of infectious diseases. Although the risk is low, several zoonoses, or animal-transmitted infections, can occur. Seek the assistance of a veterinarian to identify the risks for specific types of infections and measures to prevent them. Infection risk can be reduced by making sure each animal is clean, vaccinated, and healthy; keeping the animal out of the areas where food is prepared and served; and having residents wash their hands after the animal visits. Products can be sprayed on the animal's fur to reduce the risk of an allergic reaction (Friedmann & Son, 2009).

"No pets" policies may not be applied to service animals. Hospitals, medical offices, laboratories, imaging services, day care centers, schools, restaurants, and others are covered under the Americans with Disabilities Act (ADA). The ADA requires that places of public accommodation modify their policies and practices to permit the use of a service animal by a person with a disability, unless doing so would create a direct threat to the safety of others or the facility. There is no legal requirement that a service animal wear special equipment or tags. Facilities are advised to accept the verbal reassurance of the person that he or she has a disability and that the animal is a service animal. Requiring "proof" is prohibited by the ADA.

If you are a pet owner, you can consider becoming a pet therapy volunteer. Many long-term care facilities encourage regular visits from people with trained and screened animals. Increasingly, these pets are also welcome at hospitals, cancer clinics, and hospices. This type of personal involvement in animal-assisted therapy can be wonderfully rewarding.

Very new to the use of animals in health care are the Mexican hairless breed known as Xolos (pronounced show-low). These dogs cuddle up to their owners and project the same amount of heat as a heating pad. This seems to work wonders for people with arthritis or fibromyalgia. The body temperature is the same as all dogs, 102 °F, but the lack of hair means the body heat is transferred directly to the surface the dog is touching. A nonprofit group, Xolos for Chronic Pain Relief, matches dogs with pain sufferers.

As a nurse you have wonderful opportunities to incorporate AAT in your work with people infected with human immunodeficiency virus (HIV) and those with acquired immune deficiency syndrome (AIDS). In the past, these individuals have been told to give up their pets for fear that their compromised immune system would place them at high risk for zoonotic infections. The reality is that people are more likely to contract zoonotic infections from contaminated food, water, soil, or even other people than from pets. You may need to explain to some clients that the HIV only infects humans and other primates and, therefore, cannot be spread from or to dogs, cats, birds, or even fish. With this understanding, you can become an advocate for the physical, emotional, and psychological benefits of pet companionship for those with HIV/AIDS.

With proper care and understanding and a healthy pet, the potential health risks of pet companionship are minimal and the benefits may far outweigh the risks. People living with HIV often deal with feelings of isolation, rejection, and lack of purpose. For such people, companion animals offer purpose, a feeling of being needed, a way to increase socialization, and a constant source of unconditional affection. If clients are selecting a new pet, they should consider one whose temperament, energy level, and environmental needs match their own. An older pet may be more appropriate than a young one. Box 27.1 describes the client-teaching you should do with any clients who are ill or immunosuppressed as a result of a disorder, chemotherapy, or organ transplants. The precautions are designed to protect people from acquiring secondary infections.

A number of communities provide services to enable people who are ill to keep their pets. Volunteers provide dog-walking services for people physically unable to walk their dogs, deliver pet food and supplies, clean litter boxes and bird cages, provide in-home care for cats whose owners must go to the hospital, and foster care for dogs in the same situation. You could volunteer your time and energy to this type of program, or if your community has no such program, you could establish one.

The Eden Alternative is a new way of thinking about long-term care facilities. Nurses are in an extraordinary position to teach others about what the Eden Alternative is, and how they can use it to transform the facilities in which they practice. Before you can educate others, it is important that you become familiar with the concepts and the 10 principles of the Eden Alternative. The principles, developed by Eden Alternative founder, William Thomas, MD (1996, 1998) and his wife, Judith, are as follows:

1. Understand that loneliness, helplessness, and boredom account for the bulk of suffering among our frail elders.
2. Surrender the institutional point of view and adopt the Human Habitat model that makes pets, plants, and children the axis around which daily life turns.

BOX 27.1

Client Teaching: Pet Owners Experiencing Illness

Veterinary Care

- Have your veterinarian examine your pet initially and then at least once a year.
- Keep your pet up to date on annual shots and rabies vaccination.
- Seek veterinary care immediately for sick pets.
- Street animals that are "adopted" should first be checked by a veterinarian before being brought into your home.

Pet Care

- Keep your pet clean and well groomed with short, blunt toenails.
- Keep the pet's living and feeding areas clean.
- Keep your cat's litter box out of the kitchen; use a litter box liner and change it daily.
- Always walk your pet on a leash and minimize the pet's contact with other animals and garbage.
- Cats should be kept indoors and be prevented from hunting birds and rodents.
- Feed your pet only commercially prepared pet foods; never feed raw meat or unpasteurized milk.
- Do not allow birds to fly free in your home; you must avoid their droppings.

General Hygiene

- Wash your hands frequently, especially before eating, smoking, or attending to open wounds.
- Keep your cat off all kitchen surfaces. If that is not possible, be sure to wipe down, with a gentle disinfectant, any surface on which food may be placed.
- Do not allow your dog to drink out of the toilet because it is a place of many germs.
- Try to avoid contact with your pet's bodily fluids. Gloves and a face mask should be worn for cleanup, including cleaning a litter box, aquarium, or bird cage.

Sources: POWARS, New York, NY; PAWS, San Francisco, CA; The Delta Society, Renton, WA; Action AIDS, Philadelphia, PA.

---

3. Provide easy access to companionship by promoting close and continuing contact between the elements of the Human Habitat and the people who live and work within it.
4. Create opportunities to give as well as receive care by promoting our elders' participation in the daily round of activities that are necessary to maintain the Human Habitat.

5. Imbue daily life with variety and spontaneity by creating an environment in which unexpected and unpredictable interactions and happenings can take place.
6. Deemphasize the programmed activities approach to life and devote these resources to the maintenance and growth of the Human Habitat.
7. Deemphasize the role of prescription drugs in our elders' daily life and commit these resources to the maintenance and growth of the Human Habitat.
8. Deemphasize top-down bureaucratic authority in the facility and seek instead to place the maximum possible decision-making authority in the hands of those closest to those for whom we care.
9. Understand that Edenizing is a never-ending process, *not* a program, and that the Human Habitat, once created, should be helped to grow and develop like any other living thing.
10. Appoint leadership that places the need to improve resident quality of life over and above the inevitable objections to change. Leadership is the lifeblood of the Edenizing process, and for it there is no substitute.

Miriam Stermer, a Certified Eden Associate from Charlotte, North Carolina, has further expanded these principles to enable you to evaluate the environment in which you practice or the environment in which your family elder may be living and what changes you might advocate to move in the direction of Edenizing the long-term care facility.

- What kind of companionship is provided for residents?
- How many and what kinds of animals live in the facility?
- What are the gardening opportunities?
- What opportunities do residents have to provide care rather than just receive care? Are residents encouraged to provide care for their plants and animals?
- Are children part of everyday life? Are there opportunities for one-to-one relationships?
- Are chemical restraints recognized as such? Does the facility pursue a restraint-free environment? Are problem behaviors approached in a holistic manner?
- Are planning teams consisting of residents, family members, staff, and community members in place?
- Has the facility committed time, money, and energy to making the approach an ongoing, continuing process?
- Does the administrator understand the Eden alternative philosophy and is she or he a leader in this process?

As the number of elderly persons increases in the United States, not only will the demand for more assisted living and long-term care facilities increase, but also will the demand for alternatives to the traditional systems. As Thomas (1996) describes it:

> As it stands now, nursing homes deliver a low perceived value at a high cost. To make matters worse, this situation is compounded by

TRY THIS

Interacting with Your Pet

When you are feeling tense or anxious and if you have a dog or a cat to whom you are attached, try this:

- Note your physical and emotional signs of tension: Are your hands clenched? Body trembling? Are you restless? Unable to relax? Mouth dry? Stomach upset? Breathing rapidly? Unable to concentrate? Worrying?
- Do something with your pet for at least 20 minutes: Play, groom, or talk.
- Conduct another self-assessment. What, if anything, has changed?

If you have a dog or a cat to whom you are attached, try this:

- Have a friend take your pulse and blood pressure.
- Gently play with your pet, stroke, pet, and talk to your animal for 15 minutes.
- Have your friend take your pulse and blood pressure again and compare the results to those taken prior to the interaction.

social trends that are weakening the sense of obligation across the generations. Ultimately, the elderly must depend on this sense of obligation for protection and sustenance. (p. 14)

Animal contact contributes to self-concept, social interaction, a decrease in loneliness and anxiety, and in general contributes to physical, psychological, and spiritual well-being. Nurses can and should be at the forefront of designing and supporting more humane approaches to those in our care.

References

Adamle, K. N., Riley, T. A., & Carlson, T. (2009). Evaluating college student interest in pet therapy. *Journal of American College Health*, 57(5): 545–548.

Balseiro, S. C., & Correia, H. R. (2006). Is olfactory detection of human cancer by dogs based on major histocompatibility complex-dependent odor components? *Medical Hypotheses*, 66(2): 270–272.

Berget, B., Ekeberg, O., & Braastad, B. O. (2008). Attitudes to animal-assisted therapy with farm animals among health staff and farmers. *Journal of Psychiatric and Mental Health Nursing*, 15: 576–581.

Cole, K. M., Gawlinski, A., Steers, N., & Kotlerman, J. (2007). Animal-assisted therapy in patients hospitalized with heart failure. *American Journal of Critical Care*, 16(6): 575–585.

Fine, A. H. (2006). *Handbook on Animal-Assisted Therapy*, 2nd ed. London: Academic Press.

Friedmann, E., & Son, H. (2009). The human-companion animal bond. *The Veterinary Clinics of North America. Small Animal Practice*, 39(2): 293–326.

Furst, G. (2006). Prison-based animal programs: A national survey. *The Prison Journal*, 86(4): 407–430.

Hakanson, M., Moller, M., Lindstrom, I., & Mattsson, B. (2009). The horse as the healer—A study of riding in patients with back pain. *Journal of Bodywork and Movement Therapies*, 13(1): 43–52.

Hume, L. (2002). Animal facilitation in occupational and physical therapy sessions. www.northeastrehab.com/features/animal-facilitated-therapy. Accessed April 10, 2009.

Johnson, R. A., Meadows, R. L., Haubner, J. S., & Sevedge, K. (2008). Animal-assisted activity among patients with cancer: Effects on mood, fatigue, self-perceived health, and sense of coherence. *Oncology Nursing Forum*, 35(2): 225–232.

King, L. (2007). *Animal Assisted Therapy*. Bloomington, IN: AuthorHouse.

Nightingale, F. (1969). *Notes on Nursing*. New York: Dover Publishing.

Perkins, J., Bartlett, H., Travers, C., & Rand, J. (2008). Dog-assisted therapy for older people with dementia: A review. *Australasian Journal on Ageing*, 27(4): 177–182.

Phillips, B. (2008). Does swimming with dolphins have any health benefits for children with cerebral palsy? *Archives of Disease in Childhood*, 93(11): 994–995.

Sockalingam, S., Li, M., Krishnadev, U., Hanson, K., Balaban, K., Pacione, L. R., et al. (2008). Use of animal-assisted therapy in the rehabilitation of an assault victim with a concurrent mood disorder. *Issues in Mental Health Nursing*, 29: 73–84.

Thomas, W. H. (1996). *Life Worth Living*. Acton, MA: VanderWyk & Burnham.

Thomas, W. H. (1998). *Open Hearts, Open Minds*. Acton, MA: VanderWyk & Burnham.

Turner, W. E. (2007). The experiences of offenders in a prison canine program. *Federal Probation*, 71(1): 38–43.

Resources

American Hippotherapy Association
136 Bush Rd.
Damascus, PA 18415
888.851.4592
www.americanhippotherapyassociation.org

Canine Assistants
3160 Francis Rd.
Milton, GA 30004
800.771.7221
www.canineassistants.org

The Delta Society
875 124th Ave., NE, Suite 101
Bellevue, WA 98005
425.679.5500
www.deltasociety.org

The Eden Alternative
14500 RR12, Suite 2
Wimberley, TX 78676
512.847.6061
www.edenalt.com

Federation of Riding for the Disabled International
P.O. Box 293
Nunawading, Vic, Australia 3131
61.3.9877.7172
www.frdi.net

Psychiatric Service Dog Society
P.O. Box 754
Arlington, VA 22216
517.216.1589
www.psychdog.org

Puppies Behind Bars
10 East 40th St., 19th Floor
New York, NY 10016
212.680.9562
www.puppiesbehindbars.com

St. John Ambulance Therapy Dog
Program
www.sja.ca/Ontario/
CommunityServices/Programs/
Pages/TherapyDogsServices.aspx

Therapet
15632 Hwy 110 S., Suite 7
Whitehouse, TX 75791
www.therapet.com

Therapy Dogs International
88 Bartley Rd.
Flanders, NJ 07836
973.252.9800
www.tdi-dog.org

APPENDIX

Alternative Therapies for Common Health Problems

This appendix is meant to provide education relating to the management of minor health problems. These types of problems often respond well to alternative therapies and lifestyle modification. If in doubt about the seriousness of symptoms, see your health care practitioner. A number of suggestions are given for various problems. Select one that seems to be the most appropriate for your situation, and keep notes on what seems to work and what does not. Modify these suggestions according to your individual needs.

ABRASIONS, SCRAPES

- Aromatherapy: After washing with soap and water, apply 1–3 drops of lavender or tea tree to wound; reapply oil 2 times a day until healed.
- To disinfect, pour 3% hydrogen peroxide into the wound and let it foam up.
- Apply the skin of a freshly peeled banana to the affected area, or cut a thin slice of raw potato and tape it over the affected area.
- Herbs: Sprinkle goldenseal powder in wound. Crushed garlic mixed with honey makes a soothing salve: spread on a piece of clean gauze and cover the injured area.

ACNE

- Aromatherapy: Bergamot, cedarwood, chamomile, clary sage, lemon grass, melissa, patchouli, rosemary, sandalwood, tea tree, thyme, ylang-ylang can be made into a facial mask, compress, or topical cream. Tea tree oil and lavender can be applied directly to blemishes.
- Herbs: arnica, borage, calendula skin products, tea tree oil
- Supplements: vitamin A, vitamin B6, zinc, or evening primrose oil

AIDS

- Acupuncture
- Herbs: curcumin, extract of boxwood plant, Echinacea, licorice, goldenseal, garlic, Chinese bitter melon
- Hyperbaric oxygen
- Massage
- Supplements: iron; vitamins C, E, and B; beta-carotene; glutamine; selenium

ALCOHOL ABUSE

- Acupuncture
- Antioxidants: selenium, zinc, vitamins C and E
- Bach flower essence, chrysanthemum, milkweed
- Herbs: milk thistle, kudzu, oatstraw, skullcap; evening primrose oil for withdrawal
- Meditation
- Megavitamin therapy: B vitamins
- Therapeutic Touch, Healing Touch
- Yoga

ALLERGIES

- Applied Kinesiology
- Herbs: Stinging nettles to lessen runny nose and sneezing. Teas made from chamomile, elder, or yarrow flowers can reduce reactions.
- Homeopathy: allium cepa (onion); windflower; for swelling in the face: 1 tablet of apis every 15 minutes—maximum 6 doses.
- Supplements: Vitamin C to decrease histamine production.
- Water: Important to keep well hydrated; 64–96 ounces of water a day.

ALZHEIMER'S DISEASE (DEMENTIA)

- Reflexology
- Supplements: zinc, selenium, evening primrose oil, fish oil, coenzyme Q10; vitamins B_6, C, and E

AMPUTATIONS: PHANTOM PAIN

- Magnets: Improve blood flow to stump and cause phantom pain to disappear.
- Massage

ANXIETY

- Acupressure: Press center of inside wrist 1 inch above crease toward elbow.
- Animal-assisted therapy
- Aromatherapy: basil, bergamot, chamomile; frankincense deepens breathing to induce calmness, green apple, juniper, lemon balm, orange, neroli for panic attacks
- Biofeedback
- Flower essences: aspen, mimulus, red chestnut
- Herbs: valerian, passion flower, lemon balm, chamomile, ylang-ylang
- Homeopathy: St. Ignatius bean, arsenic, Rescue® Remedy

- Massage
- Meditation
- Reiki
- Relaxation techniques
- Therapeutic Touch, Healing Touch
- Performance anxiety: hypnosis, guided imagery, Alexander Technique

ARTHRITIS

- Aromatherapy: cedarwood, coriander, cypress massage or cold compress, compress of rosemary to swollen joints, ginger and orange oil massage
- Acupuncture
- Alexander Technique: to relieve muscular tension and uneven weight bearing
- Bioelectromagnetics
- Chiropractic
- Exercise (non-weight-bearing) in water or moderate exercise as tolerated
- Feldenkrais Method
- Herbs: devil's claw, boswellia, SAMe, evening primrose oil; ginger; feverfew, capsaicin cream applied topically, glucosamine (1500 mg) and chondroitin (1200 mg) to help restore joint integrity; natural anti-inflammatories such as willowbark, turmeric, and ginger
- Homeopathy: poison ivy
- Ice joints and then rub in analgesic oils
- Magnets placed over an inflamed area on regular basis
- Reflexology: All joints of the hands and feet should be worked for pain relief and mobility of corresponding body joints.
- Rolfing
- Supplements: thiamine, vitamins B_6, B_{12}, calcium, magnesium, glucosamine, chondroitin; green tea, avocado-soybean unsaponifiables
- Therapeutic Touch
- Yoga: Practice slowly, seeing how far the affected joints can be moved without pain. Do not exercise joints when they are inflamed.

ASTHMA

- Acupuncture
- Alexander Technique: teaches a more relaxed way of breathing and enables an individual to manage better during an asthma attack
- Aromatherapy: Put several drops of cypress on a handkerchief and inhale deeply. Put frankincense on a pillow at night to slow and deepen the breathing.
- Biofeedback
- Breathing exercises
- Hypnosis

- Herbs: holy basil, elecampine, country mallow, malabar nut, bayberry. Mix 3 parts tincture of lobelia with 1 part tincture of capsicum. Take 20 drops in water at the start of an asthmatic attack. Repeat every 30 minutes for a total of 3 or 4 doses.
- Homeopathy: arsenicum album, 1 tablet 3 times daily; maximum 1 week
- Meditation
- Reflexology: During an asthma attack, work the reflexes for the diaphragm and lungs on the balls of the feet.
- Water: Drink plenty of water to keep the respiratory tract secretions fluid.
- Yoga: Focus on expansive postures and breathing practices designed to increase the length of the exhalation.

ATHLETE'S FOOT

- Acupressure: Do full foot or hand acupressure massage sessions twice a week to stimulate the immune and endocrine systems. Do not press on broken, sore, or cracked skin areas.
- Aromatherapy: cedarwood, lemon balm, rosemary. Mix 2 drops lavender oil and 1 drop tea tree oil and apply between toes.
- Herbs: bitter orange. Apply black walnut tincture directly to fungus patches and drink a tea of green crushed walnut hulls for fungus anywhere in body.
- Naturopathy: kyolic garlic tablets. Dust your feet and shoes with garlic powder.
- Supplements: Take B-complex vitamins, 50–100 mg, thrice a day, with meals. Dust vitamin C powder directly onto affected area. Zinc may help clear the skin and boost the immune system.

ATTENTION DEFICIT HYPERACTIVITY DISORDER

- Aromatherapy: lavender, rosemary, valerian
- Diet change from "junk foods" high in artificial flavors, preservatives, and sucrose to nutrient-dense foods
- Herbs: chamomile
- Homeopathy
- Massage
- Meditation
- Neurofeedback
- Supplements: B vitamins, iron, magnesium, omega-3
- Yoga

BACK PAIN

- Acupuncture
- Alexander Technique: teaches a more balanced use of body since muscular imbalance often contributes to back pain

- Applied Kinesiology
- Biofeedback
- Chiropractic
- Equine-assisted therapy
- Herbs: valerian, nutmeg, gotu kola. To ease local discomfort, soak a compress in 1/2 cup hot water containing 1 tsp camp bark and 1 tsp. cinnamon tinctures.
- Homeopathy: 4 tablets of arnica as soon as possible after an injury and repeat every hour for the first day while awake; second day: 4 tablets every 2 hours; third day: 4 tablets four times a day
- Hydrotherapy: For acute back pain, use an ice pack on affected area for 20 minutes every 1–2 hours.
- Magnets: Place small magnets over area of muscle spasm in back.
- Massage with warm oil.
- Reflexology: Work the spinal reflexes, especially the tender points, on the medial longitudinal arches of the feet (the bony ridges on the inside).
- Sleep on back with pillows under knees or on side with pillow between bent knees.
- Yoga: Lie down with legs bent, feet flat on floor, exhale fully and slowly for at least 12 breaths. Long-term yoga practice can strengthen back muscles.

BALANCE PROBLEMS

- Alexander Technique
- Equine-assisted therapy
- Qigong
- T'ai chi

BEE STINGS/INSECT BITES

- Aromatherapy: tea tree, basil, bergamot, lavender, thyme, ylang-ylang
- Add enough water to baking soda or meat tenderizer to make a paste and apply it to the sting.
- Cover affected area with a small amount of mashed fresh papaya.
- Herbs: Apply fresh aloe vera sap directly to the bite. If bite becomes infected, bathe with marigold or echinacea tea. Apply a fresh slice of onion to both bee and wasp stings. A mixture of honey and crushed garlic makes a soothing ointment.
- Homeopathy: apis, 1 tablet every 30 minutes, maximum 6 doses for burning and swelling

BONES (BROKEN)

- Aromatherapy: Massage in elemi oil prior to casting.
- Bioelectromagnetics: Place magnets into the dressings over fractures.
- Healing Touch

- Reiki
- Therapeutic Touch

BRUISES

- Aromatherapy: cypress. Combine 1 drop of chamomile with 2 tsp. of ice cold water. Soak a cotton pad in this mixture and apply to affected area.
- Herbs: witch hazel (topical), arnica tablets or massage tincture of arnica into bruised area; 200–400 mg 3 times a day of bromelain on an empty stomach
- Homeopathy: aconite, 1 or 2 doses only over 15 minutes immediately for the "shock" of the injury
- Hydrotherapy: cold compresses for first 12 hours with occasional breaks to prevent excessive chilling
- Supplements: 2000 mg vitamin C, 3 times a day, for people who bruise easily. Drink pineapple juice because enzymes speed the rate at which the blood causing the bruise dissolves.

BURNS (MINOR)

- Aromatherapy: For pain relief: chamomile, eucalyptus, geranium, lavender. To reduce inflammation: chamomile, clary sage, geranium, lavender, myrrh, tea tree. To regenerate skin: chamomile, clary sage, eucalyptus, geranium, myrrh, rose, tea tree
- Herbs: aloe vera sap, calendula lotion, or raw honey
- Hydrotherapy: Immediately immerse the affected part in ice water for 5–10 minutes with brief break during the first 20 minutes after the injury.
- Magnets: Place over site of injury to control pain and speed healing.

CANCER

- Acupuncture to treat side effects and symptoms
- Antineoplaston therapy: under investigation with FDA-approved clinical trials
- Antioxidants: vitamins A, C, and E; co-enzyme 10
- Faith and prayer
- Herbs: betulinic acid from birch trees, thuja tincture, bromelain, gotu kola, essiac, green or black tea, maitake mushroom, selenium
- Imagery
- Massage
- Meditation
- Qigong
- Shark cartilage: works best against solid tumors, especially ovarian and prostate tumors

- Shark liver oil may help people tolerate chemotherapy and radiation.
- Supplements: reishi mushroom
- Yoga

CANKER SORES

- Herbs: licorice root gel, echinacea tincture, butternut, comfrey. Gargle with a mixture of 1 cup of warm water with 1/4 tsp. of salt and 1/2 tsp. of goldenseal powder.
- Supplements: Vitamin A (25,000–50,000 IU daily) prevents infection from spreading. B-complex (50–100 IU TID); vitamin E (400–800 IU daily); selenium (200 mcg daily); acidophilus, 4 capsules, 4–6 times per day

CARPAL TUNNEL SYNDROME

- Acupressure: Firmly press (for 2 minutes) on point on inside surface of forearm about 1 inch up from wrist fold. Also press on point on out-side surface of forearm one-third of way up between wrist fold and elbow.
- Chiropractic
- Herbs: ginger compress
- Hydrotherapy: contrast applications
- Magnets: Place over the front and back of the wrist to control symptoms.
- Massage
- Pressure point therapies

CHEST CONGESTION

- Aromatherapy: cedarwood, steam inhalation of eucalyptus, frankin-cense. Massage chest with lavender. Inhale marjoram, peppermint, euca-lyptus, or rosemary. Place drops of tea tree on handkerchief.
- Herbs: tea made with peppermint and yarrow (1/2 tsp. each). Mix sage or eucalyptus leaves in a bowl of steaming water and inhale with a towel draped over the head.
- Magnets: Wear on chest over bronchial tubes and at equal level on the back. Sleeping on a magnetic mattress pad can be helpful.

CHOLESTEROL (HIGH)

- Herbs: garlic, ginger, green tea, Indian gooseberry, soy, artichoke leaf ex-tract
- Meditation
- Supplements: Profibe (grapefruit fiber), oatmeal
- Yoga

CHRONIC FATIGUE SYNDROME

- Acupuncture
- Herbs: acute phase—echinacea, goldenseal, licorice; chronic phase—goldenseal, astragalus, Siberian ginseng
- Supplements: beta-carotene, vitamin C, zinc

CIRCULATION (POOR)

- Aromatherapy: rosemary (increases circulation to skin), vetiver
- Biofeedback: Increases circulation to specific areas of the body.
- Exercise
- Herbs: ginkgo, garlic, cayenne, hawthorn, bilberry
- Hypnosis
- Imagery
- Magnets
- Massage
- Therapeutic Touch
- Yoga

COLD SORES

- Aromatherapy: Apply tea tree oil at onset and continue until cleared.
- Herbs: Echinacea or goldenseal, L-lysine. Lemon-balm tea shows significant antiviral activity against herpes simplex.
- Hydrotherapy: For early stages, use ice application—on the sore for 10 minutes, off for 5 minutes.
- Supplements: vitamins C, B-complex, E

COLIC

- Aromatherapy: chamomile (rubbed on abdomen), coriander, orange, peppermint
- Chiropractic
- Massage abdomen. Massage bottom of feet with warmed sesame oil.

COMMON COLD

- Acupressure: if sinuses become blocked or painful
- Aromatherapy: Inhale lavender, eucalyptus, or peppermint oil in steam vaporizer to speed recovery and lessen stuffiness. Add 3 drops lemon oil, 2 drops each of thyme and tea tree oil, and 1 drop eucalyptus into hot bath.
- Herbs: tea from fresh ginger and brown sugar; echinacea at the first sign of a cold; astragalus, garlic, goldenseal, eyebright, elecampane

- Homeopathy: allium cepa (onion), monkshood, aconite or natrum muriaticum
- Reflexology: Work the fingers and thumbs, the webs between the fingers, the pads beneath the fingers, and the spaces on the back of the hands for the reflexes of the head, lungs, and upper lymphatics.
- Supplements: vitamins A and C, zinc lozenges; selenium for 3 days to help resist a cold

CONSTIPATION

- Aromatherapy: Massage abdomen in a clockwise direction with orange, black pepper, ginger, or marjoram mixed in a carrier oil.
- Biofeedback of pelvic floor muscles
- Exercise, especially activities that work the abdominal muscles such as rowing, swimming, walking, or sit-ups
- Herbs: dandelion root, chicory root, angelica root, cascara sagrada, senna. Psyllium can be used for several days; long-term use can be damaging.
- Homeopathy: bryonia (wild hops) or nux vomica
- Reflexology: areas for the colon on the soles of both feet
- Water: Drink 6–8 glasses daily.
- Yoga: Twisting postures and forward bends are often helpful.

CORNS

- Aromatherapy: Mix 2 drops each of orange, lemon, and lavender oils in a basin of warm water and soak feet for at least 15 minutes per day.
- Hydrotherapy: hot Epsom salts foot bath, then rub corns with fresh lemon juice
- Reflexology: around and directly on the corns

COUGH

- Aromatherapy: cedarwood. Place several drops of cypress or tea tree on handkerchief and inhale deeply. Add 3 drops eucalyptus and 2 drops thyme oil to 2 tsp. vegetable oil. Massage into neck and chest. Do steam inhalation using sandalwood, benzoin, eucalyptus, frankincense, or peppermint.
- Herbs: licorice, wild cherry bark, thyme; tincture of mullein in warm water 3 times a day; horehound
- Homeopathy: bryonia (wild hops), monkshood, rumex, stannum
- Reflexology: Work the lung and diaphragm reflexes on and beneath balls of feet and webs between big toes and second toes.

DEPRESSION

- Acupuncture
- Animal-assisted therapy
- Aromatherapy: bergamot, geranium, jasmine, lemon balm, rose, ylang-ylang. Add 15 drops geranium, 10 drops of bergamot, and 5 drops of lavender to bath.
- Exercise
- Flower essences: gentian, hornbeam, mustard, gorse, sweet chestnut
- Herbs: St. John's wort, SAMe, valerian
- Homeopathy: Rescue Remedy
- Hypnotherapy
- Meditation
- Neurofeedback
- Reiki
- Supplements: B vitamins, omega-3
- T'ai chi
- Therapeutic Touch
- Transcranial magnetic stimulation
- Yoga

DIABETES

- Aromatherapy: Using a carrier oil, rub juniper or cedar oil over spleen and pancreas area.
- Biofeedback
- Exercise
- Herbs: blueberry leaf tea, 2 cups a day on a regular basis; 100–200 mg of co-enzyme Q every day for at least 3 months to stabilize blood sugar; gymnesly, green tea, ginger, ginseng, goldenseal
- Supplements: vitamins B_6, C, and E, chromium, magnesium, essential fatty acids, flaxseed oil
- Yoga

DIARRHEA

- Aromatherapy: Gently massage abdomen with coriander, chamomile, neroli, lavender, or peppermint in carrier oil.
- Herbs: 2 tsp. per cup of boiling water to make tea of black pepper, chamomile, coriander, rosemary, sandalwood, or thyme
- Homeopathy: podophyllum—1 tablet hourly until improved, then every 4 hours—maximum 5 days
- Supplements: zinc
- Replace lost fluids.

DRUG ADDICTION

- Bach flower essence: California poppy, morning glory, chrysanthemum
- Biofeedback
- Herbs: chamomile and ginseng (cocaine withdrawal); valerian (benzodiazepine withdrawal)

EAR INFECTIONS

- Acupressure: Massage just behind the tip of the mastoid bone at the bottom of the back of the ear to relieve pain.
- Aromatherapy: Put a drop of lavender on cotton and put it in the ear. Use a chamomile tea bag that has been infused for a few minutes and place it on the side of the face or over the ear while it is still warm.
- Chiropractic
- Craniosacral manipulation
- Ear candles
- Herbs: warm mullein oil drops in ear
- Homeopathy: pulsatilla, belladonna, or aconite
- Reflexology: Work all fingers and toes, paying close attention to the webs between the fingers and toes, especially between the third, fourth, and fifth digits.

ECZEMA

- Aromatherapy: bergamot, chamomile, lavender, Melissa, neroli, eucalyptus, geranium, juniper
- Flower essences: Rescue Remedy, crab apple
- Herbs: evening primrose oil applied directly
- Hydrotherapy: heat compresses once a day

EMOTIONAL DISTRESS

- Aromatherapy: chamomile, frankincense (deepens breathing to induce calmness), marjoram
- Breathing exercises
- Gratitude exercises
- Positive affirmations

ENERGY IMBALANCE

- Applied Kinesiology
- Magnets
- Polarity Therapy

- Pressure point therapies
- Reiki
- Shiatsu massage
- Thai massage
- Therapeutic Touch

FATIGUE

- Aromatherapy: Peppermint, rose, rosemary, and basil stimulate the brain. Lemon grass and rosemary are best for physical fatigue. Use these oils in the bath, in massage oils, in vaporizers, or on a handkerchief. Do not use peppermint or rosemary at night because they are too stimulating. Rosemary should not be used by people with hypertension or epilepsy.
- Herbs: ginseng, especially for people over the age of 40
- Qigong
- Reflexology: a brisk complete foot treatment for more energy or a slow complete foot treatment to induce sleep
- Supplements: zinc, co-enzyme Q
- Yoga: Start with relaxation and gentle movements on your back, progressing to kneeling, standing, and/or seated postures.

FEET (TIRED)

- Aromatherapy: Mix 2 drops each of rosemary, sage, and peppermint oils in basin of hot water and soak feet for at least 15 minutes. Rosemary (20 drops), sage (15 drops), and peppermint (10 drops) mixed in oil base can be applied directly to feet.
- Massage
- Reflexology: Massage entire foot.

FEVER

- Aromatherapy: Tea tree and juniper encourage the body to sweat. Lavender and peppermint are cooling. Chamomile is soothing and calming, and can be used either in a bath or in cool water to sponge the body.
- Herbs: white willow. To a large mug of boiling water, add juice of 1 lemon, 2 tsp. honey, 1 tsp. grated ginger, 1/2 tsp. cinnamon, 1/2 tsp. nutmeg, and 1 tsp brandy or whisky.
- Homeopathy: belladonna, aconite, ferrum phosphoricum, gelsemium

FIBROMYALGIA

- Acupuncture
- Biofeedback
- Herbs: topical capsaicin; 1 tsp. TID of equal parts of echinacea, black cohosh, devil's claw, licorice, dandelion, and celery

- Hypnotherapy
- Magnets: Sleep on a magnetic mattress and use a magnetic pillow. Magnets can also be placed over painful areas during the day.
- Massage
- Supplements: magnesium, malic acid, vitamins E and C, fish oil, selenium, zinc, SAMe

FLUID RETENTION (EDEMA)

- Herbs: dandelion leaf (diuretic and replaces potassium)
- Massage feet and ankles.
- Reflexology: lymph system, kidneys, adrenals points on the feet
- Elevate legs

HEADACHE (TENSION)

- Acupressure: Press pressure points between eyebrows or at bottom of web between thumb and first finger.
- Alexander Technique: helps improve posture to avoid buildup of tension in neck and shoulders
- Aromatherapy: basil, chamomile; massage lavender, peppermint, or eucalyptus around temples; rose compress to eyes
- Chiropractic
- Herbs: ginseng, chamomile, turmeric, valerian, willow bark; 1/2 tsp. each of betony and skullcap made into tea
- Homeopathy: bryonia (wild hops), windflower, yellow jasmine, nux vomica
- Neurofeedback
- Pulsating electromagnetic fields
- Relaxation techniques
- Therapeutic Touch
- Yoga

HEART DISEASE

- Animal-assisted therapy
- Aromatherapy: to strengthen the heart muscle—garlic, lavender, peppermint, marjoram, rose, rosemary
- Biofeedback
- Exercise
- Herbs: garlic, ginger; 1–2 capsules of hawthorn 4 times a day for mild angina
- Meditation
- Supplements: vitamins E, C, B_6, and B_{12}, L-carnitine, co-enzyme Q to improve utilization of oxygen at cellular level, beta-carotene, selenium,

magnesium, calcium, fish oil, plant sterols/stanols, black, green, oolong, white tea
- T'ai chi, qigong

HEAT RASH

- Herbs: Sprinkle arrowroot powder on affected area. Place 1/2 cup of freshly grated ginger into a quart of boiling water, remove from heat immediately, and steep for 5 minutes, then cool and sponge ginger water onto affected areas and let it dry.

HEMORRHOIDS

- Aromatherapy: Massage geranium, chamomile, or lavender oil, mixed with a carrier oil, into the rectal area as needed.
- Herbs: Apply aloe vera gel to relieve itching. Use compresses of witch hazel to clean area after bowel movement.
- Homeopathy: aesculus, aloe, or hamamelis
- Hydrotherapy: Sit in warm bath for 15 minutes several times a day.

HICCUPS

- Acupressure: Place your middle and index fingers behind each earlobe. Apply light to firm pressure on the neck for 2 minutes as you concentrate on breathing slowly and deeply.
- Reflexology: diaphragm and stomach points on the feet

HYPERTENSION

- Animal-assisted therapy
- Aromatherapy: ylang-ylang, clary sage, lavender, marjoram
- Biofeedback
- Chiropractic
- Exercise
- Herbs: garlic, hawthorn, olive leaf extract, maitake mushroom, reishi mushroom, evening primrose oil, ginger, goldenseal
- Hypnotherapy
- Massage
- Meditation
- Qigong
- Supplements: vitamin C, magnesium, flaxseed oil; calcium for pregnancy-induced hypertension
- T'ai chi
- Yoga

IMMUNE ENHANCEMENT

- Aromatherapy: elemi, eucalyptus
- Herbs: echinacea, goldenseal, astragalus
- Massage
- Qigong
- Supplements: vitamins E and C, beta-carotene, garlic

INDIGESTION

- Aromatherapy: Use basil, chamomile, coriander, ginger, or peppermint as a tea or in massage oil or warm compress over stomach area.
- Herbs: chamomile, peppermint, ginger as a tea; for heaviness after a meal, chew on cardamom or fennel seeds
- Homeopathy: windflower; nux vomica—1 tablet hourly for 6 doses, then 3 times daily—maximum 1 week

INFECTION (BACTERIAL)

- Aromatherapy: calendula, geranium, rosemary, tea tree, lavender, eucalyptus, thyme, niaouli, bergamot. These oils work by attacking the organisms themselves, by killing airborne germs, and by strengthening the immune system.
- Herbs: echinacea at first sign of infection; echinacea may be combined with goldenseal; garlic in capsules
- Supplements: medicinal honey—manuka from New Zealand or medi-honey from Australia

INFECTION (FUNGAL)

- Aromatherapy: calendula, lemon balm, rosemary
- Herbs: garlic, tea tree oil (topical)

INFECTION (VIRAL)

- Aromatherapy: eucalyptus, lemon balm
- Herbs: goldenseal, echinacea, garlic, tea tree oil (topical)
- Supplements: zinc, selenium

INFERTILITY

- Meditation for unexplained infertility
- Supplements: zinc for men
- Acupuncture immediately after in vitro fertilization

INFLAMMATION

- Aromatherapy: benzoin, birch, chamomile, clary sage, elemi, fennel, geranium, helichrysum, jasmine, myrrh, patchouli, rose, sandalwood
- Bee venom may slow down the body's inflammatory response by inhibiting the amount of free radicals or by stimulating the adrenal glands to release cortisol.
- Homeopathy: belladonna
- Hydrotherapy: applications of heat and cold
- Magnets

INSOMNIA

- Acupuncture
- Aromatherapy: chamomile, which can also be used with children; clary sage, lavender, marjoram, neroli, or vetiver in bath or a pillow or as a room fragrance
- Exercise: not later than early evening
- Herbs: valerian, lemon balm, catnip, hops, passion flower, skullcap teas (If taste is unpleasant, add sugar, honey, or lemon.)
- Homeopathy: windflower, nux vomica, arsenicum album
- Hydrotherapy: warm baths
- Light therapy—full spectrum lights for 30 minutes a day
- Magnets: Use magnetic pillow or pad for sedating effect.
- Meditation
- Neurofeedback
- Supplements: melatonin

IRRITABLE BOWEL SYNDROME

- Biofeedback
- Exercise
- Herbs: eneric-coated peppermint oil, ginger, chamomile, valerian, rosemary, lemon balm
- Hypnotherapy
- Meditation
- Yoga

JET LAG

- Herbs: melatonin
- Drink fluids and avoid alcohol. Do in-flight stretches.

LIVER DISEASE

- Herbs: milk thistle, dandelion root tea
- Hydrotherapy: Take steam baths or saunas frequently to help body eliminate toxins.

MACULAR DEGENERATION

- Herbs: ginko, bilberry, blackberry, cranberry, raspberry
- Supplements: antioxidants, zinc, fish oil

MEMORY PROBLEMS

- Aromatherapy: basil, black pepper, coriander, ginger, peppermint, rosemary, thyme
- Exercise
- Supplements: vitamin B_6, green tea

MENOPAUSE

- Aromatherapy: geranium, rose, chamomile, yuzu, sandalwood, lavender, bergamot, fennel in bath or in body creams
- Herbs: black cohosh (estrogen enhancer, hot flashes), chasteberry (hormone balancing), St. John's wort (mood swings), motherwort (palpitations and hot flashes), skullcap (anxiety), dong quai (estrogen enhancer), wild yam as tea; Chinese tonic of He Shou Wu, red clover, licorice
- Homeopathy: pulsatilla (mood changes), sulfur (hot flashes)
- Hypnotherapy
- Meditation
- Supplements: vitamin E, soy protein, calcium, magnesium, flaxseed, evening primrose oil

MENSTRUAL DISCOMFORT

- Aromatherapy: basil. Massage abdomen and lower back with lavender, clary sage, and rose mixed in carrier oil.
- Herbs: tea of agnus castus with rosemary for premenstrual water retention; black haw for cramps—4 tsp. in glass of warm water, repeat after 4 hours if necessary; Chinese tonic of dong quai, dandelion leaf for water retention
- Homeopathy: viburnum, magnesium phosphate, sepia, lachesis
- Hydrotherapy: warm compresses
- Reflexology: Massage uterine reflexes below inside ankle bones and ovarian reflexes beneath outside ankle bones.
- Supplements: calcium and manganese, fish oil, parsley, celery, and dandelion leaves are all mild diuretics
- Yoga stretches; more relaxation and breathing exercises

MIGRAINE HEADACHES

- Aromatherapy: Green apple (inhalant), lavender, Melissa, or peppermint can be put on a facecloth with cool water and used as a compress on the forehead or back of the neck.

- Herbs: feverfew (prophylaxis), ginkgo
- Homeopathy: iris, sanguinaria, glonoine
- Hypnotherapy
- Neurofeedback
- Pressure point therapies
- Pulsating electromagnetic fields
- Spiritual meditation

MUSCLE SORENESS

- Aromatherapy: chamomile, juniper
- Herbs: Rub in wintergreen oil or capsicum cream.
- Hydrotherapy: spa
- Massage
- Movement therapy: t'ai chi, qigong, Feldenkrais
- Yoga

NAUSEA

- Acupressure: wristband—small weights that exert pressure on a specific pressure point on the wrist
- Aromatherapy: ginger, lavender, peppermint used as a compress and as teas
- Healing Touch
- Herbs: ginger
- Homeopathy: ipecacuanha, sepia, clossypium
- Imagery
- Reiki
- Therapeutic Touch

OSTEOPOROSIS

- Exercise: weight bearing unless advanced stage of disease
- Herbs: a tea of stinging nettles, alfalfa, or sage, horsetail, dandelion root
- Supplements: calcium, vitamins D and C, magnesium, natural hormone therapy, soy

PAIN

- Acupuncture
- Alexander Technique
- Biofeedback
- Chiropractic
- Herbs: feverfew, devil's claw
- Hydrotherapy: hot water packs, cold applications

- Hypnotherapy
- Guided imagery
- Magnets
- Pressure point therapies
- Reiki
- Sports massage
- Therapeutic Touch
- Trager Approach
- Trigger point massage

PHYSICAL DISABILITIES

- Balance difficulties—t'ai chi, yoga, equine-assisted therapy

POISON IVY AND POISON OAK

- Rinse the exposed area with soap and cold water. Mix baking soda with water to form a paste and apply it to skin. Once the paste has hardened, remove with cool water and apply a thin layer of honey to the area.
- aloe; For itching and discomfort, grind 1 cup raw, whole oats to a fine powder and add to tepid bath—soak for 20–30 minutes.
- Homeopathy: Rhus tox

PREGNANCY

Although not a health care problem, it is included here for relief of some of the discomfort.

Morning Sickness

- Acupressure: wristband—small weights that exert pressure on a specific pressure point on the wrist
- Herbs: peppermint, catnip, ginger, chamomile, cinnamon, red raspberry leaf teas

Labor

- Acupuncture and moxibustion for breech presentation
- Aromatherapy: Blend of clary sage, rose, and ylang-ylang can be used for massage. Deep massage of lower back and hips during contractions—between contractions, massage shoulders, back, hands, and feet; if contractions are lagging, a light massage of the breasts may stimulate activity.
- Herbs: red raspberry tea, black cohosh tea, blue cohosh, bethroot
- Hydrotherapy: water birth
- Hypnotherapy

Postpartum
- Herbs: lavender oil or aloe for perineal discomfort; cabbage leaves, mother's milk, alfalfa to encourage lactation
- Reflexology to encourage lactation

PREMENSTRUAL SYNDROME
- Acupuncture
- Aromatherapy: Massage or warm bath with rose oil, clary sage, ylang-ylang, lavender, lemon grass, sandalwood, jasmine, bergamot. One will have to decide, by trial and error, which of these oils best suits the individual.
- Deep breathing exercises for a least 20 minutes a day
- Exercise
- Herbs: vitex, black cohosh extract, agnus-castus, chasteberry, Helonias, evening primrose oil, Chinese tonic of dong quai
- Homeopathy: windflower, pulsatilla, lachesis
- Massage
- Meditation
- Reflexology: Massage uterine reflexes below inside ankle bones and ovarian reflexes beneath outside ankle bones.
- Supplements: vitamins A, E, B, and B_6; 2–3 g capsule of combined fish oil and evening primrose oil, magnesium, zinc, calcium

PROSTATE ENLARGEMENT (BENIGN)
- Herbs: saw palmetto, pygeum africanum, stinging nettle root tea
- Supplements: vitamins C, E, and B_3, zinc, manganese. Add soy foods to diet.

PSORIASIS
- Aromatherapy: bergamot (heal skin plaques), lavender (itching), Melissa or geranium (irritated skin), jasmine (dry skin)
- Diet: Include foods with zinc, beta-carotene, vitamin D, and omega-3 fatty acids. Avoid liver and other organ meats, which are foods that aggravate psoriasis.
- Flower essences: Rescue Remedy cream, crab apple
- Herbs: evening primrose oil, echinacea, licorice, milk thistle. Apply aloe vera extract topically 3 times a day. Do not cover.
- Homeopathy: sepai, arsenicum iodatum, petroleum
- Take 2 tsp almond oil. Add 2 drops calendula oil and 1 drop lavender oil to it and then massage area with this.
- Sunshine on the skin is helpful.

RINGWORM

- Aromatherapy: rosemary, tea tree oil, lavender, geranium, peppermint, thyme
- Herbs: Apply a paste made of equal parts of myrrh powder and goldenseal powder mixed with a little water. A thin slice of garlic bandaged directly over the skin lesion and left for several days has a powerful antifungal effect.
- Homeopathy: sepia, arsen alb, graphites

SCIATICA

- Acupuncture
- Applied Kinesiology
- Chiropractic
- Herbs: willow bark, black cohosh, chamomile, fenugreek, juniper berries, parsley, rosemary, skullcap
- Homeopathy: colocynth, viscum album, lachesis, rhus tox, aconite, belladonna
- Hydrotherapy: warm water jets
- Reflexology: hip, sciatic, knee, lower spine, shoulder points on feet

SEXUAL DYSFUNCTION

- Acupuncture
- Herbs: ginkgo for erectile problems; ashwaganda
- Hypnotherapy
- Imagery

SHINGLES

- Aromatherapy: eucalyptus, tea tree oil, lavender, chamomile, bergamot. Smooth the oil gently over the affected areas and down either side of the spine; if body is too painful to touch, add oils to a water spray or use in a bath
- Flower essences: Rescue Remedy, crab apple
- Herbs: Echinacea, St. John's wort tea. Apply aloe vera gel to blistering area.
- Hydrotherapy: body temperature bath for 30 minutes

SINUS PROBLEMS

- Acupuncture
- Aromatherapy: Put basil, marjoram, or eucalyptus on handkerchief, or use with a vaporizer.

- Herbs: ephedra, goldenseal, yarrow, coltsfoot. Make a tea using 2 tsp. of herb per cup. Use herbs in cream or oil, and massage the sinus areas.
- Homeopathy: hydrastis, kali bichromicum, arsenicum album, silicea
- Hydrotherapy: hot and cold compresses, steam inhalation, nasal lavage
- Reflexology: Massage the sinus reflexes on the tips of the fingers and toes.

SKIN (DRY)

- Aromatherapy: Mix 2 drops each of sandalwood, rose, and geranium oil with a tsp of almond oil. Use as a topical evening moisturizer. Other oils good for dry skin include jasmine, orange, and ylang-ylang used in a moisturizer or in a bath.

SORE THROAT

- Aromatherapy: Take several drops of sandalwood on handkerchief, or mix with carrier oil and massage into throat area. Then wrap something warm around the throat.
- Herbs: Gargle with 1 cup of warm water with 1/4; to 1 tsp. of salt and 1/2 tsp. of goldenseal powder.
- Homeopathy: monkshood, poison ivy, belladonna
- Hydrotherapy: contrast applications to neck and throat; heat compresses
- Reflexology: Massage the throat reflexes around the "neck" of the big toes and thumbs.

SPRAIN AND STRAINS

- Aromatherapy: chamomile, ginger, lavender as massage to area
- Herbs: Mix 1/4 cup each of dry mustard powder and flour with warm water to make a thick paste, spread the paste onto cheesecloth or gauze, roll it up, and apply to the strained area.
- Homeopathy: poison ivy
- Hydrotherapy: cold compresses to reduce swelling first 24 hours; then warm compresses to increase circulation
- Magnets: Cover area with magnetic pad and secure with an Ace bandage. Put it on for 12 hours then off for 12 hours.
- Myofascial release
- Pressure point therapies
- Reiki
- Therapeutic Touch

STRESS

- Acupuncture
- Aromatherapy: juniper, lavender, vetiver, ylang-ylang. Use jasmine in massage oil or put in bath.
- Breathing exercises; alternate nostril breathing (pranayama)
- Exercise
- Herbs: chamomile tea, passionflower, valerian, ginseng
- Humor and laughter
- Massage
- Meditation
- Music therapy
- Progressive relaxation
- Qigong
- Yoga: Focus on slow movements and long exhalations.

SUNBURN

- Aromatherapy: Spray or rub with lavender and chamomile.
- Herbs: Soak a soft cloth in cooled black or green tea and spread over the burned area. Leave on 15–30 minutes. Apply aloe vera sap to area.
- Hydrotherapy: cold compresses. Soak in a bath of tepid water and baking soda (1 pound) for 20–30 minutes; later that day or next take a tepid bath with 1 or 2 cups of milk added.
- Grated potato applied directly to the skin will decrease pain and prevent blistering; wrap in place with a clean cloth.

SURGERY

- Hypnotherapy and visualization before surgery
- Magnets: Place magnets over the incision site for 24 to 48 hours before surgery to improve postoperative recovery. Place magnets over wound after surgery.
- Meditation before and after surgery

TENSION

- Aromatherapy: hot bath or massage using one of the following oils—bergamot, rose, cedarwood, chamomile, geranium, lavender, melissa, orange, or sandalwood
- Feldenkrais Method
- Herbs: valerian, passion flower, chamomile, ginseng as teas
- Massage

- Meditation
- Reiki
- Therapeutic Touch

TINNITUS

- Acupuncture
- Herb: ginko
- Homeopathy: saliclicum acidum, chenopodium, cinchona officinalis
- Supplement: vitamin B_{12}

URINARY INCONTINENCE

- Biofeedback of pelvic floor muscles

URINARY TRACT INFECTION

- Aromatherapy: bergamot, sandalwood, lavender, or juniper in bath water
- Herbs: uva ursi, goldenseal; saw palmetto for men
- Homeopathy: pulsatilla, sepia, nux vomica
- Hydrotherapy: contrast sitz baths
- Supplements: unsweetened cranberry juice (300 mL daily); vitamins A and C
- Urinate after sexual activity.
- Drink plenty of water.

WARTS

- Aromatherapy: 1 drop each of lemon, thyme, and tea tree oil mixed in a base oil and swabbed 2 times a day.
- Duct tape: Cover the warts with duct tape and leave undisturbed for several days.
- Hypnotherapy
- Imagery
- Supplements: vitamins A, C, B-complex, and E, zinc, L-cysteine

WEIGHT CONTROL

- Aromatherapy: green apple, fennel, juniper, rosemary, bitter orange
- Exercise
- Herb: evening primrose oil
- Supplements: 2.5 g of vitamin B_5, 4 times a day; calcium, chromium, conjugated linoleic acid (CLA)
- Yoga

WOUNDS

- Aromatherapy: To disinfect: bergamot, chamomile, clary sage, jasmine, juniper, lavender, rose, tea tree. To relieve pain: bergamot, chamomile, geranium, jasmine, lavender, rosemary. To stop bleeding: cypress, geranium, rose. To reduce inflammation: chamomile, geranium, helichrysum, jasmine, patchouli. To promote formation of scar tissue: bergamot, chamomile, helichrysum, jasmine
- Bioelectromagnetics
- Herbs: echinacea, goldenseal
- Homeopathy: calendula, hypericum, ledum
- Hydrotherapy: warm water irrigation
- Unprocessed honey may help to disinfect wounds, sores, and actively promote wound healing.

INDEX